Obsessive-Compulsive Disorder

World Psychiatric Association Evidence and Experience in Psychiatry Series

Series Editor: Michelle Riba, WPA Secretary for Publications, Department of Psychiatry, University of Michigan

Post-Traumatic Stress Disorders
Edited by Dan Stein, Matthew Friedman and Carlos Blanco
ISBN: 9780470688977

Substance Abuse Disorders
Edited by Hamid Ghodse, Helen Herrman, Mario Maj and Norman Sartorius
ISBN: 9780470745106

Depressive Disorders, 3e
Edited by Helen Herrman, Mario Maj and Norman Sartorius
ISBN: 9780470987209

Schizophrenia 2e
Edited by Mario Maj, Norman Sartorius
ISBN: 9780470849644

Dementia 2e
Edited by Mario Maj, Norman Sartorius
ISBN: 9780470849637

Obsessive-Compulsive Disorders 2e
Edited by Mario Maj, Norman Sartorius, Ahmed Okasha, Joseph Zohar
ISBN: 9780470849668

Bipolar Disorders
Edited by Mario Maj, Hagop S Akiskal, Juan José López-Ibor, Norman Sartorius
ISBN: 9780471560371

Eating Disorders
Edited by Mario Maj, Kathrine Halmi, Juan José López-Ibor, Norman Sartorius
ISBN: 9780470848654

Phobias
Edited by Mario Maj, Hagop S Akiskal, Juan José López-Ibor, Ahmed Okasha
ISBN: 9780470858332

Personality Disorders
Edited by Mario Maj, Hagop S Akiskal, Juan E Mezzich
ISBN: 9780470090367

Somatoform Disorders
Edited by Mario Maj, Hagop S Akiskal, Juan E Mezzich, Ahmed Okasha
ISBN: 9780470016121

Current Science and Clinical Practice Series

Series Editor: Michelle Riba, WPA Secretary for Publications, Department of Psychiatry, University of Michigan

Obsessive-Compulsive Disorder
Edited by Joseph Zohar
ISBN: 9780470711255

Schizophrenia
Edited by Wolfgang Gaebel
ISBN: 9780470710548

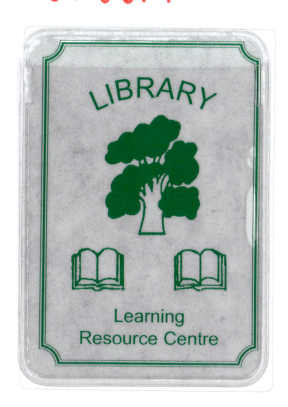
Obsessive-Compulsive Disorder
Current Science and Clinical Practice

Editor

Joseph Zohar
Tel Aviv University, Tel Aviv, Israel

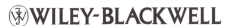
WILEY-BLACKWELL

A John Wiley & Sons, Ltd., Publication

Library of Congress Cataloging-in-Publication Data

Obsessive-compulsive disorder : current science and clinical practice / editor, Joseph Zohar.
    p. ; cm.
  Includes bibliographical references and index.
  Summary: "A clear summary of what is known about a highly prevalent and debilitating disorder that affects nearly as many people as asthma. Expert authors review the biological basis for the disorder and describe both pharmacological and psychological approaches to treatment"–Provided by publisher.
  ISBN 978-0-470-71125-5 (cloth)
  I. Zohar, Joseph.
  [DNLM: 1. Obsessive-Compulsive Disorder–diagnosis. 2. Obsessive-Compulsive Disorder–drug therapy. 3. Obsessive-Compulsive Disorder–therapy. WM 176]
  616.85′227–dc23

2012009775

A catalogue record for this book is available from the British Library.

Wiley also publishes its books in a variety of electronic formats. Some content that appears in print may not be available in electronic books.

Set in 11/13pt Times by Aptara Inc., New Delhi, India
Printed and bound in Malaysia by Vivar Printing Sdn Bhd
First Impression 2012

Contents

SECTION 2   CLINICAL SPOTLIGHTS

List of Contributors

Anat Abudy
Psychiatry Department A, Division of Psychiatry
Chaim Sheba Medical Center
Tel Hashomer, Israel

Rianne M. Blom
Department of Psychiatry
Academic Medical Center
University of Amsterdam
Amsterdam, The Netherlands

Ashley R. Brown
Clinical and Research Program in Pediatric Psychopharmacology
Department of Psychiatry
Massachusetts General Hospital
Boston, MA, USA

Andrea Cantisani
Department of Psychiatry
University of Florence
Florence, Italy

Samuel R. Chamberlain
Department of Psychiatry
University of Cambridge
Addenbrooke's Hospital
Cambridge, UK

Eric H. Decloedt
Department of Medicine
Division of Clinical Pharmacology
University of Cape Town
Cape Town, South Africa

Damiaan Denys
Department of Psychiatry
Academic Medical Center
University of Amsterdam
Amsterdam, The Netherlands;
The Netherlands Institute for Neuroscience
Amsterdam, The Netherlands

Phillip C. Easter
Department of Psychiatry and Behavioral Neurosciences
Wayne State University School of Medicine
University Health Center
Detroit, MI, USA

Alyssa L. Faro
Clinical and Research Program in Pediatric Psychopharmacology
Department of Psychiatry
Massachusetts General Hospital
Boston, MA, USA

Martijn Figee
Department of Psychiatry
Academic Medical Center
University of Amsterdam
Amsterdam, The Netherlands

Naomi A. Fineberg
National OCD Treatment Service
Hertfordshire Partnership NHS Foundation Trust
Queen Elizabeth II Hospital
Welwyn Garden City, UK
and University of Hertfordshire, College Lane
Hatfield UK

Martin E. Franklin
University of Pennsylvania School of Medicine
Philadelphia, PA, USA

Daniel A. Geller
Clinical and Research Program in Pediatric Psychopharmacology
Department of Psychiatry
Massachusetts General Hospital
Boston, MA, USA;
Harvard Medical School
Boston, MA, USA

Adriel Gerard
Montefiore Medical Center
University Hospital of Albert Einstein College of Medicine
Bronx, NY, USA

Addie Goss
Bryn Mawr College
Bryn Mawr, PA, USA

Giacomo Grassi
Department of Psychiatry
University of Florence
Florence, Italy

Eric Hollander
Montefiore Medical Center
University Hospital of Albert Einstein College of Medicine
Bronx, NY, USA

Alzbeta Juven-Wetzler
Psychiatry Department A, Division of Psychiatry
Chaim Sheba Medical Center
Tel Hashomer, Israel

Hannah C. Levy
Department of Psychology
Concordia University
Montreal, QC, Canada

John S. March
Department of Psychiatry and Behavioral Sciences
Duke University Medical Center
Durham, NC, USA

Jose M. Menchon
Department of Psychiatry
Hospital Universitari de Bellvitge-IDIBELL
Hospitalet de Llobregat Barcelona;
Department of Clinical Sciences
School of Medicine
Universitat de Barcelona;
Centro de Investigación Biomédica en Red de Salud Mental (CIBERSAM)
Instituto de Salud Carlos III
Ministry of Science and Innovation
Barcelona, Spain

Lara Menzies
Department of Psychiatry
University of Cambridge
Addenbrooke's Hospital
Cambridge, UK

Georgia Michalopoulou
Wayne State University School of Medicine;
Children's Hospital of Michigan
Department of Psychiatry and Psychology
Detroit, MI, USA

Stefano Pallanti
Department of Psychiatry
Mount Sinai School of Medicine
New York, NY, USA;
Department of Psychiatry
University of Florence
Florence, Italy;
Institute of Neuroscience
Florence, Italy

David L. Pauls
Psychiatric and Neurodevelopmental Genetics Unit
Center for Human Genetic Research
Massachusetts General Hospital
Harvard Medical School
Boston, MA, USA

Steven Poskar
Montefiore Medical Center
University Hospital of Albert Einstein College of Medicine
Bronx, NY, USA

Samar Reghunandanan
National OCD Treatment Service
Hertfordshire Partnership NHS Foundation Trust
Queen Elizabeth II Hospital
Welwyn Garden City
UK

David R. Rosenberg
Children's Hospital of Michigan;
Wayne State University School of Medicine
Department of Psychiatry
University Health Center
Detroit, MI, USA

Rachel Sonnino
Psychiatry Department A, Division of Psychiatry
Chaim Sheba Medical Center
Tel Hashomer, Israel

Dan J. Stein
Department of Psychiatry
University of Cape Town
Cape Town, South Africa

Nienke Vulink
Department of Psychiatry
Academic Medical Center
University of Amsterdam
Amsterdam, The Netherlands

Joseph Zohar
Psychiatry Department A, Division of Psychiatry
Chaim Sheba Medical Center
Tel Hashomer, Israel

Introduction

During my career, I have witnessed two revolutions in obsessive-compulsive disorder (OCD).

As a resident in psychiatry (in the late 1970s), I asked my supervisor for advice, having examined a patient with OCD; his response was that there was very little that could be done for these rare cases. He was right; at that time, OCD was considered a rare disorder of psychological origin, and refractory to treatment. The first revolution in OCD overturned all three of these conceptions. The seminal work of M.M. Weissman reported a lifetime prevalence of about 2%. Pioneering double-blind, placebo-controlled work at the National Institute of Mental Health (NIMH) raised the curtain on the specific response to serotonergic medication, highlighted the serotonergic basis and gave initial hints for the relevant brain regions involved in OCD.

The second revolution in OCD is taking place right now. It is composed of building blocks such as neurocognitive endophenotypes (see Chapter 12), genetics (Chapter 11), sophisticated brain imaging (Chapter 10), daring conceptual challenges (Chapter 6), and venturing beyond the conventional serotonin hypothesis (Chapter 9).

To help us build these new, improved, contemporary understandings of OCD and OC spectrum disorders, we use better assessment tools (Chapter 1), and utilize much more sophisticated methodological techniques (Chapter 8). All of this provides us with sharper pharmacological tools (Chapter 2) and psychological interventions (Chapter 3), for adult patients as well as for children (Chapter 7). Moreover, it enables us to embark on new therapeutic approaches (Chapter 5), including new physical interventions (Chapter 4).

This book is a sort of celebration of the emergence of the second revolution in OCD, and I hope that the reader will feel the enthusiasm shared by all the contributors about the promising present and the bright future of OCD.

Joseph Zohar
2012

Assessment and Treatment

CHAPTER 1

Assessment

Jose M. Menchon

*Department of Psychiatry, Hospital Universitari de Bellvitge-IDIBELL,
Hospitalet de Llobregat (Barcelona), Universitat de Barcelona,
CIBERSAM, Spain*

INTRODUCTION

Many people have some obsessions during their lives: it is estimated that more than one-quarter of people experience obsessions or compulsions at some time [1], and a substantial proportion of them will meet the criteria for obsessive-compulsive disorder (OCD). The lifetime prevalence of OCD is about 2–2.5%, and the annual prevalence is 1–2% among the general population [1,2]. The male to female ratio is approximately unity, with some studies finding a slightly higher prevalence in women, while in the child and adolescent populations males show a higher prevalence.

The hallmark of OCD is the presence of either obsessions or compulsions. According to the *Diagnostic and Statistical Manual of Mental Disorders, 4th Edition, Text Revision* (DSM-IV-TR) [3] diagnostic criteria, the obsessions are defined by the following four criteria:

1. Recurrent and persistent thoughts, impulses or images that are experienced, at some time during the disturbance, as intrusive and inappropriate and that cause marked anxiety or distress.
2. The thoughts, impulses or images are not simply excessive worries about real-life problems.
3. The person attempts to ignore or suppress such thoughts, impulses or images, or to neutralize them with some other thought or action.
4. The person recognizes that the obsessional thoughts, impulses or images are a product of his or her own mind (not imposed from without as in thought insertion).

Obsessive-Compulsive Disorder: Current Science and Clinical Practice, First Edition. Edited by Joseph Zohar.
© 2012 John Wiley & Sons, Ltd. Published 2012 by John Wiley & Sons, Ltd.

Compulsions are defined as: '1) repetitive behaviors (e.g., hand washing, ordering, checking) or mental acts (e.g., praying, counting, repeating words silently) that the person feels driven to perform in response to an obsession, or according to rules that must be applied rigidly, and 2) the behaviors or mental acts are aimed at preventing or reducing distress or preventing some dreaded event or situation; however, these behaviors or mental acts either are not connected in a realistic way with what they are designed to neutralize or prevent or are clearly excessive.' Hence, obsessions and compulsions are repetitive, unpleasant and intrusive (although recognized as own thoughts), and usually the individual considers that the obsessions or compulsions are excessive or irrational, demonstrated by the subject's attempts to resist them. While obsessions are considered phenomena that increase anxiety or discomfort, compulsions are behaviours that are aimed at reducing it.

Obsessions and compulsions are very diverse and have been grouped into various types. Table 1.1 shows the percentage of obsessions and compulsions in adult OCD samples reported in several studies. Such diversity in the clinical manifestations of OCD has led researchers to examine whether the different obsessions and compulsions seen in patients could be related and grouped into a few subtypes or dimensions; for instance, a recent meta-analysis [10] has derived four main factors: symmetry, forbidden thoughts, cleaning and hoarding. Apart from its descriptive utility, this kind of approach has heuristic value since it allows examination of the possible heterogeneity of OCD in terms of neurobiology, genetics or

Table 1.1 Percentage of obsessions and compulsions in OCD adult samples reported in various studies.

Study	[4] (n = 560)	[5] (n = 354)	[6] (n = 180)	[7] (n = 293)	[8] (n = 485)	[9] (n = 343)
Obsessions						
Aggressive	31	44	56	71	58	36
Contamination	50	35	60	58	59	48
Sexual	24	15	17	13	26	10
Hoarding		18	11	29	34	12
Religious		22	22	26	31	8
Symmetry	32	36	32	48	50	42
Somatic	33	23	26	26	40	12
Compulsions						
Washing/cleaning	50	35	59	60	59	47
Checking	61	43	72	69	73	47
Repeating rituals		42	58	56	52	31
Counting	36	29	16	26	34	14
Ordering	28	29	25	43	50	22
Hoarding	18	16	13	28	36	12

Numbers in brackets refer to the relevant reference.

Table 1.2 Components in the assessment of OCD.

Clinical Assessment
    Present obsessive-compulsive symptoms: subtype/dimensions of symptoms;
      severity; degree of insight
    Risk of suicide
    Cognitive biases and behavioural analysis (how does the patient behave in
      response to obsessions? What kind of obsessions elicits compulsions? How
      much associated anxiety is there? Is there any resistance to and control over
      compulsions?)
    Neuropsychological dysfunctions

Conditions associated with the onset and course of the symptoms: past or present
    history of tics or Tourette disorder; possible history of PANDAS (Pediatric
    Autoimmune Neuropsychiatric Disorders Associated with Streptococcal
    infections); relationship of the disorder with reproductive events (onset or
    worsening of symptoms at the menarche, pregnancy and other reproductive
    events); relationship with life events

Course of the disorder: age at onset of the first symptoms and of the disorder,
    degree of stability of the subtype of symptoms (have always been the same
    type of symptoms?), age at first treatment, type of evolution (episodic, chronic
    or fluctuating, progressive improvement or worsening), degree of functional
    impairment

Personality traits or disorders

Differential diagnosis of other disorders and comorbidities: organic brain
    disorders, schizophrenia, depression, hypochondriasis, phobias, Tourette or tic
    disorder, obsessive-compulsive personality disorder, body dysmorphic
    disorders, grooming disorders (trichotillomania, skin picking disorder),
    hoarding, presence of other obsessive-compulsive spectrum disorders

Family assessment: family history of psychiatric disorders, degree of support from
    relatives, degree of understanding of the disorder by relatives, ability of the
    relatives to participate in the treatment

Treatment: previous drug treatments (doses and duration), previous psychological
    therapies, response to previous treatments (remission, partial response, no
    response)

treatment response, among other aspects [11]. This issue is reviewed in detail in Chapter 6 of this book.

The assessment of OCD includes the usual elements involved in the psychiatric assessment of mental disorders, although there are also specific issues related to this condition. Relevant issues in the OCD assessment are (Table 1.2):

- the instruments for detecting and diagnosing the disorder;
- the examination of the obsessive-compulsive (OC) symptoms: the severity and type of symptoms, the level of insight, cognitive biases and behavioural analysis;

- the assessment of the suicide risk;
- the appraisal of neuropsychological functions;
- differential diagnosis;
- the presence of comorbid and related/spectrum disorders;
- the review of the course of the disorder: age of onset of OC symptoms, age at which the subject met diagnostic criteria for OCD, type of course of the disorder (e.g. episodic, chronic with or without fluctuations, progressive worsening);
- the analysis of the response to previous treatments, including both clinical outcome and degree of disability of the patient's functioning.

Given that some of the components of the assessment are examined in other chapters, the present review will focus on the detection of OCD, the clinical rating of OC symptoms, the assessment of insight and the suicide risk, the differential diagnosis, and OC related and spectrum disorders.

DETECTING OCD

Many OCD sufferers experience shame about their symptoms or think that these will be misunderstood as 'madness', while others may even be afraid that their symptoms do actually mean that they are becoming 'mad'. For some patients these symptoms may be stigmatizing while others do not view their symptoms as a disorder, lacking insight of their morbid nature; others may think that they do not require treatment. All these beliefs and attitudes reduce the likelihood of disclosing their OCD symptoms to their physicians. A study of attitudes towards OCD symptoms [12] showed that the attitudes may vary across the different symptoms of the disorder, finding that obsessions related to harm were the most feared and unacceptable, followed by the washing behaviour, and then the checking behaviour. Therefore, fear of the meaning of the obsessions/compulsions, embarrassment about reporting them, viewing them as stigmatizing, or lacking insight into their nature, may all delay seeking help for them. This delay was evident in the study by Pinto *et al.* [7], which found that the time elapsed between the first symptoms and the first treatment was 17 years, and that between meeting the diagnostic criteria for OCD and the first treatment was 11 years.

The importance of adequate recognition of OCD is reflected in a study in which only 30.9% of severe OCD cases received a specific OCD treatment [1], although 93% of the patients reported that they were receiving mental health treatment in some kind of health setting (general medical, mental health settings, human services or complementary/alternative medicine). The data were more striking in patients with moderate OCD, since only 2.9% of this group of patients were on specific OCD treatment while 25.6% of this group were receiving mental health treatment.

These data regarding attitudes to OCD symptoms, and therefore the delay in both receiving an OCD diagnosis and starting an adequate treatment, emphasize the importance of the strategies to detect OCD.

Screening in clinical interview

Some patients with OCD will describe their symptoms quite well, and diagnosing OCD will not be difficult provided that the physician knows the disorder. However, other patients will display other symptoms that may not be so apparently related to OCD, thereby making it more difficult to reach the diagnosis. For instance, some patients may describe general complaints of anxiety or depression, avoidance of specific situations, or excessive concerns about illnesses. In some cases, the presence of hand dermatitis may suggest repetitive hand washing due to contamination obsessions. Indeed, it is not unusual that patients see non-psychiatrist doctors such as dermatologists for dermatitis or trichotillomania, neurologists for tics, plastic surgeons for concerns about appearance (typically in body dysmorphic disorder), or other physicians for fear of cancer or HIV infection [13]. Therefore, it is useful to have some easy screening questions to detect OCD if the doctor suspects it during the clinical interview.

One of the most useful sets of screening questions are those derived from the Zohar–Fineberg Obsessive Compulsive Screen (ZF-OCS) [14], which are also recommended by the National Institute for Health and Clinical Excellence (NICE) guideline [15]:

1. Do you wash or clean a lot?
2. Do you check things a lot?
3. Is there any thought that keeps bothering you that you'd like to get rid of but can't?
4. Do your daily activities take a long time to finish?
5. Are you concerned about orderliness and symmetry?
6. Do these problems trouble you?

These questions have good sensitivity and specificity for detecting OCD. Using the Mini International Neuropsychiatric Interview (MINI, see below for full description) as the criterion, the five first questions showed a sensitivity of 94.4% and a specificity of 85.1%, with a kappa agreement of 0.66, in a sample of 92 referred dermatology patients [14].

Several OCD guidelines propose similar questions to detect OCD. The American Psychiatric Association guideline [16] suggests the following screening questions to detect OCD:

- Do you have unpleasant thoughts you can't get rid of?
- Do you worry that you might impulsively harm someone?

- Do you have to count things, or wash your hands, or check things over and over?
- Do you worry a lot about whether you performed religious rituals correctly or have been immoral?
- Do you have troubling thoughts about sexual matters? Do you need things arranged symmetrically or in a very exact order?
- Do you have trouble discarding things, so that your house is quite cluttered?
- Do these worries and behaviours interfere with your functioning at work, with your family, or in social activities?

The Canadian Psychiatric Association [17] recommends essentially two questions to detect obsessions and compulsions:

- *Obsessions:* Do you experience disturbing thoughts, images or urges that keep coming back to you and that you have trouble putting out of your head? For example, being contaminated by something, something terrible happening to you or someone you care about, or of doing something terrible?
- *Compulsions:* Do you ever have to perform a behaviour or repeat some action that doesn't make sense to you or that you don't want to do? For example, washing or cleaning excessively, checking things over and over, counting things repeatedly?

When a doctor in a clinical setting suspects OCD all these screening questions may be very useful since they are quick and easy to ask.

Structured interviews

Apart from screening questions, OCD diagnosis may also be examined through more formal clinical interviews. In fact, the most widely used structured clinical interviews contain some questions or a section for the diagnosis of OCD. The structured clinical interviews most used for diagnosing OCD are the following.

- *Anxiety Disorders Interview Schedule for DSM-IV (ADIS-IV).* The ADIS provides information about the presence or absence of a given diagnosis, as well as information about subthreshold symptom levels or the severity of the disorder. The ADIS-IV [18] is a semi-structured interview designed to assess the DSM anxiety disorders and other often comorbid DSM-IV disorders as well as disorders that are usually screened in research trials. The ADIS should be administered by trained clinicians. There are lifetime and child versions. With regard to OCD, it provides more information than the SCID (see below), since it assesses severity of obsessive-compulsive symptoms, insight, resistance and avoidance. It has good psychometric properties but it is time-consuming, being more used in research than in clinical practice.

- *Structured Clinical Interview for DSM-IV-TR Axis I Disorders (SCID-I).* The SCID-I [19,20] is a semi-structured interview that provides a broad assessment of major DSM Axis I disorders. Like the ADIS, it should be administered by experienced clinicians or trained mental health professionals. In general, SCID has good psychometric properties although the data specifically for OCD are more moderate. For instance, reliability studies (including studies for both DSM-III-R and DSM-IV) selected in the SCID website show coefficients ranging from 0.40 to 0.70 [21].
- *Composite International Diagnostic Interview (CIDI).* The CIDI is a comprehensive, fully structured interview designed to be used by trained lay interviewers for the assessment of mental disorders according to the definitions and criteria of the *International Classification of Diseases, Tenth Revision* (ICD-10) and DSM-IV. It is intended for use in large epidemiological and cross-cultural studies as well as for clinical and research purposes [22]. The CIDI is an expansion of the Diagnostic Interview Schedule (DIS) that was developed under the auspices of the World Health Organization (WHO) to address the problem that DIS diagnoses were exclusively based on the definitions and criteria of the DSM, and therefore to generate diagnoses based on the definitions and criteria of the WHO ICD. This is a very lengthy interview since it can take an average of approximately 2 hours to administer. Therefore, using CIDI to detect OCD requires administration specifically of the module with OCD.
- *Mini International Neuropsychiatric Interview (MINI).* The MINI was designed as a structured interview for the major Axis I psychiatric disorders in DSM-IV and ICD-10. The administration of the MINI usually takes 15–20 minutes. Although its administration is short, the MINI covers the following disorders: panic disorder, agoraphobia, social phobia, OCD, specific phobia, generalized anxiety disorder (GAD), posttraumatic stress disorder (PTSD), major depressive disorder, dysthymic disorder, suicidality, mania, alcohol dependence, alcohol abuse, drug dependence (non-alcohol), drug abuse (non-alcohol), psychotic disorder, anorexia nervosa, bulimia and antisocial personality disorder. The MINI has been shown to have good concordance with other diagnostic measures [23]. The MINI also has good interrater reliability, with κ coefficients ranging between 0.88 and 1.0, and good test-retest reliability, with coefficients ranging between 0.76 and 0.93 [24,25].

CLINICAL ASSESSMENT OF OBSESSIVE-COMPULSIVE SYMPTOMS

The assessment and rating of OCD symptoms to establish the severity of the disorder has been complex due to the nature of the disorder. For instance, the severity of the disorder could be interpreted differently depending on whether the assessment is based on the number of obsessions or compulsions, or the distress that they cause, or the degree of interference associated with them. Some subjects may have many obsessions and compulsions without these being too disabling, while other subjects with notably fewer obsessions may experience them as much more distressing or as severely interfering with their daily functioning. There are also many types of obsessions and compulsions, which are not always specified in the rating scales and which may be very particular to a given individual. In other subjects, the obsessions may not have all their usual characteristics, for instance in subjects lacking insight into their symptoms. As a result, many different scales that try to capture the severity of the OC symptoms have been developed and used for the assessment of OCD. Those used most widely are described below.

Yale–Brown Obsessive-Compulsive Scale

The Yale–Brown Obsessive-Compulsive Scale (Y–BOCS) [26,27] is probably the most widely used scale for measuring the severity of obsessive-compulsive symptoms and has become the 'gold standard' for OCD assessment. The scale was designed to assess OCD severity independently of the number and type of the obsessive and compulsive symptoms.

The Y–BOCS includes two primary sections: the Symptom Checklist and the Severity Scale. The Symptom Checklist examines the current (within the past week) and past presence of 64 obsessions and compulsions. These obsessions and compulsions are arranged into 13 specific (plus two miscellaneous) categories. Within the obsessions, the following categories are examined: aggressive, contamination, sexual, hoarding/saving, religious, need for symmetry or exactness, somatic and miscellaneous obsessions. The categories examined for compulsions are: cleaning/washing, checking, repeating rituals, counting, ordering/arranging, hoarding/collecting and miscellaneous compulsions. A substantial number of studies on its factor structure have been carried out providing solutions with between three and five factors. A recent meta-analysis of 21 factor analytic studies [10] yielded four main factors: hoarding, symmetry, forbidden thoughts and cleaning.

The Severity Scale is a semi-structured clinician-administered scale that assesses the presence and severity of obsessive-compulsive symptoms over the past week. It contains 10 items that assess separately several features of the obsessions (five items) and compulsions (five items). The five items for obsessions and compulsions are similar: time occupied by obsessive thoughts or compulsions; interference due to obsessions or compulsions; distress related to obsessions or not performing compulsions; efforts to resist obsessions or compulsions; and degree of control over obsessions or compulsions.

In addition to these sections, there is a target symptom list and a number of supplemental items that assess symptoms or behaviours that may be present but which are not included in the definition of OCD and are not used in the Y–BOCS scoring. The target symptom list refers to the patient's three most impairing or distressing obsessions, compulsions and avoidance behaviours. The supplemental items comprise insight, avoidance, indecisiveness, sense of responsibility, pervasive slowness and pathological doubt.

The Y–BOCS provides three summary scores: the severity score for obsessions (range 0–20), for compulsions (range 0–20), and a total score, which is the sum of all items (range 0–40). Y-BOCS scores of 0–7 are considered to indicate subclinical OCD symptoms; scores of 8–15, mild symptoms; 16–23, moderate symptoms; 24–31, severe symptoms; and 32–40, extreme severity.

The scale has good psychometric properties. The intraclass correlation coefficients reported are 0.81–0.97 for the test-retest reliability, 0.80–0.99 for the interrater reliability, and an internal consistency (Cronbach's alpha) ranging from 0.69 to 0.91. The convergent validity has been found to be good, although the discriminant validity has been more discrete, with large correlations with depression and anxiety [28–30]. The Y–BOCS has been shown to be sensitive to treatment-induced change and has become one of the most widely used scales in clinical trials [31]. There is also a self-report version, a computerized version and a child version.

A new version of the Y–BOCS, the Y–BOCS-II, has been developed [32] to improve some areas that had certain limitations. Several changes have been proposed. One of them has been to replace the item 4, 'resistance to obsessions', on the severity scale, which has a low correlation with the total severity score, by an item called 'obsession-free interval'. Another change concerns increasing the scoring range of the scoring of all items from 5-point (0–4) to 6-point (0–5), since it had been observed that the scale was less sensitive to change in patients with very high scores. In order to emphasize the assessment of avoidance behaviours, changes have also been made to two of the compulsion items ('distress if compulsions (or avoidance) prevented' and 'interference from compulsions') and one obsession item ('interference'). Finally, some modifications have been made to the wording and content of the Symptom Checklist.

Dimensional Yale–Brown Obsessive-Compulsive Scale (DY–BOCS)

The DY–BOCS [33] was developed from the theoretical rationale that OCD may be a heterogeneous disorder given its clinical diversity, and the number of genetic and treatment studies that support this view. Assessment of different symptom dimensions yields more homogeneous subgroups that may allow a better understanding of OCD's complexity and provide a valuable approach to elucidating genetic and neurobiological mechanisms underlying the heterogeneous OCD presentations, through identification of more robust endophenotypes as well as comorbidity or treatment outcome studies [11]. The DY–BOCS was initially developed at Yale University and refined in other centres of the United States, Brazil and Japan. The DY–BOCS is based on the Y–BOCS and is composed of semi-structured scales for assessing the presence and severity of OC symptom dimensions. The DY–BOCS includes a self-report instrument and a clinician-administered instrument. The self-report instrument consists of an 88-item checklist of obsessions and compulsions, divided into six dimensions:

1. obsessions about harm due to aggression/injury/violence/natural disasters and related compulsions;
2. sexual/moral/religious obsessions and related compulsions;
3. obsessions about symmetry/'just-right' perceptions, and compulsions to count or order/arrange;
4. contamination obsessions and cleaning compulsions;
5. obsessions and compulsions related to hoarding; and
6. miscellaneous obsessions and compulsions that relate to somatic concerns and superstitions, among other symptoms.

The clinician-administered scales can be used to assess the presence and severity of each of the above symptom dimensions. Each of these scales consists of three items (frequency, distress and interference) measured on a 0–5 scale, yielding a total score ranging from 0 to 15. Further, the rater estimates the global symptom severity scale using the same three ordinal scales (frequency, distress and interference; score range 0–15) and an impairment score to assess the overall level of current impairment due to OC symptoms on a scale (range 0–15). The total global score is obtained by combining the sum of the global severity scores and the impairment score, yielding a maximum total global severity score of 30. The psychometric properties of the DY–BOCS are good: interrater reliability showed intraclass correlation coefficients greater than 0.98 for each component score of the DY–BOCS, the levels of agreement between self-report and expert ratings had Pearson correlation coefficients of 0.75–0.87 for each dimension, the internal consistency showed a Cronbach's alpha of 0.94–0.95 for each dimension, and it has also showed good construct and divergent validity in both child and adult populations [33,34].

Leyton Obsessional Inventory (LOI)

The LOI [35] had been a commonly used scale before the appearance of the Y–BOCS, and the Child Version of the scale is still often used. The original LOI is a 69-item scale designed as a card sorting, or 'post-box', activity that measures obsessional symptoms and traits in a yes/no type of response. Two other subscales scored from 0 to 3 are 'resistance' and 'interference', which should help to differentiate between obsessional symptoms and traits. Several versions of the LOI have been developed, such as a pencil-and-paper version [36], the Leyton Obsessional Inventory – Child Version [37] and a shortened 10-item version, the Lynfield Obsessional Compulsive Questionnaire [38]. Evidence for reliability and validity is limited. The main limitations found are that the questionnaire is biased towards domestic topics such as cleanliness or tidiness (in fact, the original study was done in a group of 'house-proud' mothers) while other kind of symptoms, such as aggressive or other unacceptable thoughts, are not well represented. The scale is not very sensitive to treatment-induced change, and the administration of the original version is very lengthy.

Maudsley Obsessional-Compulsive Inventory (MOCI)

The MOCI [39] is a 30-item self-rated questionnaire that yields a score on four factorially derived subscales: checking, cleaning, doubting and slowness. Each item is rated dichotomously as true or false and, therefore, the total score range is 0–30. Due to the type of items included in the scale, patients with checking or cleaning symptoms will tend to score higher than will other patients with different kinds of obsessions with few symptoms or behaviours, even if they are very severe. Its reliability and validity are acceptable and it is easily administered. However, not all kinds of obsessions/compulsions are represented and its sensitivity to treatment-induced change is limited.

Padua Inventory (PI)

The PI [40] is a 60-item self-report questionnaire that measures OCD severity. The design of the inventory was addressed to measure obsessional complaints and intrusive phenomena not well covered by former OCD measures. It covers common obsessional and compulsive behaviour and identifies four factors underlying OCD: impaired control of mental activities, becoming contaminated, checking behaviours, and urges and worries about losing control over motor behaviours. One of the limitations of the scale is that its items do not adequately differentiate obsessions from worries [41].

Several revisions of the scale have been published. The Padua Inventory – Washington State University Revision (PI–WSUR) [42] aims to achieve a better differentiation between worries and obsessional symptoms. It has 39 items that cover five content categories relevant to obsessions and compulsions: obsessional thoughts about harm to self/others; obsessional impulses to harm self/others; contamination obsessions and washing rituals; checking compulsions; and dressing/grooming rituals.

The Padua Inventory – Revised (PI–R) [43] was derived from a factor-analytic study which found a five-factor structure instead of the original four factors. It is a 41-item scale that assesses five subscales: Impulses, Washing, Checking, Rumination and Precision.

A recently proposed revision, the Padua Inventory – Palatine Revision (PI–PR) [44], with 24 items, was derived from the study of the factor structure of the previous two revisions (PI–R and PI–WSUR) in OCD, anxiety and depression samples, and assesses six subscales: contamination and washing; checking; numbers; dressing and grooming; rumination; and harming obsessions and impulses.

Obsessive Compulsive Inventory (OCI)

The OCI [45] was developed to address the problems inherent in the available instruments for diagnosing and determining the severity of OCD. It is a self-report inventory and consists of 42 items comprising seven subscales: washing, checking, doubting, ordering, obsessing (i.e. having obsessional thoughts), hoarding and mental neutralizing. Each item is rated on a five-point (0–4) Likert scale for both frequency and distress. Psychometric properties are generally strong, although less so for the hoarding subscale. It has been translated into several languages. A child version has recently been developed [46]. A shorter, 18-item version, the revised OCI (OCI–R) has also been developed [47]. This shorter version improves on the previous version in that it eliminates the redundant frequency scale, simplifies the scoring of the subscales, and reduces overlap across subscales, all while retaining good psychometric properties.

INSIGHT

Although a main feature of OCD is that the person recognizes that the obsessional thoughts, impulses or images are a product of his or her own mind, in some cases there is poor or even a lack of insight into their symptoms. This feature that is observed in some patients is explicitly recorded in DSM-IV as a specifier. In fact, the only specifier of OCD that was established in DSM-IV is 'with poor insight', which is defined as: 'when, for most of the time during the current episode, the individual does not recognize that the obsessions or compulsions are excessive or unreasonable' [48]. The presence of overvalued ideation denotes poor insight while a degree of delusional intensity corresponds to a lack of insight. However, in cases where the ideation is considered to achieve the degree of delusional intensity, DSM-IV proposes the use of the diagnostic categories 'delusional disorder' or 'psychotic disorder not otherwise specified'. However, this suggestion has been called into question since those patients who are diagnosed with delusional disorder due to the lack of insight on their obsessions may not have a disorder that is distinct from OCD [49,50].

One issue that in some cases may become difficult is differentiating an overvalued ideation from delusions and from obsessions. Overvalued ideas may be considered as strongly held unreasonable beliefs, accompanied by strong affect. Overvalued ideas are not felt to be as intrusive as an obsession, are not considered by the individual as senseless, are egosyntonic and, hence, there is neither resistance nor struggle against them. They are held strongly, although with less than delusional intensity, and their content may not be as bizarre as in some delusions. Compared to delusions, they may lead to repeated action that is considered justified [51]. However, the concept of insight, particularly in OCD, and related concepts such as poor insight or overvalued ideation, has been the subject of different definitions and considerations. There is no unique definition for overvalued ideation, nor is there an operationalized definition. DSM-IV acknowledges the difficulty in clinical practice to distinguish an overvalued idea from a delusion, and places it on a continuum based on the intensity of the belief. While a delusion is defined as a 'false personal belief based on an incorrect inference about external reality and firmly sustained in spite of what almost everyone else believes', DSM-IV describes overvalued ideation as 'an unreasonable and sustained belief that is maintained with less than delusional intensity (i.e., the person is able to acknowledge the possibility that the belief may or may not be true). The belief is not one that is ordinarily accepted by other members of the person's culture or sub-culture' [48]. The general view is that there is a continuum from an obsession, with full or good insight at one end of the continuum, to a poorer insight with overvalued ideation in the middle, and a delusional intensity of belief at the other extreme.

The diagnostic criteria of DSM-IV require that 'at some point during the course of the disorder, the person has recognized that the obsessions or compulsions are excessive or unreasonable' (criterion B). This criterion may be considered to reflect the insight quality of the obsessional symptoms but there is no clear and operationalized definition of what 'excessive or unreasonable' means, and this aspect may be interpreted in different ways by clinicians [50]. This lack of a definite meaning of 'excessive and unreasonable' in the diagnostic criteria of DSM-IV has led to the suggestion of deleting criterion B and expanding the specifier 'with poor insight' to include a broader range such as 'good or fair insight', 'poor insight' and 'lack of insight' in DSM-5 [50].

Rating insight

Since insight is an important feature of OCD, its measurement has become an important issue, and several scales have been designed to assess the degree of insight. Insel and Akiskal [52] had already studied insight in 23 patients using a scale that explored different aspects, such as the perceived validity, strength of belief in the feared consequences, resistance and bizarreness of the obsessions. Subsequently, other more formal scales have been developed.

- *Brown Assessment of Beliefs Scale (BABS).* One of the most widely used scales for the assessment of insight is the BABS [53]. The BABS is a semi-structured, clinician-administered, seven-item scale with specific probes and five anchors for each item, designed to assess insight/degree of delusionality during the past week in a variety of psychiatric disorders. It assumes that insight exists on a continuum and that insight itself consists of a number of components. The components covered by the scale are conviction (how convinced the person is that his/her belief is accurate); perception of others' views (how certain the person is that most people think the belief makes sense); explanation of differing views (the person's explanation for the difference between his/her and others' views of the belief); fixity (whether the person could be convinced that the belief is wrong); attempt to disprove beliefs (how actively the person tries to disprove his/her belief); insight (whether the person recognizes that the belief has a psychiatric/psychological cause); and referential thinking (an optional item that assesses ideas/delusions of reference). Each of the first six items is rated from 0 to 4 and the total score is the sum of these six items. The psychometric properties of this scale are well established, with a strong internal consistency (Cronbach's alpha $= 0.87$) and strong interrater (intraclass correlation coefficient (ICC) for total $= 0.96$) and retest reliability (ICC for total $= 0.95$). The BABS is sensitive to treatment-induced changes.
- *Overvalued Ideas Scale (OVIS).* Another scale used to measure insight is the OVIS [54]. This is a nine-item clinician-administered scale designed to quantitatively assess levels of overvalued ideas in OCD. The components that form the scale are: bizarreness, belief accuracy, fixity, reasonableness, effectiveness of compulsions, pervasiveness of belief, reasons others do not share the belief, and two items assessing stability of belief. One study [54] found the scale to show adequate internal consistency reliability (alpha coefficient $= 0.88$ at baseline), test-retest reliability ($r = 0.86$) and interrater reliability ($r = 0.88$). Moderate to high levels of convergent validity were found with measures of obsessive-compulsive symptoms, a single-item assessment of overvalued ideas and psychotic symptoms. This study also obtained medium levels of discriminant validity with respect to measures of anxiety and depression. Individuals regarded as having high OVIS scores showed greater stability of this pathology than did those with lower OVIS scores, suggesting that overvalued ideas are stable for extreme scorers.
- *Fixity of Beliefs Scale.* This is a five-item instrument designed to measure patients' degree of recognition that their obsessive-compulsive beliefs are unreasonable [55]. The items rate the patients' beliefs about the feared consequences of not performing their compulsions. The items assess: (1) patients' confidence that the harmful consequence will happen; (2) patients' recognition of the

disparity of their beliefs from conventional beliefs; (3) patients' understanding of why they have unrealistic beliefs; (4) flexibility in changing mistaken beliefs; and (5) bizarreness of obsessive ideas. Foa *et al.* [56] found that two items, presence of feared consequences and certainty that the feared consequence will occur, predicted treatment outcome for OCD.

Patients with OCD with poor insight have been reported to suffer a more severe form of the disorder, with higher Y–BOCS scores and a greater number of symptoms [57–62], although some studies have not found this association [63,64]. However, the greater severity found in some studies could be at least partially explained by the higher scores on specific items (lack of resistance and lack of control) that are assigned to these patients on the Y–BOCS scale given that poor insight involves the absence of struggle against obsessions and rituals that are not considered senseless [62]. Poor insight has also been associated with a poorer response to treatment [60,65], although not all studies have confirmed this relationship [66].

In summary, poor insight is a phenomenon that has been reported in 15–36% of obsessive patients [51,52,57–59,62,63,67,68]. In some cases, the distinction among obsessions, overvalued ideas and delusions may be complex and part of this complexity may stem from the definition of the nature of insight. A recent review [69] considers that insight could be best conceived as a dynamic mental state rather than a symptom or a component of the symptoms, and it would be independent of the disorder itself. Notwithstanding, the assessment of insight is essential because of the clinical, diagnostic and outcome issues that may be associated with poor or lack of insight.

ASSESSMENT OF THE RISK OF SUICIDE

Traditionally, suicidal behaviour in OCD has been estimated to be infrequent. Patients with OCD have classically been considered to be at low risk for suicide, with reports of completed suicides in less than 1% [70], and a history of suicide attempts in 3–4% of patients [71–73]. However, more recent studies have found higher rates of suicidal behaviour, suggesting that 10–27% of those suffering from an OCD may attempt suicide at least once in their life [74–76]. Kamath *et al.* [75] have reported that OCD is associated with high rates of both suicide attempts (27%) and suicidal ideation (59% of patients at any time in their life). A Brazilian study [76] found that 46% of OCD patients surveyed had suicidal thoughts, 20% had made suicidal plans and 10% had attempted suicide. The Brown Longitudinal Obsessive Compulsive Study [7] has studied 293 OCD patients and found a reported rate of suicidal ideation in 52% of them, while a history of at least one suicide attempt was found in 15% of them. Another study [77] followed-up 216 OCD patients for 1 to 6 years and found persistent suicidal ideation in 8% of the sample (persistent defined as being present in three consecutive assessments, each carried out every

3 months), while 5% of the sample attempted suicide and two patients (0.9%) actually committed suicide during the follow-up. The most frequent factor found to be associated with suicidal behaviour has been severity of depression. Other factors found in studies have been hopelessness, being non-married, and symmetry/ordering obsessions and compulsions. Some limitations of these studies are that many of them have recorded the information retrospectively and consequently only a few factors have been examined for their association with suicidal behaviour.

Suicidality is not usually related to compulsive behaviours. When suicidal ideation is present, it may be related to hopelessness due to a chronic and highly invalidating OCD disorder, or to the presence of comorbid disorders such as depression, substance abuse/dependence (including alcohol), or other mental disorders with a high risk of suicide. Although the rates for completed suicide in OCD are lower than those found in some other mental disorders such as depression or schizophrenia, the risk of suicide in OCD deserves specific evaluation. In fact, suicidal ideation and suicide attempts are more frequent among OCD patients than in the general population and they may be the steps prior to a completed suicide.

DIFFERENTIAL DIAGNOSIS, COMORBIDITIES AND RELATED DISORDERS

The assessment of OCD involves screening for the presence of other disorders. Several disorders may exhibit obsessive or compulsive symptoms as part of their manifestations, and a differential diagnosis from OCD must therefore be carried out. Furthermore, some of these disorders show a high comorbidity with OCD and their detection is important. A subgroup of these disorders that show either certain similarities or comorbidity with OCD have been included within the term 'OC spectrum disorders'.

Although distinct from OCD, they seem to be related and it has been proposed that they could be best considered as belonging to an OC spectrum [78]. The disorders that have been ascribed to the OC spectrum are diverse and have numbered from 10 to 20. Some of these disorders are more neurological disorders – such as Tourette disorder or autism – while others are associated with bodily preoccupation – such as body dysmorphic disorder, anorexia nervosa or hypochondriasis – and even others belong to impulse control disorders –such as pathological gambling, kleptomania or trichotillomania [79]. More recently, Phillips *et al.* [80], in an article that was commissioned by the DSM-V Anxiety, Obsessive-Compulsive Spectrum, Posttraumatic, and Dissociative Disorders Work Group, have proposed that these disorders be considered according to three groups:

1. motoric or lower-order repetitive behaviours (e.g. trichotillomania, skin-picking disorder);

2. cognitive or higher-order OC symptoms (e.g. body dysmorphic disorder, hypochondriasis); and
3. impulse control disorders or behavioural addictions (e.g. pathological gambling).

The assessment of the presence of OC spectrum disorders is relevant because of their similarities with OCD which may pose issues in the differential diagnosis, or their comorbidity with OCD that some of them have.

The differential diagnosis of OCD includes organic brain disorders, schizophrenia, depression, hypochondriasis, phobias, Tourette disorder and tic disorders, obsessive-compulsive personality disorder, body dysmorphic disorder and hoarding.

Organic brain disorders

As is the case with other mental symptoms, the clinician should rule out brain diseases that may underlie OC symptoms. The presence of OC symptoms may result from brain disturbances, either focal or diffuse, that can affect brain areas or circuits involved in OCD. In fact, the hypothesis that a biological substrate might underlie obsessions and compulsions was supported by the observation of the presence of OC symptoms in patients affected by the lethargic encephalitis pandemic between 1917 and 1926 [81,82]. Currently, different brain areas and circuits have been related to OCD, more specifically the cortico-subcortical-thalamic-cortical circuits, particularly the orbitofrontal circuit that involves the orbitofrontal cortex, areas of the basal ganglia and thalamus. Diseases or lesions that may affect these areas and circuits or others related to them, may result in obsessive symptoms either as one of the first expressions of an underlying disease or as a residual symptom after the injury. OC symptoms have been reported in different kinds of injuries and diseases [83], such as traumatic brain injury [84], cerebrovascular accidents [85,86], brain tumours [87], temporal lobe epilepsy (in 14–22% of patients with this disease) [88,89], frontotemporal dementia [90,91], progressive supranuclear palsy [92], neuroacanthocytosis [93], brain infections (encephalitis and postencephalitic states, acquired inmunodeficiency syndrome) [94], manganese intoxication [95] or brain surgery [96]. Huntington's chorea may also show OC symptoms in 22–50% of the cases, and this may be difficult to distinguish from primary OCD [97–99]. Usually, these neurological disorders will have associated specific neurological symptoms – apart from the obsessional ones – which will help in making the differential diagnosis.

One particular case concerns patients with Parkinson's disease who are treated with dopamine agonists and who may show compulsive behaviours that are usually linked to impulse control disorders. A recent study of 3090 patients with Parkinson's disease found that 17% of those taking dopamine agonists had at least one impulse control disorder (gambling, compulsive sexual behaviour, compulsive buying, binge-eating disorder) [100]. The mechanism has been related to dysfunctions in reward processing [101].

Schizophrenia

The distinction between OCD and schizophrenia is not usually difficult to make since subjects with OCD usually recognize the absurdity of their symptoms, even in some cases in which the obsessional thoughts and the behaviours associated with them may be quite bizarre. In patients with OCD with poor insight the distinction may be more complex, but the absence of typical schizophrenic features can help in the differentiation. There is another group of patients in whom the initial manifestations are OC symptoms but who eventually go on to develop typical symptoms of schizophrenia. Furthermore, OCD will be comorbid in a substantial group of patients with schizophrenia. Several studies [102–109] have found that about 25–35% of subjects with schizophrenia have OC symptoms, and even around 15–25% meet criteria for OCD, although the figures differ among studies. Although antipsychotic treatment, particularly clozapine, may be a factor that accounts for the appearance of OC symptoms in some cases, in others the comorbidity between these two disorders cannot be explained by these drugs.

Depression

Depression, either as a full-blown syndrome or in the form of depressive symptoms, is a condition very often associated with OCD. It has been estimated that about 60–70% of OCD patients may have a comorbid lifetime diagnosis of major depression [7,102]. In many cases depressive symptoms are related to the distress and disability due to OCD, which is the primary disorder. Reciprocally, obsessive symptoms may also appear in about 20% of cases of a primary depressive disorder [110,111]. In those patients in whom both the obsessional symptoms and depressive symptoms appear it may be difficult to distinguish between a primary OCD and secondary obsessions due to a depressive disorder. Depression as a primary diagnosis usually has a later onset than OCD, and show an episodic course, with a remission of the obsessional symptoms during the interepisodic periods; the ruminations are more centred on past events (whereas in OCD concerns are more focused on present or future threats) and are more egosyntonic.

Hypochondriasis

Fear of becoming ill is a common preoccupation in both OCD and hypochondriasis. But patients with OCD tend to have less intensity in their conviction of having an illness and they may have other obsessions and rituals not related to bodily health. In hypochondriasis the beliefs are more egosyntonic and subjects may experience somatic sensations. About 10% of OCD patients could also meet criteria for hypochondriasis [112,113].

Phobias

In some cases OC symptoms, particularly contamination obsessions and fear of losing control, may be confounded with phobias. Genuine phobias are usually more circumscribed to specific stimuli, there are no rituals associated, and the avoidance behaviours are very efficacious in relieving anxiety.

Tourette disorder and tic disorders

These disorders are considered to be closely related to OCD. About 30% of OCD patients have comorbid lifetime tic disorders [114]. With Tourette disorder, OC symptoms are present in about 40% of the patients and OCD in 20% of them [115]. It is usually easy to distinguish between tics and compulsions, but it may be more difficult in some complex tics. OCD compulsions usually have an obsessional thought associated with them and are more goal-directed, whereas the premonitory experiences in tics are more sensorial or perceived as urges and with fewer associated cognitions [116,117]. Finally, patients with both OCD and tics may represent a particular subgroup since several differences have been reported in this group, such as an earlier age of onset [118], feelings of incompleteness, a need for things to be 'just right', and more aggressive and symmetry obsessions [115,119].

Obsessive-compulsive personality disorder (OCPD)

Obsessive-compulsive personality disorder is characterized by excessive preoccupation with orderliness, perfectionism, and mental and interpersonal control, symptoms that may resemble the compulsivity in OCD. There is also a certain comorbidity between OCD and OCPD: about 30% of patients with OCD also show OCPD [7,120,121] and OCD is present in approximately 20% of OCPD subjects [122]. An important difference between OCD and OCPD is that in OCD the symptoms are experienced as egodystonic (i.e. not acceptable by the individual) whereas in OCPD they are egosyntonic. Further, the degree of functional impairment in OCPD is significantly lower than in OCD.

Body dysmorphic disorder (BDD)

In BDD repetitive behaviours may emerge in response to an excessive preoccupation with an imagined defect in appearance or a slight physical anomaly [123].

About one-third of subjects with BDD will meet OCD criteria [124]. Insight is poorer in BDD than in OCD, there is no feeling of incompletion, and the behaviour is related to the preoccupations about appearance.

Hoarding

Although hoarding is a typical OCD symptom that is present in 15–40% of OCD patients [5,55,125], it may also appear independently of OCD. This has led to the proposal that hoarding syndrome could be considered as a different disorder [126,127]. In those cases in which hoarding is related to OCD, this behaviour can be explained as a consequence of the patients' obsessions (e.g. items not discarded due to fear of catastrophic consequences, complicated rituals before discarding items that lead to avoidance of discarding), the hoarded items may be more bizarre, and the behaviour is more usually experienced as egodystonic [128]. Hoarding behaviour may also be associated with severe neurological conditions (e.g. dementia, brain lesions) and other psychiatric disorders (e.g. alcoholism, schizophrenia, schizotypal or obsessive personality disorders) [129].

Other disorders

Other psychiatric disorders may also show obsessive symptoms or compulsivity, like anxiety, impulse control disorders or behavioural addictions (e.g. pathological gambling, compulsive buying), autism, or disorders related to grooming, such as trichotillomania or skin picking disorders. In general, the specific behaviours and symptoms associated with the definition of these conditions will permit the differential diagnosis from OCD.

CONCLUSIONS

The assessment of OCD follows the general procedure that is carried out in other disorders, but there are also specific characteristics to be examined which may be relevant to treatment decisions and to general management of an individual OCD case. As studies have found that the time elapsed between the first OCD symptoms and the diagnosis is very long, screening procedures for the detection of OCD can be used in the general assessment of cases in which OCD may be suspected. Apart from the more formal structured clinical interviews, several researchers have proposed a few easy questions to detect the disorder. Early detection may help to prevent functional impairment and improve the long-term prognosis.

OCD is a complex disorder with very different clinical manifestations, courses and outcomes, which has led to discussion of the possible heterogeneity of the disorder. Studies have identified a number of characteristics (Table 1.2) that are useful to consider when assessing an OCD patient. Regarding OC symptoms, many clinical scales have been designed to capture the severity and diversity of them. Among the clinical features, the assessment of insight is one of the most important since it may have a critical bearing on the adherence to treatment and outcome. Although suicide in OCD is less common than in some other mental disorders, the assessment of this risk should always be included. The relationship of OCD to other disorders is also complex. Differential diagnosis must be carried out for a number of organic and mental disorders but OCD can also be comorbid with some of them. Indeed, the identification of these disorders is essential for an adequate approach. Other characteristics reviewed in other chapters that deserve to be examined are those related to previous treatments and the previous course of the disorder. The assessment of these clinical factors and comorbid conditions may be essential since they have been associated with different clinical clusters, neurobiological factors and outcomes, and the assessment of these features may allow a more personalized management.

REFERENCES

1. Ruscio AM, Stein DJ, Chiu WT, Kessler RC. The epidemiology of obsessive-compulsive disorder in the National Comorbidity Survey Replication. *Mol Psychiatry* 2010;**15**:53–63.
2. Robins LN, Helzer JE, Weissman MM *et al*. Lifetime prevalence of specific psychiatric disorders in three sites. *Arch Gen Psychiatry* 1984;**41**:949–958.
3. American Psychiatric Association. *Diagnostic and Statistical Manual of Mental Disorders*, 4th edn, Text Revision. Washington, DC: American Psychiatric Association, 2000.
4. Rasmussen SA, Eisen JL. Clinical and epidemiologic findings of significance to neuropharmacologic trials in OCD. *Psychopharmacol Bull* 1988;**24**:466–470.
5. Mataix-Cols D, Rauch SL, Manzo PA, Jenike MA, Baer L. Use of factor-analyzed symptom dimensions to predict outcome with serotonin reuptake inhibitors and placebo in the treatment of obsessive-compulsive disorder. *Am J Psychiatry* 1999;**156**:1409–1416.
6. Cavallini MC, Di Bella D, Siliprandi F, Malchiodi F, Bellodi L. Exploratory factor analysis of obsessive-compulsive patients and association with 5-HTTLPR polymorphism. *Am J Med Genet* 2002;**114**:347–353.
7. Pinto A, Mancebo MC, Eisen JL, Pagano ME, Rasmussen SA. The Brown Longitudinal Obsessive Compulsive Study: clinical features and symptoms of the sample at intake. *J Clin Psychiatry* 2006;**67**:703–711.
8. Pinto A, Greenberg BD, Grados MA *et al*. Further development of YBOCS dimensions in the OCD Collaborative Genetics study: symptoms vs. categories. *Psychiatry Res* 2008;**160**:83–93.
9. Matsunaga H, Hayashida K, Kiriike N, Maebayashi K, Stein DJ. The clinical utility of symptom dimensions in obsessive-compulsive disorder. *Psychiatry Res* 2010;**180**:25–29.

10. Bloch MH, Landeros-Weisenberger A, Rosario MC, Pittenger C, Leckman JF. Meta-analysis of the symptom structure of obsessive-compulsive disorder. *Am J Psychiatry* 2008;**165**:1532–1542.

11. Mataix-Cols D, Rosario-Campos MC, Leckman JF. A multidimensional model of obsessive-compulsive disorder. *Am J Psychiatry* 2005;**162**:228–238.

12. Simonds LM, Thorpe SJ. Attitudes toward obsessive-compulsive disorders: an experimental investigation. *Soc Psychiatry Psychiatr Epidemiol* 2003;**38**:331–336.

13. Heyman I, Mataix-Cols D, Fineberg NA. Obsessive-compulsive disorder. *Brit Med J* 2006;**333**:424–429.

14. Fineberg NA, O'Doherty C, Rajagopal S, Reddy K, Banks A, Gale TM. How common is obsessive-compulsive disorder in a dermatology outpatient clinic? *J Clin Psychiatry* 2003;**64**:152–155.

15. National Institute for Health and Clinical Excellence. Obsessive-compulsive disorder: core interventions in the treatment of obsessive-compulsive disorder and body dysmorphic disorder. Clinical guideline 31. London: NICE, 2006.

16. American Psychiatric Association. Practice guideline for the treatment of patients with obsessive-compulsive disorder. Arlington, VA: American Psychiatric Association, 2007.

17. Canadian Psychiatric Association. Clinical Practice Guidelines. Management of Anxiety Disorders. 6. Obsessive-compulsive disorder. *Can J Psychiatry* 2006;**51**(Suppl. 2):43s–49s.

18. Brown TA, Di Nardo PA, Barlow DH. *Anxiety Disorders Interview Schedule for DSMIV*. San Antonio, TX: The Psychological Corporation, 1994.

19. First MB, Spitzer RL, Gibbon M, Williams JBW. *Structured Clinical Interview for DSM-IV Axis I Disorders, Clinician Version (SCID-CV)*. Washington, DC: American Psychiatric Press, Inc., 1996.

20. First MB, Spitzer RL, Gibbon M, Williams JBW. *Structured Clinical Interview for DSM-IV-TR Axis I Disorders, Research Version, Patient Edition (SCID-I/P)*. New York: Biometrics Research, New York State Psychiatric Institute, 2002.

21. Official website for Structured Clinical Interview for DSM disorders (SCID). What is the Reliability of the SCID-I? http://www.scid4.org/psychometric/scidI_reliability.html. Accessed 4 August 2010.

22. Kessler RC, Ustun TB. The World Mental Health (WMH) Survey Initiative version of the World Health Organization (WHO) Composite International Diagnostic Interview (CIDI). *Int J Methods Psychiatr Res* 2004;**13**:93–121.

23. Lecrubier Y, Sheehan DV, Weiller E *et al.* The Mini International Neuropsychiatric Interview (MINI): a short diagnostic structured interview: reliability and validity according to the CIDI. *Eur Psychiatry* 1997;**12**:224–231.

24. Sheehan DV, Lecrubier Y, Sheehan KH *et al.* The validity of the Mini International Neuropsychiatric Interview (MINI) according to the SCID-P and its reliability. *Eur Psychiatry* 1997;**12**:232–241.

25. Sheehan DV, Lecrubier Y, Sheehan KH *et al.* The Mini-International Neuropsychiatric Interview (MINI): the development and validation of a structured diagnostic psychiatric interview for DSM-IV and ICD-10. *J Clin Psychiatry* 1998;**59**(Suppl. 20):22–33.

26. Goodman WK, Price LH, Rasmussen SA *et al.* The Yale-Brown Obsessive Compulsive Scale: I. Development, use, and reliability. *Arch Gen Psychiatry* 1989; **46**:1006–1011.

27. Goodman WL, Price LH, Rasmussen SA, Mazure C. The Yale-Brown obsessive compulsive scale (Y-BOCS): Validity. *Arch Gen Psychiatry* 1989;**46**:1012–1016.

28. Taylor S. Assessment of obsessive-compulsive disorder. In: Swinson RP, Antony MM, Rachman S, Richter MA (eds), *Obsessive-Compulsive Disorder: Theory, Research and Treatment.* New York: Guilford Press, 1998; pp. 229–257.

29. St Clare T. Assessment procedures. In: Menzies RG, De Silva P (eds), *Obsessive-Compulsive Disorder: Theory, Research and Treatment.* Chichester: John Wiley & Sons, Ltd, 2003; pp. 239–257.

30. Mataix-Cols D, Fullana MA, Alonso P, Menchón JM, Vallejo J. Convergent and discriminant validity of the Yale-Brown Obsessive-Compulsive Scale Symptom Checklist. *Psychother Psychosom* 2004;**73**:190–196.

31. Tolin DF, Abramowitz JS, Diefenbach GJ. Defining response in clinical trials for obsessive-compulsive disorder: a signal detection analysis of the Yale-Brown obsessive compulsive scale. *J Clin Psychiatry* 2005;**66**:1549–1557.

32. Storch EA, Rasmussen SA, Price LH, Larson MJ, Murphy TK, Goodman WK. Development and psychometric evaluation of the Yale-Brown Obsessive-Compulsive Scale, Second Edition. *Psychol Assess* 2010;**22**:223–232.

33. Rosario-Campos MC, Miguel EC, Quatrano S *et al.* The Dimensional Yale-Brown Obsessive-Compulsive Scale (DY-BOCS): an instrument for assessing obsessive-compulsive symptom dimensions. *Mol Psychiatry* 2006;**11**:495–504.

34. Pertusa A, Fernández de la Cruz L, Alonso P, Menchón JM, Mataix-Cols D. Independent validation of the Dimensional Yale-Brown Obsessive Compulsive Scale (DY-BOCS). *European Psychiatry* 12 May 2011 (epub ahead of print). Accessed at http://dx.doi.org/10.1016/j.eurpsy.2011.02.010, on 26th January 2012.

35. Cooper J. The Leyton obsessional inventory. *Psychol Med* 1970;**1**:48–64.

36. Snowdon J. A comparison of written and postbox forms of the Leyton Obsessional Inventory. *Psychol Med* 1980;**10**:165–170.

37. Berg CJ, Rapoport JL, Flament M. The Leyton Obsessional Inventory – Child Version. *J Am Acad Child Psychiatry* 1986;**25**:84–91.

38. Allen JJ, Tune GS. The Lynfield Obsessional/Compulsive Questionnaires. *Scott Med J* 1975;**20**(1 Suppl.):21–24.

39. Hodgson RJ, Rachman S. Obsessive compulsive complaints. *Behav Res Ther* 1977;**15**:389–395.

40. Sanavio E. Obsessions and compulsions: the Padua inventory. *Behav Res Ther* 1988;**26**:169–177.

41. Freeston MH, Ladouceur R, Rhéaume J, Letarte H, Gagnon F, Thibodeau N. Self-report of obsessions and worry. *Behav Res Ther* 1994;**32**:29–36.

42. Burns GL, Keortge SG, Formea GM, Sternberger LG. Revision of the Padua Inventory of obsessive compulsive disorder symptoms: distinctions between worry, obsessions, and compulsions. *Behav Res Ther* 1996;**34**:163–173.

43. van Oppen P, Hoekstra RJ, Emmelkamp PMG. The structure of obsessive-compulsive symptoms. *Behav Res Ther* 1995;**33**:15–23.

44. Gönner S, Ecker W, Leonhart R. The Padua Inventory: do revisions need revision? *Assessment* 2010;**17**:89–106.

45. Foa EB, Kozak MJ, Salkovskis PM, Coles ME, Amir N. The validation of a new obsessive-compulsive disorder scale: the obsessive-compulsive inventory. *Psychol Assess* 1998;**10**:206–214.

46. Foa EB, Coles M, Huppert JD, Pasupuleti RV, Franklin ME, March J. Development and validation of a child version of the obsessive compulsive inventory. *Behav Ther* 2010;**41**:121–132.
47. Foa EB, Huppert JD, Leiberg S *et al.* The Obsessive-Compulsive Inventory: development and validation of a short version. *Psychol Assess* 2002;**14**:485–496.
48. American Psychiatric Association. *Diagnostic and Statistical Manual of Mental Disorders*, 4th edn. Washington, DC: American Psychiatric Association, 1994.
49. Stein DJ, Denys D, Gloster AT *et al.* Obsessive-compulsive disorder: diagnostic and treatment issues. *Psychiatr Clin North Am* 2009;**32**:665–685.
50. Leckman JF, Damiaan Denys D, Blair Simpson H *et al.* Obsessive-compulsive disorder: a review of the diagnostic criteria and possible subtypes and dimensional specifiers for DSM-V *Depress Anx* 2010;**27**:507–527.
51. Veale D. Over-valued ideas: A conceptual analysis. *Behav Res Ther* 2002;**40**:383–400.
52. Insel TR, Akiskal HS. Obsessive-compulsive disorder with psychotic features: a phenomenologic analysis. *Am J Psychiatry* 1986;**143**:1527–1533.
53. Eisen JL, Phillips KA, Baer L, Beer DA, Atala KP, Rasmussen SA. The Brown Assessment of Beliefs Scale – reliability and validity. *Am J Psychiatry* 1998;**155**:102–108.
54. Neziroglu F, McKay D, Yaryura-Tobias JA, Stevens KP, Todaro J. The Overvalued Ideas Scale: development, reliability and validity in obsessive-compulsive disorder. *Behav Res Ther* 1999;**37**:881–902.
55. Foa EB, Kozak MJ, Goodman WK, Jenike MA, Hollander E, Rasmussen S. DSM IV field trial: obsessive-compulsive disorder. *Am J Psychiatry* 1995;**152**: 90–96.
56. Foa EB, Abramowitz JS, Franklin ME, Kozak MJ. Feared consequences, fixity of belief, and treatment outcome in patients with obsessive-compulsive disorder. *Behav Ther* 1999;**30**:717–724.
57. Matsunaga H, Kiriike N, Matsui T, *et al.* Obsessive-compulsive disorder with poor insight. *Compr Psychiatry* 2002;**43**:150–157.
58. Türksoy N, Tükel R, Özdemir O, Karali A. Comparison of clinical characteristics in good and poor insight obsessive-compulsive disorder. *J Anxiety Disord* 2002;**16**:413–423.
59. De Berardis D, Campanella D, Gambi F *et al.* Insight and alexithymia in adult outpatients with obsessive compulsive disorder. *Eur Arch Psychiatry Clin Neurosci* 2005;**255**:350–358.
60. Ravi V, Kishore R, Samar R, Janardhan YC, Reddy CR, Chandrasekhar K. Clinical characteristics and treatment response in poor and good insight obsessive-compulsive disorder. *Eur Psychiatry* 2004;**19**:202–208.
61. Solyom L, DiNicola VF, Phil M, Sookman D, Luchins D. Is there an obsessive psychosis? Aetiological and prognostic factors of an atypical form of obsessive-compulsive neurosis. *Can J Psychiatry* 1985;**30**:372–380.
62. Alonso P, Menchón JM, Segalàs C *et al.* Clinical implications of insight assessment in obsessive-compulsive disorder. *Compr Psychiatry* 2008;**49**:305–312.
63. Marazziti D, Dell'Osso L, Di Nasso E *et al.* Insight in obsessive-compulsive disorder: a study of an Italian sample. *Eur Psychiatry* 2002;**17**:407–410.
64. Eisen JL, Phillips KA, Coles ME, Rasmussen SA. Insight in obsessive-compulsive disorder and body dysmorphic disorder. *Compr Psychiatry* 2004;**45**:10–15.
65. Catapano F, Sperandeo R, Perris F, Lanzaro M, Maj M. Insight and resistance in patients with obsessive-compulsive disorder. *Psychopathology* 2001;**34**:62–68.

66. Eisen JL, Rasmussen SA, Phillips KA *et al*. Insight and treatment outcome in obsessive-compulsive disorder. *Compr Psychiatry* 2001;**42**:494–497.

67. Eisen JL, Rasmussen SA. Obsessive-compulsive disorder with psychotic features. *J Clin Psychiatry* 1993;**54**:373–398.

68. Foa EB, Kozak MJ, Goodman WK, Hollander E, Jenike MA, Rasmussen SA. DSM-IV field trial: obsessive-compulsive disorder. *Am J Psychiatry* 1995;**152**:90–96.

69. Marková IS, Jaafari N, Berrios GE. Insight and obsessive-compulsive disorder: a conceptual analysis. *Psychopathology* 2009;**42**:277–282.

70. Goodwin DW, Guze SB, Robins E. Follow-up studies in obsessional neurosis. *Arch Gen Psychiatry* 1969;**20**:182–187.

71. Coryell W. Obsessive-compulsive disorder and primary unipolar depression. Comparisons of background, family history, course and mortality. *J Nerv Ment Dis* 1981;**169**:220–224.

72. Koran LM, Thienemann ML, Davenport R. Quality of life for patients with obsessive-compulsive disorder. *Am J Psychiatry* 1996;**153**:783–788.

73. Khan A, Leventhal RM, Khan S, Brown WA. Suicide risk in patients with anxiety disorders: a meta-analysis of the FDA database. *J Affect Disord* 2002;**68**:183–190.

74. Torres AR, Prince MJ, Bebbington PE *et al*. Obsessive-compulsive disorder: prevalence, comorbidity, impact, and help-seeking in the British National Psychiatric Morbidity Survey of 2000. *Am J Psychiatry* 2006;**163**:1978–1985.

75. Kamath P, Reddy YC, Kandavel T. Suicidal behavior in obsessive-compulsive disorder. *J Clin Psychiatry* 2007;**68**:1741–1750.

76. Torres AR, de Abreu Ramos-Cerqueira AT, Torresan RC, de Souza Domingues M, Hercos AC, Guimaraes AB. Prevalence and associated factors for suicidal ideation and behaviors in obsessive-compulsive disorder. *CNS Spectrums* 2007;**12**:771–778.

77. Alonso P, Segalàs C, Real E *et al*. Suicide in patients treated for obsessive-compulsive disorder: a prospective follow-up study. *J Affect Disord* 2010;**124**:300–308.

78. Hollander E. *Obsessive-Compulsive Related Disorders*. Washington, DC: American Psychiatric Press, 1993.

79. Hollander E. Treatment of obsessive-compulsive spectrum disorders with SSRIs. *Br J Psychiatry Suppl* 1998;**173**(Suppl. 35):7–12.

80. Phillips KA, Stein DJ, Rauch SL *et al*. Should an obsessive-compulsive spectrum grouping of disorders be included in DSM-V? *Depress Anxiety* 2010;**27**:528–555.

81. Mayer-Gross W, Steiner G. Encephalitis lethargica in der Selbstbeobachtung. *Z ges Neurol Psychiat* 1921;**73**:283–286.

82. Schilder P. The organic background of obsessions and compulsions. *Am J Psychiatry* 1938;**94**:1397–1416.

83. Coetzer BR. Obsessive-compulsive disorder following brain injury: a review. *Int J Psychiatry Med* 2004;**34**:363–377.

84. Grados MA. Obsessive-compulsive disorder after traumatic brain injury. *Int Rev Psychiatry* 2003;**15**:350–358.

85. Rodrigo Escalona P, Adair JC, Roberts BB, Graeber DA. Obsessive-compulsive disorder following bilateral globus pallidus infarction. *Biol Psychiatry* 1997;**42**:410–412.

86. Carmin CN, Wiegartz PS, Yunus U, Gillock KL. Treatment of late-onset OCD following basal ganglia infarct. *Depress Anxiety* 2002;**15**:87–90.

87. Mordecai D, Shaw RJ, Fisher PG, Mittelstadt PA, Guterman T, Donaldson SS. Case study: suprasellar germinoma presenting with psychotic and obsessive-compulsive symptoms. *J Am Acad Child Adolesc Psychiatry* 2000;**39**:116–119.

88. Isaacs KL, Philbeck JW, Barr WB, Devinsky O, Alper K. Obsessive-compulsive symptoms in patients with temporal lobe epilepsy. *Epilepsy Behav* 2004;**5**:569–574.

89. Monaco F, Cavanna A, Magli E *et al*. Obsessionality, obsessive-compulsive disorder, and temporal lobe epilepsy. *Epilepsy Behav* 2005;**7**:491–496.

90. Mendez MF, Perryman KM, Miller BL, Swartz JR, Cummings JL. Compulsive behaviors as presenting symptoms of frontotemporal dementia. *J Geriatr Psychiatry Neurol* 1997;**10**:154–157.

91. Rosso SM, Roks G, Stevens M *et al*. Complex compulsive behaviour in the temporal variant of frontotemporal dementia. *J Neurol* 2001;**248**:965–970.

92. O'Sullivan SS, Djamshidian A, Ahmed Z *et al*. Impulsive-compulsive spectrum behaviors in pathologically confirmed progressive supranuclear palsy. *Mov Disord* 2010;**25**:638–642.

93. Wyszynski B, Merriam A, Medalia A, Lawrence C. Choreoacanthocytosis. *Neuropsychiatry Neuropsychol Behav Neurol* 1989;**2**:137–144.

94. McDaniel JS, Johnson KM. Obsessive-compulsive disorder in HIV disease. Response to fluoxetine. *Psychosomatics* 1995;**36**:147–150.

95. Bowler RM, Mergler D, Sassine MP, Larribe F, Hudnell K. Neuropsychiatric effects of manganese on mood. *Neurotoxicology* 1999;**20**:367–378.

96. Caplan R, Comair Y, Shewmon DA, Jackson L, Chugani HT, Peacock WJ. Intractable seizures, compulsions, and coprolalia: a pediatric case study. *J Neuropsychiatry* 1992;**4**:315–319.

97. Cummings JL, Cunningham K. Obsessive-compulsive disorder in Huntington's disease. *Biol Psychiatry* 1992;**31**:263–270.

98. Marder KS, Zhao H, Myers R *et al*. (Huntington Study Group). Rate of functional decline in Huntington's disease. *Neurology* 2000;**54**:452–458.

99. Anderson KE, Louis ED, Stern Y, Marder KS. Cognitive correlates of obsessive and compulsive symptoms in Huntington's disease. *Am J Psychiatry* 2001;**158**:799–801.

100. Weintraub D, Koester J, Potenza MN *et al*. Impulse control disorders in Parkinson disease: a cross-sectional study of 3090 patients. *Arch Neurol* 2010;**67**:589–595.

101. Voon V, Pessiglione M, Brezing C *et al*. Mechanisms underlying dopamine-mediated reward bias in compulsive behaviors. *Neuron* 2010;**65**:135–142.

102. Karno M, Golding JM, Sorenson SB, Burnam MA. The epidemiology of obsessive-compulsive disorder in five US communities. *Arch Gen Psychiatry* 1988;**45**:1094–1099.

103. Berman I, Merson A, Viegner B, Losonczy MF, Pappas D, Green AI. Obsessions and compulsions as a distinct cluster of symptoms in schizophrenia: a neuropsychological study. *J Nerv Ment Dis* 1998;**186**:150–156.

104. Dominquez RA, Backman KE, Lugo SC. Demographics, prevalence and clinical features of the schizo-obsessive subtype of schizophrenia. *CNS Spectrums* 1999;**12**:50–56.

105. Poyurovsky M, Fuchs C, Weizman A. Obsessive-compulsive disorder in patients with first-episode schizophrenia. *Am J Psychiatry* 1999;**156**:1998–2000.

106. Bermanzohn PC, Porto L, Arlow PB, Pollack S, Stronger R, Siris SG. Hierarchical diagnosis in chronic schizophrenia: a clinical study of co-occurring syndromes. *Schizophr Bull* 2000;**26**:517–525.

107. Tibbo P, Kroetsch M, Chue P, Warneke L. Obsessive-compulsive disorder in schizophrenia. *J Psychiatr Res* 2000;**34**:139–146.

108. Lysaker PH, Bryson GJ, Marks KA, Greig TC, Bell MD. Association of obsessions and compulsions in schizophrenia with neurocognition and negative symptoms. *J Neuropsychiatry Clin Neurosci* 2002;**14**:449–453.

109. Ohta M, Kokai M, Morita Y. Features of obsessive-compulsive disorder in patients primarily diagnosed with schizophrenia. *Psychiatry Clin Neurosci* 2003;**57**: 67–74.

110. Videbech T. The psychopathology of anancastic endogenous depression. *Acta Psychiatr Scand* 1975;**52**:336–373.

111. Chen YW, Dilsaver SC. Comorbidity for obsessive-compulsive disorder in bipolar and unipolar disorders. *Psychiatry Res* 1995;**59**:57–64.

112. Abramowitz JS, Brigidi BD, Foa EB. Health concerns in patients with obsessive-compulsive disorder. *J Anxiety Disord* 1999;**13**:529–539.

113. Bienvenu OJ, Samuels JF, Riddle MA *et al.* The relationship of obsessive-compulsive disorder to possible spectrum disorders: results from a family study. *Biol Psychiatry* 2000;**48**:287–293.

114. Richter MA, Summerfeldt LJ, Antony MM, Swinson RP. Obsessive-compulsive spectrum conditions in obsessive-compulsive disorder and other anxiety disorders. *Depress Anxiety* 2003;**18**:118–127.

115. Leckman JF, Walker DE, Goodman WK, Pauls DL, Cohen DJ. "Just right" perceptions associated with compulsive behavior in Tourette's syndrome. *Am J Psychiatry* 1994;**151**:675–680.

116. Leckman JF, Walker DE, Cohen DJ. Premonitory urges in Tourette's syndrome. *Am J Psychiatry* 1993;**150**:98–102.

117. Miguel EC, Coffey BJ, Baer L *et al.* Phenomenology of intentional repetitive behaviors in obsessive-compulsive disorder and Tourette's disorder. *J Clin Psychiatry* 1995;**56**:246–255.

118. Rosario-Campos MC, Leckman JF, Mercadante MT *et al.* Adults with early-onset obsessive-compulsive disorder. *Am J Psychiatry* 2001;**158**:1899–1903.

119. Miguel EC, do Rosário-Campos MC, Prado HS *et al.* Sensory phenomena in obsessive-compulsive disorder and Tourette's disorder. *J Clin Psychiatry* 2000;**61**:150–156.

120. Samuels J, Nestadt G, Bienvenu OJ *et al.* Personality disorders and normal personality dimensions in obsessive-compulsive disorder. *Br J Psychiatry* 2000;**177**:457–462.

121. Coles ME, Pinto A, Mancebo MC, Rasmussen SA, Eisen JL. OCD with comorbid OCPD: a subtype of OCD? *J Psychiatr Res* 2008;**42**:289–296.

122. Mancebo MC, Eisen JL, Grant JE, Rasmussen SA. Obsessive compulsive personality disorder and obsessive compulsive disorder: clinical characteristics, diagnostic difficulties, and treatment. *Ann Clin Psychiatry* 2005;**17**:197–204.

123. Phillips KA, Wilhelm S, Koran LM *et al.* Body dysmorphic disorder: some key issues for DSM-V. *Depress Anxiety* 2010;**27**:573–591.

124. Gunstad J, Phillips KA. Axis I comorbidity in body dysmorphic disorder. *Compr Psychiatry* 2003;**44**:270–276.
125. Rasmussen SA, Eisen JL. The epidemiology and clinical features of obsessive compulsive disorder. *Psychiatr Clin North Am* 1992;**15**:743–758.
126. Saxena S. Is compulsive hoarding a genetically and neurobiologically discrete syndrome? Implications for diagnostic classification. *Am J Psychiatry* 2007;**164**:380–384.
127. Mataix-Cols D, Frost RO, Pertusa A *et al.* Hoarding disorder: a new diagnosis for DSM-V? *Depress Anxiety* 2010;**27**:556–572.
128. Pertusa A, Frost RO, Fullana MA *et al.* Refining the diagnostic boundaries of compulsive hoarding: a critical review. *Clin Psychol Rev* 2010;**30**:371–386.
129. Pertusa A, Fullana MA, Singh S, Alonso P, Menchón JM, Mataix-Cols D. Compulsive hoarding: OCD symptom, distinct clinical syndrome, or both? *Am J Psychiatry* 2008;**165**:1289–1298.

Pharmacotherapy of Obsessive-Compulsive Disorder

Eric H. Decloedt[1] and Dan J. Stein[2]

[1]*Department of Medicine, Division of Clinical Pharmacology, University of Cape Town, South Africa;* [2]*Department of Psychiatry, University of Cape Town, South Africa*

INTRODUCTION

Since the serendipitous discovery of the efficacy of clomipramine in the late 1960s, there have been significant advances in the pharmacotherapy of obsessive-compulsive disorder (OCD). The evidence base has gradually grown to the point that many dozens of clinical trials in OCD are available. This chapter attempts to summarize and synthesize some of this work in an evidence-based manner, with the emphasis on a practical perspective for the busy clinician.

Our approach was to collate the evidence on the pharmacotherapy of OCD by doing a systematic search of the electronic database MEDLINE, using the MeSH (Medical Subject Headings) term 'obsessive-compulsive disorder'. Subheadings of particular classes and names of drugs were selected to refine the search. The focus included randomized or controlled trials, systematic reviews and meta-analyses.

In clinical practice, the response of OCD patients to pharmacological interventions can be measured using a range of scales (a detailed discussion can be found in Chapter 1, 'Assessment'). The Yale–Brown Obsessive-Compulsive Scale score (Y–BOCS), ranging from 0 to 40, is the most widely used clinician-rated severity scale in OCD research [1]. The Clinical Global Impression scale (CGI) rates patients according to severity of illness, global improvement and efficacy of treatment, and is a clinically useful measure [2]. We will refer to both measures throughout.

Obsessive-Compulsive Disorder: Current Science and Clinical Practice, First Edition. Edited by Joseph Zohar.
© 2012 John Wiley & Sons, Ltd. Published 2012 by John Wiley & Sons, Ltd.

We begin with the question, 'What is the first-line pharmacotherapy intervention in OCD?' In order to address this question, we will discuss the evidence base for the pharmacotherapy of OCD, focusing on placebo-controlled trials of the different serotonin reuptake inhibitors (SRIs), and then go on to discuss meta-analyses comparing different pharmacotherapeutic agents for OCD.

PLACEBO-CONTROLLED STUDIES OF CLOMIPRAMINE

The discovery of the first agent for OCD was serendipitous. In searching for more effective treatments for depression, Ciba-Geigy chlorinated imipramine in 1964 [3]. Although chlorimipramine (clomipramine) did not prove to be a superior antidepressant, it turned out to have a therapeutic effect on obsessive-compulsive symptoms. One of the first anecdotal reports on this was published in 1967 by the Spanish psychiatrists Fernandez and Lopez-Ibor [4,5].

Subsequently, clomipramine was thoroughly studied and became the first drug approved by the US Food and Drug Administration (FDA) for the treatment of OCD. Early, small, randomized, placebo-controlled trials found that clomipramine was efficacious [6,7]. A large ($n = 520$) placebo-controlled study confirmed these data [8]. While the placebo-treated participants achieved a maximum mean decrease of 5% reduction in Y–BOCS score at 10 weeks, clomipramine-treated participants experienced symptomatic improvement of up to 44% on the Y–BOCS [9].

The discovery that clomipramine was effective for OCD was important not only because there was now a registered treatment, but also because the selective efficacy of this agent led to a serotonin hypothesis of OCD. Thus, for example, clomipramine but not more noradrenergic agents such as nortriptyline and desipramine, were superior to placebo in OCD [10]. Similarly in placebo-controlled trials, clomipramine showed superiority compared to clorgyline, as well as D-amphetamine [11,12].

The serotonin hypothesis, together with the fact that tricyclic antidepressants are poorly tolerated because they act on a range of neuroreceptors, gave impetus to the study of more selective serotonin reuptake inhibitors (SSRIs) in OCD [13,14]. One of the first of these agents was fluvoxamine, which we discuss next.

PLACEBO-CONTROLLED STUDIES OF FLUVOXAMINE

Fluvoxamine acts primarily on the serotonin transporter inhibitor, although it also has effects at sigma 1 sites [15]. Sixteen outpatients were studied in the first fluvoxamine double-blind placebo-controlled OCD study [16]. After 20 weeks of treatment, 13 patients improved on fluvoxamine compared to 3 on placebo. A larger ($n = 42$) trial found that 9 of 21 participants on fluvoxamine responded while none of the placebo-treated participants did [17]. Another 10-week trial ($n = 38$) showed superiority of fluvoxamine for two out of three measures of OCD symptom improvement [18]. Cottraux *et al.* found that fluvoxamine had superior efficacy compared to placebo over both the short term (week 8) and the longer term (week 24) [19].

By the end of 1994, fluvoxamine was registered by the FDA for the treatment of OCD. Indeed, a large ($n = 78$) randomized multicentre study by Goodman *et al.* (1996) confirmed the superiority of fluvoxamine on all outcome measures used. The percentage of participants classified as responders was significantly higher in the fluvoxamine group from week 6 onwards, with 33.3% fluvoxamine-treated participants responding compared to only 9.0% of those treated with placebo [20].

Controlled-release (CR) and extended release (ER) fluvoxamine formulations aim to minimize the peak-to-trough plasma concentration fluctuations and improve therapeutic efficacy. Once-daily doses of fluvoxamine CR (100–300 mg) proved superior to placebo and significantly decreased Y–BOCS symptom scores, with a mean reduction of 31.7% compared to 21.2% at 12 weeks [21]. Fluvoxamine ER had a significantly greater improvement than placebo on Y–BOCS scores at 12 weeks, and also improved health-related quality of life [22].

PLACEBO-CONTROLLED STUDIES OF FLUOXETINE

Fluoxetine was the first SSRI studied in several multinational randomized controlled trials of OCD, including dose-finding studies. Fluoxetine not only increases presynaptic serotonin, but also antagonizes 5-HT$_{2C}$ receptors resulting in increased noradrenaline (norepinephrine) and dopamine activity, which may be relevant to OCD [23,24]. In an 8-week, double-blind, placebo-controlled study of 214 patients who received 20 mg, 40 mg or 60 mg fluoxetine, both the Y–BOCS total score and the responder rate improved significantly in the 60 mg group ($n = 54$), while in the 40 mg group ($n = 52$) only the responder rate was significantly higher [25]. The 20 mg dose group ($n = 52$) showed little difference compared to placebo. No differences were noted in adverse events between fluoxetine and placebo. The study period was relatively short and it is possible that the 20 mg or 40 mg patients may have responded when treated for longer.

Indeed, in a larger ($n = 355$) randomized, double-blind, parallel, 13-week, fixed-dose study, fluoxetine at all doses (20, 40 and 60 mg) proved to be superior to placebo on the Y–BOCS total score and other efficacy measures, although with a trend towards greater efficacy at 60 mg [26]. The greater efficacy at the higher dose was offset by more adverse events in the higher dose participants. Jenike and colleagues compared 80 mg fluoxetine with 60 mg of the monoamine oxidase inhibitor phenelzine and placebo; the high-dose fluoxetine once again proved to be superior compared to placebo, with no efficacy difference between phenelzine and placebo [27]. In general, many expert consensus guidelines have emphasized the potential value of increasing SSRI dose in OCD, and we will return to this issue later.

PLACEBO-CONTROLLED STUDIES OF PAROXETINE

In addition to serotonin reuptake inhibition, paroxetine has weak noradrenaline re-uptake inhibition and mild muscarinic anticholinergic effects [28]. A multinational, randomized, double-blind study of 406 subjects found paroxetine (up to 60 mg) to be significantly more effective than placebo, and as effective as clomipramine (up to 250 mg) after 12 weeks [29]. However, paroxetine had a superior tolerability profile compared with clomipramine. A small 10-week, single-blind, randomized study compared fluvoxamine ($n = 10$) (maximum dose 300 mg), paroxetine ($n = 9$) and citalopram ($n = 11$) (both at a maximum dose of 60 mg) [30]. These SSRIs were not found to have significant differences in efficacy or tolerability.

The FDA approved paroxetine in 1992. While most registration studies have taken place in the West, a recent registration study in Japanese OCD patients established efficacy and tolerability of 20–50 mg of paroxetine in a 12-week trial [31]. Hollander *et al.* established evidence of long-term efficacy of paroxetine (up to 15 months, using a relapse prevention design), with higher doses of 40–60 mg, but not 20 mg, significantly more efficacious than placebo [32].

PLACEBO-CONTROLLED STUDIES OF SERTRALINE

Sertraline is a SSRI that also inhibits the dopamine transporter and binds to the sigma 1 receptor. An 8-week trial of flexible sertraline dosing of up to 200 mg showed superior efficacy compared to placebo [33]. Subsequently, a large ($n = 324$), 12-week, fixed-dose (50, 100 and 200 mg) study confirmed the efficacy of sertraline in OCD [34]. Kronig *et al.* confirmed in a flexible-dose design with doses up to 200 mg that sertraline was more efficacious than placebo in a 12-week study ($n = 167$) [35]. A rapid (150 mg in 5 days) titration regimen showed some benefit compared to the slow (150 mg in 15 days) regimen at 4 and 6 weeks [36].

Efficacy and good tolerability were noted in a long-term trial where a 1-year double-blind placebo-controlled intervention was followed by a 1-year open-label extension [37]. An 80-week study followed and confirmed the long-term efficacy of sertraline [38]. Sertraline was well tolerated during the 28-week double-blind phase and it was of note that dropouts due to adverse events occurred at a higher rate among placebo-treated patients. The rate of sertraline dose titration made no difference to efficacy in the long term.

PLACEBO-CONTROLLED STUDIES OF CITALOPRAM/ESCITALOPRAM

Citalopram is an SSRI that consists of two enantiomers, R and S. The R-enantiomer appears to bind to the serotonin transporter without inhibiting it, reducing the ability of the *S*-enantiomer to increase synaptic serotonin. Citalopram demonstrated efficacy and good tolerability at fixed doses of 20, 40 and 60 mg in a 12-week placebo-controlled trial [39]. The 60 mg group had the highest response rate, defined as 25% improvement in Y–BOCS entry score, and also the fastest response rate. There was no difference in the rate of discontinuation between the different dosing groups and placebo.

Escitalopram is made up of only the active *S*-enantiomer. Escitalopram 10–20 mg demonstrated efficacy and good tolerability in OCD compared to placebo, with the higher dose associated with earlier and larger response rates [40]. Escitalopram-treated patients also had a lower relapse rate compared to placebo when responders to 16-week open-label escitalopram (10 or 20 mg) were randomized to active medication or placebo during longer-term treatment [41].

PLACEBO-CONTROLLED STUDIES OF VENLAFAXINE

Venlafaxine is thought to be an SSRI at lower doses and to have serotonin and noradrenaline reuptake inhibitor (SNRI) properties at higher doses. Venlafaxine has not been adequately studied in placebo-controlled trials of OCD [42]. One placebo-controlled study showed no difference, but findings are limited by many methodological shortcomings including small sample size, short study duration and lack of a standard outcome measure [43]. However, when venlafaxine titrated to 300 mg was compared with doses of up to 60 mg of paroxetine in a 12-week double-blind trial, significant efficacy or tolerability differences were noted [44].

IMPROVING EARLY RESPONSE IN OCD

Response to SSRIs in OCD may take several weeks. The $5\text{-}HT_{1A}$ receptor functions as a somatodendritic autoreceptor, and activation causes hyperpolarization of the neuronal membrane, reducing the firing rate of serotonergic neurons [45]. It has been suggested that blockade of the $5\text{-}HT_{1A}$ somatodendritic autoreceptor may accelerate the effect of antidepressants by increasing presynaptic serotonin. Pindolol is a non-selective β-blocker and a $5\text{-}HT_{1A}$ receptor partial antagonist, but in a fluvoxamine double-blind, placebo-controlled study, it failed to shorten the latency of the anti-obsessional effects of fluvoxamine [46]. The lack of effect in OCD may be due to differences in the neurobiological mechanisms underlying depression and OCD, or that currently used doses of pindolol (7.5 mg per day) only occupy 40% or less of the $5\text{-}HT_{1A}$ autoreceptors and higher doses may be required [45,46]. Strategies for reliably improving early response to OCD remain to be found.

SPECIAL POPULATIONS: CHILDREN

Paediatric OCD is covered (Chapter 7 – Pædiatric OCD: Developmental Aspects and Treatment Considerations). In brief, it is important to note that OCD often begins early in life, and that symptoms in children are quite similar to those seen among individuals who develop OCD in adulthood, although there are differences in sex ratios and patterns of comorbidity [47]. There is evidence of overlapping neurobiology and it is therefore not surprising that children respond to similar pharmacotherapy.

The pharmacokinetics of drugs in children may differ from adults for several reasons: variability due to age, gender, body composition, functionality of liver and kidneys, and the degree of maturation of enzymatic systems [48]. Furthermore, there is evidence that drug dosing relates to body weight in a non-linear relationship [49]. Drug efficacy findings and dosing in adults may therefore not simply be extrapolated to children. As paediatric OCD is covered fully elsewhere in this volume, here we cover this area only briefly.

CLOMIPRAMINE

Short-term clomipramine studies have demonstrated efficacy in the paediatric population. In a 5-week, double-blind, cross-over placebo trial involving 19 children with a mean age of 14.5 years, significant improvement was shown in response to clomipramine (mean clomipramine dosage of 141 mg/day) [50]. Similarly, in 48 children and adolescents participating in a 10-week double-blind crossover trial of clomipramine (mean dose 150 mg/day) and desipramine (mean dose 153 mg/day), clomipramine was superior [51]. Furthermore, most patients (64%) who received clomipramine as their first active treatment showed at least some sign of relapse during desipramine treatment.

Fluvoxamine

Compared to placebo, fluvoxamine dosed at 50–200 mg/day demonstrated superior efficacy and good tolerability in a multicentre, randomized, placebo-controlled trial of 120 children aged 8–17 years [52].

Fluoxetine

Three studies examined the use of fluoxetine compared to placebo in childhood OCD. A 20-week, randomized, double-blind, placebo-controlled, fixed-dose

(20 mg), crossover trial of fluoxetine in 14 children, aged 8 to 15 years, showed improvement in the CGI but not the Y–BOCS scores [53]. Y–BOCS total score decreased 44% after the initial 8 weeks of fluoxetine treatment, compared with a 27% decrease after placebo treatment. A larger 13-week placebo-controlled trial that titrated fluoxetine doses from 10 mg up to a maximum of 60 mg ($n = 103$) also showed efficacy on the Y–BOCS [54]. Liebowitz *et al.* used higher dosages of fluoxetine with fixed dosing to 60 mg for the first 6 weeks and the option of increasing to 80 mg per day [55]. Fluoxetine demonstrated superiority over placebo after 8 weeks and after 16 weeks: 57% compared to 27% placebo-treated children were responders. The high dose of fluoxetine was well tolerated.

Paroxetine

Twenty patients aged 8 to 17 years were treated with paroxetine 10 to 60 mg in a 12-week open-label trial [56]. Although no comparator was used, there was a significant decrease in CY–BOCS scores on paroxetine. A large ($n = 207$), 10-week, randomized, double-blind, placebo-controlled trial confirmed the efficacy of paroxetine [57]. Paroxetine pharmacokinetics in paediatric patients are similar to adults, with a complicated non-linear relationship between dose and exposure, as measured by area under the plasma concentration time-curve (AUC_{0-24}) and maximum observed concentration (C_{max}) [58]. Children had twice the plasma concentration at 10 mg compared to adolescents – best explained in terms of cytochrome 2D6 (CYP2D6) saturability and the ability of paroxetine to inhibit CYP2D6. Although no apparent relationship between paroxetine plasma concentrations and adverse events was found, a more conservative dosing approach might be appropriate in children, with treatment initiation of paroxetine at 5 mg.

Sertraline

A multicentre, randomized, placebo-controlled trial of 107 children and adolescents showed efficacy of sertraline from week 3 until endpoint (12 weeks) [59]. A 12-week placebo-controlled study provided reassuring cardiovascular safety data for an average dose of 167 mg in 107 children and 80 adolescents [60]. A longer 52-week open-label study with a mean sertraline dose of 161 mg confirmed efficacy (defined as a >25% decrease in CY–BOCS and a CGI-I score of 1 or 2), with response seen in 72% of children and 61% of adolescents [61]. More adverse events occurred in children compared to adolescents (14% vs 9%). The pharmacokinetics in children and adolescents differ, with children having greater C_{max} and AUC_{0-24} values accounted for by normalizing for bodyweight, indicating that dosing should probably take weight into account [62]. However, the pharmacokinetics of sertraline are similar to those in adults, allowing for adult titration schedules.

Citalopram

The clinical effectiveness and tolerability of citalopram in the long-term treatment of paediatric OCD seems to be comparable with the observations of other SSRIs [63].

META-ANALYSES

Given that a number of different SRIs (SSRIs and clomipramine) are efficacious in OCD, an immediate question is which to use first. Meta-analysis provides a quantifiable approach to compare the efficacy of different agents in the pharmacotherapy of OCD. Several meta-analyses have been undertaken, and are summarized in Table 2.1.

Early meta-analyses suggested that both SSRIs and clomipramine were more effective than placebo. Of note is that when the data for the SSRIs were compared to clomipramine, clomipramine generally had greater effect sizes. However, head-to-head studies have found similar efficacy of clomipramine and SSRIs. This may be partly explained by the fact that clomipramine studies were typically conducted earlier, patients were more likely to be treatment naive (and so perhaps more responsive), and placebo response was lower. In contrast, the SSRI studies may have included patients who had previously failed to respond to other agents, and had higher placebo responses.

As above, individual studies comparing SSRIs to clomipramine demonstrate very little difference in efficacy. In a small study, fluvoxamine (40 mg) showed similar efficacy to clomipramine (150 mg), with both treatments well tolerated [64]. Comparisons between fluvoxamine and clomipramine demonstrated equal efficacy although once again both studies were small (clomipramine dose 100–250 mg vs fluvoxamine 100–250 mg and clomipramine 150–300 mg vs fluvoxamine 150–300 mg respectively) [65,66]. In an adequately powered comparison between sertraline and clomipramine, no significant difference in efficacy was found between the treatment arms [67].

A recent Cochrane review compared differences in SSRI efficacy and tolerability in OCD [68]. The SSRIs of interest were fluoxetine, fluvoxamine, sertraline, paroxetine and citalopram. The SSRIs as a group were shown to be more efficacious for OCD symptoms compared to placebo, and individually all drugs showed effect sizes of reasonable magnitude. Narrow confidence intervals were reported for citalopram, fluvoxamine, paroxetine and sertraline, and slightly wider confidence intervals for fluoxetine studies. The overall relative risk (RR) across all five SSRI studies was 1.84 (95% confidence interval (CI) 1.56–2.17). The RR for response rate in the citalopram group was 1.58 (95% CI 1.20–2.08), fluoxetine 2.41 (95% CI 1.58–4.56), paroxetine 1.74 (95% CI 1.28 to 2.36) and sertraline 1.54

Study	n	Design (no. of trials)	Duration	Effect on OCD
Greist et al. (1995) [137]	1520	PL controlled (7) [CMI, FLX, FLV, SER]	10–13 weeks	CMI and SSRIs > PL CMI > SSRIs No significant difference in dropouts because of side effects
Piccinelli et al. (1995) [138]	1809	PL controlled (26) [CMI, FLX, FLV, SER, TCA]	5–36 weeks	CMI and SSRIs > PL CMI > SSRIs
Stein et al. (1995) [139]	1039	PL controlled (12) [FLX, FLV, SER, TRZ, CMI] Head to head (10) Open trial (6)	6–13 weeks	CMI and SSRIs > PL CMI = SER > FLX
Abramowitz (1997) [140]	20 studies with a range of 10–519 participants in each study	PL controlled (5) [FLX, FLV, SER, CMI] Head to head (4)	4–13 weeks	CMI and SSRIs > PL CMI > FLV > FLX > SER Side effects correlated with effect size
Kobak et al. (1998) [141]	4641	PL controlled (5) [FLX, FLV, SER, CMI, PAR] Head to head (7)	Not reported	CMI and SSRIs > PL CMI = FLV = FLX > other SSRIs No difference in dropout rates
Ackerman et al. (2002) [142]	1876	PL controlled (18) [CMI, FLX, FLV, SER, PAR] Head to head (8)	8–13 weeks	CMI and SSRIs > PL CMI = FLV = FLX = PAR
Soomro (2008) [68]	3097	PL controlled (17) [FLX, FLV, SER, PAR, CIT]	6–13 weeks	Overall RR 1.84 (95% CI 1.56–2.17) CIT RR 1.58 (95% CI 1.20–2.08) FLX RR 2.41 (95% CI 1.58–4.56) PAR RR 1.74 (95% CI 1.28–2.36) SER RR 1.54 (95% CI 1.20–1.99) NNT 6–12

CIT, citalopram; CMI, clomipramine; FLV, fluvoxetine; FLX, fluoxetine; NT, number needed to treat; PAR, paroxetine; PL, placebo; RR, relative risk; SER, sertraline; TCA, tricyclic antidepressants; TRZ, trazodone.

(95% CI 1.20–1.99). Citalopram, paroxetine and sertraline showed similar effect sizes of between 1.54 and 1.74, while fluvoxamine and fluoxetine showed larger effect sizes. However, lower limits of the confidence intervals of effect sizes of all five drugs individually were comparable and the residual chi-squared value indicated that the difference between the individual drugs was not significant. The numbers needed to treat were calculated assuming that a response rate without treatment may be expected to be between 10 and 20%. Should 10% of patients be expected to recover without treatment, 12 patients would need to be treated with an SSRI to achieve improvements for one additional patient, and should 20% of patients be expected to recover without treatment, six patients would need to be treated to achieve improvements for one additional patient.

The evidence does not support superior efficacy of clomipramine over the SSRIs or a more efficacious SSRI from within the SSRI drug class for the treatment of OCD. However, these various agents have differences in drug tolerability and in the potential to cause drug interactions. We review tolerability next.

TOLERABILITY OF CLOMIPRAMINE AND SEROTONIN REUPTAKE INHIBITORS

SSRIs increase synaptic availability of serotonin, and a large number of postsynaptic 5-HT receptor types, including 5-HT_3 receptors, are stimulated. Stimulation of 5-HT_3 receptors is suspected to be responsible for some adverse effects of SSRIs. Although reported adverse effect data were limited in the Cochrane review, the overall and individual adverse effects for the different SSRIs were always worse than for placebo, and in the majority of cases the difference was statistically significant [68]. Nausea, headache and insomnia were consistently reported amongst the most common adverse effects in trials of each of the drugs. SSRIs are particularly prone to cause sexual side effects, and the relative risk ranged from 5.74 to 18.64 for the individual drugs compared to placebo.

Epileptic seizures have been reported during treatment with almost all antidepressants including clomipramine and the SSRIs. Attempts to assign relative seizure risks to various antidepressants should be interpreted cautiously due to various limitations in the human studies, but the bulk of evidence suggests that clomipramine has a relatively high risk of seizure incidence, while SSRIs exhibit a lower seizure risk. The seizure risk seems to be dose related [69].

Both clomipramine and SSRIs are associated with weight gain in the long-term (more than 2 years) treatment of patients with OCD [70]. Clomipramine appears to have the greatest potential to induce weight gain, and sertraline and fluoxetine the least. Weight gain seems to be more significant for females. The small sample studied in OCD limits rigorous comparisons between SSRIs, but a meta-analysis of second-generation antidepressants for the treatment of major depressive disorder indicated that paroxetine may have the greatest propensity to cause weight gain [71].

Clomipramine blockade of muscarinic, histaminergic and adrenergic receptors decreases tolerability and safety. Common adverse effects include blurred vision, xerostomia, urinary retention, constipation, orthostatic hypotension and sedation. The major safety concern with the use of clomipramine is the drug's ability to slow cardiac conduction, which may precipitate life-threatening arrhythmias in overdose. The increased toxicity in overdose may be due to modulation of ion channel function, particularly potassium and sodium channels, within the myocardium. Mortality data show that tricyclic antidepressants are associated with a significantly higher number of accidental and intentional deaths when compared to SSRIs [72]. Clomipramine was responsible for 11 deaths per million prescriptions while SSRIs as a class were responsible for 2 deaths per million prescriptions, confirming that SSRIs are rarely fatal in overdose. When death occurred, the SSRI was mostly found in combination with other drugs, particularly tricyclic antidepressants (TCAs). Very high doses of SSRIs (>75 times the normal daily dose) may cause more serious adverse events, including seizures and decreased consciousness [73].

In head-to-head studies clomipramine discontinuation rates were greater than those for SSRIs. When fluvoxamine was compared to clomipramine, fluvoxamine was better tolerated, with clomipramine having double the amount of withdrawals due to adverse side effects [66]. In an adequately powered comparison between sertraline and clomipramine, significantly more patients withdrew from the clomipramine group due to adverse side effects [67].

SSRI adverse event frequency also differs between age groups, with hyperactivity and vomiting two- to three-fold more prevalent in children than in adolescents, and the rate lowest in adults [74]. Somnolence frequency increases with advancing age, while insomnia and nausea are common across all ages.

Taken together, the evidence strongly indicates that SSRIs have a more favourable tolerability profile than clomipramine.

OPTIMAL DOSE OF TREATMENT

There is evidence to suggest that the OCD drug response is better at higher doses [75]. Paroxetine was shown to have a positive dose–response relationship, with higher doses of 40 mg and 60 mg more effective than placebo [76]. Similarly, when fluoxetine was evaluated in three fixed doses (20, 40, 60 mg), all doses were effective but the highest dose tended to give the greatest benefit [77]. A dose-finding study of escitalopram in OCD suggested a dose–response effect, with escitalopram 20 mg numerically more robust than escitalopram 10 mg on some secondary measures [40].

Mundo et al. noted, however, that lower doses are adequate for treatment maintenance [78]. Successfully treated clomipramine and fluvoxamine patients were enrolled in a double-blind study and examined for clinical deterioration when drug treatment doses were decreased. Over a 102-day period, patients either received no reduction, one-third or two-thirds reduction in drug dose. There were no significant differences in the cumulative proportions of patients from each treatment group who did not worsen, suggesting that long-term maintenance therapy for OCD may be provided with lower doses of the anti-obsessional drug, with clear advantages for tolerability and compliance.

Success with SSRI doses greater than noted in the SPCs (summary of product characteristics) has been shown in treatment-refractory patients. A multicentre, randomized, double-blind, non-placebo trial was performed to evaluate the efficacy and safety of 12 additional weeks of high-dose sertraline (250–400 mg, mean 357 mg) in 30 OCD patients who had failed to respond to 16 weeks of standard-dose sertraline treatment [79]. High doses of sertraline resulted in significantly greater and more rapid improvement in OCD symptoms compared to the maximal labelled dose of sertraline (200 mg). The higher doses of sertraline were well tolerated, although patients had increased rates of tremor and agitation on these doses. Pampaloni *et al.* described retrospective outcomes of high doses of SSRIs in treatment-refractory patients [80]. Patients on high-dose treatment showed significant within-group improvements although endpoint scores for the high-dose group remained significantly higher than those of control patients treated for a matched period, suggesting enduring treatment resistance. No differences were found between the cases and controls with regards to the side effects. There is also evidence for the efficacy of high-dose escitalopram in treatment-refractory OCD patients (see below). Currently, however, expert consensus guidelines typically recommend gradually increasingly the SSRI dose to maximum, and are somewhat wary of recommending doses above the SPC limit. Should patients not respond after an adequate medication trial, medication should be changed or augmented with another agent [81,82].

DURATION OF TREATMENT

OCD is a chronic illness, and while most studies have focused on the acute treatment of OCD, the evidence base for long-term treatment is less clear. A series of controlled studies has demonstrated that discontinuation of treatment is associated with symptomatic relapse, irrespective of treatment duration. In a double-blind treatment discontinuation study, of the 21 patients who manifested sustained improvement during 5 to 27 months of clomipramine treatment, 16 had substantial recurrence of OC symptoms by the end of the 7-week placebo period [83].

In a 52-week follow-up study, responders on various doses of fluoxetine were randomly assigned to receive continued treatment of fluoxetine or placebo after 20 weeks [84]. Fluoxetine-treated patients had numerically lower relapse rates compared to their placebo-treated counterparts, although the difference was not significant at 31.9% and 20.6% respectively. Only patients who continued treatment with fluoxetine at doses of 60 mg had significantly lower rates of relapse compared to those switched to placebo.

Koran *et al.* randomized sertraline responders to 28 weeks of double-blind 50–200 mg of sertraline or placebo and measured full relapse, dropout due to relapse or insufficient response, or acute exacerbation of OCD symptoms [38]. A relapse was similarly specified as in the Romano *et al.* [84] study and monitored over a 1-month interval to differentiate relapse from routine oscillations. Sertraline-treated patients had significantly better results than placebo-treated patients on two of the three primary outcomes: study discontinuation due to relapse or insufficient clinical response (9% vs 24% respectively) and acute exacerbation of OCD symptoms (12% vs 35%), but not full relapse.

Responders ($n = 105$) to open-label paroxetine randomized to 6-months of either double-blinded placebo or paroxetine, demonstrated a greater proportion of relapse in placebo (59%) than paroxetine (38%) treated patients [32]. Paediatric patients responding to paroxetine after 16-weeks of treatment were randomized to 16 weeks of either paroxetine or placebo; paroxetine-treated patients had reduced relapse rates irrespective of baseline comorbid disorders [85].

Only a relatively small proportion of OCD patients ordinarily show remission in response to SRIs. For example, a prospective 2- to 7-year follow-up study after initial clomipramine treatment of 54 children and adolescents showed significant long-term improvements, but only 6% were in complete remission. Although 38 patients (70%) continued to take clomipramine at follow-up, 10 patients (19%) had worse or unchanged OCD symptoms [86]. We discuss the treatment of refractory OCD next.

REFRACTORY OCD

Despite the substantial clinical improvements provided by the pharmacological treatment of OCD with clomipramine and SSRIs, 40–60% of patients do not respond completely [87]. Various alternative strategies have been proposed for the pharmacotherapy of treatment-resistant OCD. As these are covered in more depth in Chapter 5, here we cover them only briefly.

Increased dose of SSRI

As mentioned above, SSRIs have been used beyond the recommended maximum dose for patients who respond poorly to treatment and who tolerate suprathera-peutic doses. An open-label, prospective, 16-week, high-dose escitalopram study demonstrated statistically significant improvement in Y–BOCS score compared to baseline in patients receiving high treatment doses [88]. Patients with resistant

OCD received a mean dose of 33.8 mg escitalopram, which was well tolerated with no treatment discontinuations. In a multicentre, double-blind trial, non-responders to 16 weeks of 50–200 mg sertraline were randomized to 200 and 250–400 mg of sertraline daily. The high-dose group demonstrated significantly greater improvement compared to the 200 mg daily group. None of the patients in the high-dose group discontinued due to side effects [79].

A retrospective folder review matched 192 patients receiving high-dose SSRIs (fluoxetine, citalopram, fluvoxamine, paroxetine, sertraline and escitalopram) with a matched number of cases receiving the standard-dose treatment [80]. Patients on the high-dose treatment showed significant within-group improvements (Y–BOCS 25.35 vs 20.95), although endpoint scores for the high-dose group remained significantly higher than the control patients for a matched period suggesting enduring treatment resistance. The frequency of adverse effects did not significantly differ between the two groups.

Augmentation of SSRI treatment with antipsychotics

Haloperidol addition was found to be particularly efficacious in SRI-refractory OCD patients with comorbid chronic tic disorders, such as Tourette's disorder, although of little benefit in patients without tics [89].

A randomized placebo-controlled trial by McDougle and colleagues demonstrated a 50% response, as defined by a ≥35% reduction in Y–BOCS score and 'improved' or 'much improved' CGI score, in patients receiving a 6-week augmentation course of risperidone, an atypical antipsychotic agent with potent dopaminergic and serotonergic antagonist activity [90]. Erzegovesi and colleagues investigated fluvoxamine-refractory patients: five of ten patients randomized to risperidone augmentation and two of nine patients receiving placebo had a significant response [91].

Results of placebo-controlled trials with olanzapine are conflicting: Shapira *et al.* found no additional advantage of adding olanzapine in OCD patients refractory to fluoxetine, compared with extending the monotherapy trial, while Bystritsky and D'Amico concluded that adding olanzapine to SRIs is potentially efficacious in the short-term treatment of patients with refractory OCD [92–94].

A randomized placebo-controlled trial of quetiapine augmentation demonstrated significant improvement in the quetiapine arm with 64% (9/14) of refractory patients scoring a significant improvement on the Y–BOCS [95]. Seven of ten patients who received quetiapine in addition to an SSRI for 8 weeks, showed a response, with a mean reduction of their Y–BOCS score of 35.4% [96]. A subsequent larger randomized placebo-controlled trial, including 40 patients with treatment-resistant OCD, demonstrated a significant improvement in Y–BOCS scores with quetiapine compared to placebo. Eight patients in the quetiapine group compared to two in the placebo group had ≥35% decrease in their Y–BOCS score after 8 weeks of treatment [97]. Carey *et al.* found no difference in patients augmented with placebo or quetiapine, but pointed out that their findings may reflect a shorter trial of an SSRI before quetiapine augmentation and lower doses of quetiapine compared to other trials [98]. The largest quetiapine placebo-controlled trial ($n = 66$) to date concluded that quetiapine was significantly superior to placebo on Y–BOCS and CGI scales [99].

Clozapine failed to show benefit when used as an augmentation agent in OCD [100].

Until recently all studies of atypical antipsychotic augmentation in OCD investigated only short-term response. A long-term follow-up, of at least $1\frac{1}{2}$ years, of patients receiving atypical antipsychotic augmentation raised concerns about the efficacy and metabolic effects of atypical antipsychotics [101]. Compared to SSRI responders, total Y–BOCS scores in those who required atypical antipsychotic augmentation were initially higher, and they remained at levels higher than those of SRI responders after 1 year of the treatment. Patients who received atypical antipsychotic augmentation had significant increases in body mass index and fasting blood glucose and demonstrated a trend towards increased cholesterol and triglyceride.

A Cochrane review of the pharmacotherapy of treatment-resistant anxiety disorder concluded that more than twice as many resistant OCD patients respond to augmentation than to placebo (31.8% vs 13.6%). The number needed to treat was found to be a clinically acceptable 5.5, and pharmacological augmentation was tolerable insofar as there was no difference between medication and placebo dropout rate. Overall, the superiority of a variety of drugs compared to placebo was demonstrated, with a relative risk of non-response of 3.16 (95% CI 1.08–9.23). A substantial proportion of the efficacy evidence was for the augmentation with antipsychotics [102].

Other drugs

A range of clinical trials of augmentation strategies have been negative in OCD. In a double-blind placebo-controlled trial, augmentation with lithium in treatment-resistant patients on fluvoxamine found no clinical improvement in OC symptoms [103]. Buspirone added to treatment with fluvoxamine proved to be no better than placebo in reducing symptoms [104]. Similarly, adjunctive desipramine showed no significant difference compared to placebo augmentation in ameliorating symptoms [105]. Administration of inositol, in a small open-label study, failed to produce a significant improvement in the majority of refractory patients [106]. Clonazepam augmentation of sertraline produced no benefit compared to placebo [107].

Pindolol augmentation of paroxetine compared to placebo augmentation showed a therapeutic difference in favour of pindolol after 4 weeks [108]. Morphine is a mu-receptor agonist, and in a placebo-controlled double-blind study it reduced the symptoms of OCD; however, its use raises obvious safety concerns [109]. The evidence for anticonvulsants in patients with refractory OCD is confined to anecdotal reports and uncontrolled trials [110].

Interactions with cytochrome 450 (CYP450) isoenzymes should be kept in mind when combining antidepressant treatment with other drugs, especially when augmenting treatment-resistant OCD patients. The metabolism of most antidepressants is greatly dependent on the activity of hepatic CYP450 enzymes. Some antidepressants are not only substrates for metabolism by CYP450 enzymes, but also can inhibit the metabolic clearance of other drugs, sometimes producing clinically significant drug–drug interactions [111]. Fluvoxamine is a potent inhibitor of CYP1A2 and CYP2C9, while fluoxetine and paroxetine potently inhibit CYP2D6. Citalopram and escitalopram are weak inhibitors of CYP450 isoenzymes and are less likely than other second-generation antidepressants to interact with co-administered medications [112]. Actual data for clomipramine inhibition of CYP2D6 are lacking and estimated from structurally related drugs, but inhibition of CYP2C19 may be significant [113]. Co-administration of fluvoxamine and clomipramine for treatment-resistant OCD resulted in markedly elevated clomipramine concentrations increasing the risk of cardiac and other side effects [114].

Alternative modes of administration of SSRIs

In a small study ($n = 15$), participants who received an intravenous pulse loading of clomipramine had greater immediate improvement compared to oral administration [115]. In a larger randomized placebo-controlled trial ($n = 54$), intravenous administration of clomipramine demonstrated superiority over placebo on outcome measures in patients who remained refractory to oral administration of clomipramine [116]. Intravenous citalopram studied in an open-label uncontrolled fashion appeared to be rapidly effective in treatment-resistant patients [117].

Combining SRIs

In children and young adults (9–23 years) with treatment-resistant OCD, combination treatment of clomipramine and SSRIs resulted in symptom improvement of all subjects ($n = 7$), but was associated with increased cardiovascular side effects [118].

Switching SSRIs

Switching SSRIs in treatment-resistant OCD may be a useful strategy. A double-blind trial studied switch of two SSRIs, venlafaxine and paroxetine, in non-responders of either venlafaxine or paroxetine as defined by a reduction of less than 25% in Y–BOCS [119]. Eighteen of forty-three (42%) patients benefited from a switch to the alternative SSRI, with a mean decrease in Y–BOCS of 25% after 12 weeks of treatment.

Adding psychotherapy

There are surprisingly few data to show that combining pharmacotherapy with cognitive behavioural therapy is superior to either modality alone. However, some patients resistant to treatment with pharmacotherapy may benefit from added cognitive behavioural psychotherapy (for a more detailed discussion, see Chapter 3) [120].

FUTURE THERAPEUTIC OPTIONS

New therapeutic options for OCD continue to be explored. D-cycloserine is a *N*-methyl-D-aspartic acid (NMDA) partial agonist, and NMDA receptor stimulation has been linked with amygdale neural plasticity and fear extinction effects [121,122]. D-cycloserine has been administered before an exposure task, in the hope that stimulation of the NMDA receptor may help extinguish fear. In a randomized, double-blind, placebo-controlled trial conducted on 23 OCD patients, D-cycloserine plus cognitive behavioural therapy improved OCD symptoms significantly at mid-treatment, and depressive symptoms significantly post-treatment compared to placebo [121]. In another randomized, double-blind, placebo-controlled trial conducted on 32 patients, D-cycloserine plus cognitive behavioural therapy decreased obsession-related distress significantly compared to placebo; however, after additional exposure sessions, the difference was no longer seen [123].

Numerous neuroimaging findings in patients with OCD have demonstrated increased cerebral blood flow, metabolism and activation in the cortico-striato-thalamo-cortical (CSTC) circuitry [124–128]. Glutamate- and γ-aminobutyric acid (GABA)-driven pathways are the main circuits within the CSTC circuitry, leading to the hypothesis that glutamatergic activation may contribute to the pathophysiology of OCD [129,130]. Direct evidence of raised cerebrospinal fluid glutamate concentrations in OCD patients compared to controls has been demonstrated [131]. Modulation of glutamatergic neurotransmission therefore provides a novel drug target. Riluzole, a glutamate antagonist, may hold promise for treatment of refractory patients [132].

Treatment other than pharmacotherapy or cognitive behavioural therapy has been explored in patients with resistant OCD. Deep brain stimulation involves delivering a current via an implanted electrode that is connected to a battery-powered impulse generator implanted beneath the skin in the subclavicular region. The therapeutic mechanism of action is modulation of neuronal network activity using a pulse generator surgically placed in specific target sites. Several clinical trials assessing the efficacy of deep brain stimulation in patients with OCD have been positive [133].

Transcranial magnetic stimulation (TMS) is a non-invasive technique that delivers magnetic pulses to the cortex by means of a handheld stimulating coil applied directly to the head [134]. There are ongoing trials of TMS in OCD, with some evidence from recent work that this modality may have potential in the treatment of OCD [135,136]. Such work is covered in more detail in Chapter 4.

It is notable that many published trials in OCD have been for registration purposes, and therefore do not provide data on effectiveness. For example, many of these trials include only patients without comorbidity (e.g. depressed patients are typically excluded), and with a limited range of morbidity (e.g. suicidal patients are typically excluded). In addition, most studies focus primarily on the Y–BOCS; there are few data on the differential response of symptom dimensions to pharmacotherapy, or on the disability and quality of life variables. Much further work is needed to determine the effectiveness of treatment in real-world settings.

CONCLUSION

There have been significant advances in the pharmacotherapy of OCD, but further work remains to be done. Extensive evidence exists to support the modest efficacy of clomipramine and the SSRIs in the treatment of OCD. Clomipramine and the SSRIs seem equally effective at relieving obsessions and compulsions, but superior safety and tolerability of the SSRIs makes them the treatment of choice. SSRIs are not, however, free of adverse effects and may significantly impact on patient quality of life. Treatment-refractory OCD remains an important clinical issue; antipsychotic augmentation is recommended, but these agents are effective and tolerated in only a proportion of patients. There have been significant advances in the neurobiology of OCD, and ongoing basic work may ultimately be translated into novel approaches to the pharmacotherapy of OCD [143].

REFERENCES

1. Tolin DF, Abramowitz JS, Diefenbach GJ. Defining response in clinical trials for obsessive-compulsive disorder: a signal detection analysis of the Yale-Brown obsessive compulsive scale. *J Clin Psychiatry* 2005;**66**:1549–1557.
2. Zaider TI, Heimberg RG, Fresco DM, Schneier FR, Liebowitz MR. Evaluation of the clinical global impression scale among individuals with social anxiety disorder. *Psychol Med* 2003;**33**:611–622.
3. Healy D. The marketing of 5-hydroxytryptamine: depression or anxiety? *Br J Psychiatry* 1991;**158**:737–742.

4. Capstick N. Chlorimipramine in obsessional states. (A pilot study). *Psychosomatics* 1971;**12**:332–335.
5. Fineberg NA, Gale TM. Evidence-based pharmacotherapy of obsessive-compulsive disorder. *Int J Neuropsychopharmacol* 2005;**8**:107–129.
6. Mavissakalian M, Turner SM, Michelson L, Jacob R. Tricyclic antidepressants in obsessive-compulsive disorder: antiobsessional or antidepressant agents? II. *Am J Psychiatry* 1985;**142**:572–576.
7. Jenike MA, Baer L, Summergrad P, Weilburg JB, Holland A, Seymour R. Obsessive-compulsive disorder: a double-blind, placebo-controlled trial of clomipramine in 27 patients. *Am J Psychiatry* 1989;**146**:1328–1330.
8. DeVeaugh-Geiss J, Landau P, Katz R. Preliminary results from a multicenter trial of clomipramine in obsessive-compulsive disorder. *Psychopharmacol Bull* 1989;**25**:36–40.
9. Clomipramine in the treatment of patients with obsessive-compulsive disorder. The Clomipramine Collaborative Study Group. *Arch Gen Psychiatry* 1991;**48**:730–738.
10. Thoren P, Asberg M, Cronholm B, Jornestedt L, Traskman L. Clomipramine treatment of obsessive-compulsive disorder. I. A controlled clinical trial. *Arch Gen Psychiatry* 1980;**37**:1281–1285.
11. Insel TR, Murphy DL, Cohen RM, Alterman I, Kilts C, Linnoila M. Obsessive-compulsive disorder. A double-blind trial of clomipramine and clorgyline. *Arch Gen Psychiatry* 1983;**40**:605–612.
12. Insel TR, Hamilton JA, Guttmacher LB, Murphy DL. D-amphetamine in obsessive-compulsive disorder. *Psychopharmacology (Berl)* 1983;**80**:231–235.
13. Insel TR, Zohar J, Benkelfat C, Murphy DL. Serotonin in obsessions, compulsions, and the control of aggressive impulses. *Ann N Y Acad Sci* 1990;**600**:574–85; discussion 585–586.
14. Pigott TA, Seay SM. A review of the efficacy of selective serotonin reuptake inhibitors in obsessive-compulsive disorder. *J Clin Psychiatry* 1999;**60**:101–106.
15. Hindmarch I, Hashimoto K. Cognition and depression: the effects of fluvoxamine, a sigma-1 receptor agonist, reconsidered. *Hum Psychopharmacol* 2010;**25**:193–200.
16. Perse TL, Greist JH, Jefferson JW, Rosenfeld R, Dar R. Fluvoxamine treatment of obsessive-compulsive disorder. *Am J Psychiatry* 1987;**144**:1543–1548.
17. Goodman WK, Price LH, Rasmussen SA, Delgado PL, Heninger GR, Charney DS. Efficacy of fluvoxamine in obsessive-compulsive disorder. A double-blind comparison with placebo. *Arch Gen Psychiatry* 1989;**46**:36–44.
18. Jenike MA, Hyman S, Baer L *et al.* A controlled trial of fluvoxamine in obsessive-compulsive disorder: implications for a serotonergic theory. *Am J Psychiatry* 1990;**147**:1209–1215.
19. Cottraux J, Mollard E, Bouvard M *et al.* A controlled study of fluvoxamine and exposure in obsessive-compulsive disorder. *Int Clin Psychopharmacol* 1990;**5**:17–30.
20. Goodman WK, Kozak MJ, Liebowitz M, White KL. Treatment of obsessive-compulsive disorder with fluvoxamine: a multicentre, double-blind, placebo-controlled trial. *Int Clin Psychopharmacol* 1996;**11**:21–29.
21. Hollander E, Koran LM, Goodman WK *et al.* A double-blind, placebo-controlled study of the efficacy and safety of controlled-release fluvoxamine in patients with obsessive-compulsive disorder. *J Clin Psychiatry* 2003;**64**:640–647.

22. Koran LM, Bromberg D, Hornfeldt CS, Shepski JC, Wang S, Hollander E. Extended-release fluvoxamine and improvements in quality of life in patients with obsessive-compulsive disorder. *Compr Psychiatry* 2010;**51**:373–379.

23. Fluitman SB, Denys DA, Heijnen CJ, Westenberg HG. Disgust affects TNF-alpha, IL-6 and noradrenalin levels in patients with obsessive-compulsive disorder. *Psychoneuroendocrinology* 2010;**35**:906–911.

24. Koo MS, Kim EJ, Roh D, Kim CH. Role of dopamine in the pathophysiology and treatment of obsessive-compulsive disorder. *Expert Rev Neurother* 2010;**10**:275–290.

25. Montgomery SA, McIntyre A, Osterheider M *et al.* A double-blind, placebo-controlled study of fluoxetine in patients with DSM-III-R obsessive-compulsive disorder. The Lilly European OCD Study Group. *Eur Neuropsychopharmacol* 1993;**3**:143–152.

26. Tollefson GD, Rampey AH Jr, Potvin JH *et al.* A multicenter investigation of fixed-dose fluoxetine in the treatment of obsessive-compulsive disorder. *Arch Gen Psychiatry* 1994;**51**:559–567.

27. Jenike MA, Baer L, Minichiello WE, Rauch SL, Buttolph ML. Placebo-controlled trial of fluoxetine and phenelzine for obsessive-compulsive disorder. *Am J Psychiatry* 1997;**154**:1261–1264.

28. Kapczinski F, Lima MS, Souza JS, Schmitt R. Antidepressants for generalized anxiety disorder. *Cochrane Database Syst Rev* 2003;(2):CD003592.

29. Zohar J, Judge R. Paroxetine versus clomipramine in the treatment of obsessive-compulsive disorder. OCD Paroxetine Study Investigators. *Br J Psychiatry* 1996;**169**:468–474.

30. Mundo E, Bianchi L, Bellodi L. Efficacy of fluvoxamine, paroxetine, and citalopram in the treatment of obsessive-compulsive disorder: a single-blind study. *J Clin Psychopharmacol* 1997;**17**:267–271.

31. Kamijima K, Murasaki M, Asai M *et al.* Paroxetine in the treatment of obsessive-compulsive disorder: randomized, double-blind, placebo-controlled study in Japanese patients. *Psychiatry Clin Neurosci* 2004;**58**:427–433.

32. Hollander E, Allen A, Steiner M *et al.* Acute and long-term treatment and prevention of relapse of obsessive-compulsive disorder with paroxetine. *J Clin Psychiatry* 2003;**64**:1113–1121.

33. Chouinard G, Goodman W, Greist J *et al.* Results of a double-blind placebo controlled trial of a new serotonin uptake inhibitor, sertraline, in the treatment of obsessive-compulsive disorder. *Psychopharmacol Bull* 1990;**26**:279–284.

34. Greist J, Chouinard G, DuBoff E *et al.* Double-blind parallel comparison of three dosages of sertraline and placebo in outpatients with obsessive-compulsive disorder. *Arch Gen Psychiatry* 1995;**52**:289–295.

35. Kronig MH, Apter J, Asnis G *et al.* Placebo-controlled, multicenter study of sertraline treatment for obsessive-compulsive disorder. *J Clin Psychopharmacol* 1999;**19**:172–176.

36. Bogetto F, Albert U, Maina G. Sertraline treatment of obsessive-compulsive disorder: efficacy and tolerability of a rapid titration regimen. *Eur Neuropsychopharmacol* 2002;**12**:181–186.

37. Rasmussen S, Hackett E, DuBoff E *et al.* A 2-year study of sertraline in the treatment of obsessive-compulsive disorder. *Int Clin Psychopharmacol* 1997;**12**:309–316.

38. Koran LM, Hackett E, Rubin A, Wolkow R, Robinson D. Efficacy of sertraline in the long-term treatment of obsessive-compulsive disorder. *Am J Psychiatry* 2002;**159**:88–95.

39. Montgomery SA, Kasper S, Stein DJ, Bang Hedegaard K, Lemming OM. Citalopram 20 mg, 40 mg and 60 mg are all effective and well tolerated compared with placebo in obsessive-compulsive disorder. *Int Clin Psychopharmacol* 2001;**16**:75–86.

40. Stein DJ, Andersen EW, Tonnoir B, Fineberg N. Escitalopram in obsessive-compulsive disorder: a randomized, placebo-controlled, paroxetine-referenced, fixed-dose, 24-week study. *Curr Med Res Opin* 2007;**23**:701–711.

41. Fineberg NA, Tonnoir B, Lemming O, Stein DJ. Escitalopram prevents relapse of obsessive-compulsive disorder. *Eur Neuropsychopharmacol* 2007;**17**:430–439.

42. Dell'Osso B, Nestadt G, Allen A, Hollander E. Serotonin-norepinephrine reuptake inhibitors in the treatment of obsessive-compulsive disorder: A critical review. *J Clin Psychiatry* 2006;**67**:600–610.

43. Yaryura-Tobias JA, Neziroglu FA. Venlafaxine in obsessive-compulsive disorder. *Arch Gen Psychiatry* 1996;**53**:653–654.

44. Denys D, van der Wee N, van Megen HJ, Westenberg HG. A double blind comparison of venlafaxine and paroxetine in obsessive-compulsive disorder. *J Clin Psychopharmacol* 2003;**23**:568–575.

45. Artigas F, Adell A, Celada P. Pindolol augmentation of antidepressant response. *Curr Drug Targets* 2006;**7**:139–147.

46. Mundo E, Guglielmo E, Bellodi L. Effect of adjuvant pindolol on the antiobsessional response to fluvoxamine: a double-blind, placebo-controlled study. *Int Clin Psychopharmacol* 1998;**13**:219–224.

47. Kalra SK, Swedo SE. Children with obsessive-compulsive disorder: are they just "little adults"? *J Clin Invest* 2009;**119**:737–746.

48. Cella M, Knibbe C, Danhof M, Della Pasqua O. What is the right dose for children? *Br J Clin Pharmacol* 2010;**70**:597–603.

49. Anderson BJ, Holford NH. Mechanistic basis of using body size and maturation to predict clearance in humans. *Drug Metab Pharmacokinet* 2009;**24**:25–36.

50. Flament MF, Rapoport JL, Berg CJ *et al.* Clomipramine treatment of childhood obsessive-compulsive disorder. A double-blind controlled study. *Arch Gen Psychiatry* 1985;**42**:977–983.

51. Leonard HL, Swedo SE, Rapoport JL *et al.* Treatment of obsessive-compulsive disorder with clomipramine and desipramine in children and adolescents. A double-blind crossover comparison. *Arch Gen Psychiatry* 1989;**46**:1088–1092.

52. Riddle MA, Reeve EA, Yaryura-Tobias JA *et al.* Fluvoxamine for children and adolescents with obsessive-compulsive disorder: a randomized, controlled, multicenter trial. *J Am Acad Child Adolesc Psychiatry* 2001;**40**:222–229.

53. Riddle MA, Scahill L, King RA *et al.* Double-blind, crossover trial of fluoxetine and placebo in children and adolescents with obsessive-compulsive disorder. *J Am Acad Child Adolesc Psychiatry* 1992;**31**:1062–1069.

54. Geller DA, Hoog SL, Heiligenstein JH *et al.* Fluoxetine treatment for obsessive-compulsive disorder in children and adolescents: a placebo-controlled clinical trial. *J Am Acad Child Adolesc Psychiatry* 2001;**40**:773–779.

55. Liebowitz MR, Turner SM, Piacentini J *et al*. Fluoxetine in children and adolescents with OCD: a placebo-controlled trial. *J Am Acad Child Adolesc Psychiatry* 2002;**41**:1431–1438.

56. Rosenberg DR, Stewart CM, Fitzgerald KD, Tawile V, Carroll E. Paroxetine open-label treatment of pediatric outpatients with obsessive-compulsive disorder. *J Am Acad Child Adolesc Psychiatry* 1999;**38**:1180–1185.

57. Geller DA, Wagner KD, Emslie G *et al*. Paroxetine treatment in children and adolescents with obsessive-compulsive disorder: a randomized, multicenter, double-blind, placebo-controlled trial. *J Am Acad Child Adolesc Psychiatry* 2004;**43**:1387–1396.

58. Findling RL, Nucci G, Piergies AA *et al*. Multiple dose pharmacokinetics of paroxetine in children and adolescents with major depressive disorder or obsessive-compulsive disorder. *Neuropsychopharmacology* 2006;**31**:1274–1285.

59. March JS, Biederman J, Wolkow R *et al*. Sertraline in children and adolescents with obsessive-compulsive disorder: a multicenter randomized controlled trial. *JAMA* 1998;**280**:1752–1756.

60. Wilens TE, Biederman J, March JS *et al*. Absence of cardiovascular adverse effects of sertraline in children and adolescents. *J Am Acad Child Adolesc Psychiatry* 1999;**38**:573–577.

61. Cook EH, Wagner KD, March JS *et al*. Long-term sertraline treatment of children and adolescents with obsessive-compulsive disorder. *J Am Acad Child Adolesc Psychiatry* 2001;**40**:1175–1181.

62. Alderman J, Wolkow R, Chung M, Johnston HF. Sertraline treatment of children and adolescents with obsessive-compulsive disorder or depression: pharmacokinetics, tolerability, and efficacy. *J Am Acad Child Adolesc Psychiatry* 1998;**37**:386–394.

63. Thomsen PH, Ebbesen C, Persson C. Long-term experience with citalopram in the treatment of adolescent OCD. *J Am Acad Child Adolesc Psychiatry* 2001;**40**:895–902.

64. Lopez-Ibor JJ Jr, Saiz J, Cottraux J *et al*. Double-blind comparison of fluoxetine versus clomipramine in the treatment of obsessive compulsive disorder. *Eur Neuropsychopharmacol* 1996;**6**:111–118.

65. Koran LM, McElroy SL, Davidson JR, Rasmussen SA, Hollander E, Jenike MA. Fluvoxamine versus clomipramine for obsessive-compulsive disorder: a double-blind comparison. *J Clin Psychopharmacol* 1996;**16**:121–129.

66. Mundo E, Rouillon F, Figuera ML, Stigler M. Fluvoxamine in obsessive-compulsive disorder: similar efficacy but superior tolerability in comparison with clomipramine. *Hum Psychopharmacol* 2001;**16**:461–468.

67. Bisserbe J, Lane R, Flament M. A double-blind comparison of sertraline and clomipramine in outpatients with obsessive-compulsive disorder. *Eur Psychiatry* 1997;**12**:82–93.

68. Soomro GM, Altman D, Rajagopal S, Oakley-Browne M. Selective serotonin reuptake inhibitors (SSRIs) versus placebo for obsessive compulsive disorder (OCD). *Cochrane Database Syst Rev* 2008 Jan 23;(1):CD001765.

69. Pisani F, Oteri G, Costa C, Di Raimondo G, Di Perri R. Effects of psychotropic drugs on seizure threshold. *Drug Saf* 2002;**25**:91–110.

70. Maina G, Albert U, Salvi V, Bogetto F. Weight gain during long-term treatment of obsessive-compulsive disorder: a prospective comparison between serotonin reuptake inhibitors. *J Clin Psychiatry* 2004;**65**:1365–1371.

71. Gartlehner G, Thieda P, Hansen RA *et al*. Comparative risk for harms of second-generation antidepressants : a systematic review and meta-analysis. *Drug Saf* 2008;**31**:851–865.

72. Cheeta S, Schifano F, Oyefeso A, Webb L, Ghodse AH. Antidepressant-related deaths and antidepressant prescriptions in England and Wales, 1998–2000. *Br J Psychiatry* 2004;**184**:41–47.

73. Barbey JT, Roose SP. SSRI safety in overdose. *J Clin Psychiatry* 1998;**59**(Suppl. 15):42–48.

74. Safer DJ, Zito JM. Treatment-emergent adverse events from selective serotonin re-uptake inhibitors by age group: children versus adolescents. *J Child Adolesc Psychopharmacol* 2006;**16**:159–169.

75. Bloch MH, McGuire J, Landeros-Weisenberger A, Leckman JF, Pittenger C. Meta-analysis of the dose–response relationship of SSRI in obsessive-compulsive disorder. *Mol Psychiatry* 2010;**15**:850–855.

76. Hollander E, Allen A, Steiner M *et al*. Acute and long-term treatment and prevention of relapse of obsessive-compulsive disorder with paroxetine. *J Clin Psychiatry* 2003;**64**:1113–1121.

77. Tollefson GD, Rampey AH Jr, Potvin JH *et al*. A multicenter investigation of fixed-dose fluoxetine in the treatment of obsessive-compulsive disorder. *Arch Gen Psychiatry* 1994;**51**:559–567.

78. Mundo E, Bareggi SR, Pirola R, Bellodi L, Smeraldi E. Long-term pharmacotherapy of obsessive-compulsive disorder: a double-blind controlled study. *J Clin Psychopharmacol* 1997;**17**:4–10.

79. Ninan PT, Koran LM, Kiev A *et al*. High-dose sertraline strategy for nonresponders to acute treatment for obsessive-compulsive disorder: a multicenter double-blind trial. *J Clin Psychiatry* 2006;**67**:15–22.

80. Pampaloni I, Sivakumaran T, Hawley C *et al*. High-dose selective serotonin reuptake inhibitors in OCD: a systematic retrospective case notes survey. *J Psychopharmacol* 2010;**34**:1439–1445.

81. March JS, Frances A, Kahn D, Carpenter D. The Expert Consensus Guideline: Treatment of obsessive-compulsive disorder. *Journal of Clinical Psychology* 1997;**58**(Suppl. 4):1–72.

82. Stein DJ, Ipser JC, Baldwin DS, Bandelow B. Treatment of obsessive-compulsive disorder. *CNS Spectrums* 2007;**12**(2 Suppl. 3):28–35.

83. Pato MT, Zohar-Kadouch R, Zohar J, Murphy DL. Return of symptoms after discontinuation of clomipramine in patients with obsessive-compulsive disorder. *Am J Psychiatry* 1988;**145**:1521–1525.

84. Romano S, Goodman W, Tamura R, Gonzales J. Long-term treatment of obsessive-compulsive disorder after an acute response: a comparison of fluoxetine versus placebo. *J Clin Psychopharmacol* 2001;**21**:46–52.

85. Geller DA, Biederman J, Stewart SE *et al*. Impact of comorbidity on treatment response to paroxetine in pediatric obsessive-compulsive disorder: is the use of exclusion criteria empirically supported in randomized clinical trials? *J Child Adolesc Psychopharmacol* 2003;**13**(Suppl. 1):S19–29.

86. Leonard HL, Swedo SE, Lenane MC *et al*. A 2- to 7-year follow-up study of 54 obsessive-compulsive children and adolescents. *Arch Gen Psychiatry* 1993;**50**:429–439.

87. Pallanti S, Hollander E, Bienstock C *et al.* Treatment non-response in OCD: methodological issues and operational definitions. *Int J Neuropsychopharmacol* 2002;**5**:181–191.

88. Rabinowitz I, Baruch Y, Barak Y. High-dose escitalopram for the treatment of obsessive-compulsive disorder. *Int Clin Psychopharmacol* 2008;**23**:49–53.

89. McDougle CJ, Goodman WK, Leckman JF, Lee NC, Heninger GR, Price LH. Haloperidol addition in fluvoxamine-refractory obsessive-compulsive disorder. A double-blind, placebo-controlled study in patients with and without tics. *Arch Gen Psychiatry* 1994;**51**:302–308.

90. McDougle CJ, Epperson CN, Pelton GH, Wasylink S, Price LH. A double-blind, placebo-controlled study of risperidone addition in serotonin reuptake inhibitor-refractory obsessive-compulsive disorder. *Arch Gen Psychiatry* 2000;**57**:794–801.

91. Erzegovesi S, Guglielmo E, Siliprandi F, Bellodi L. Low-dose risperidone augmentation of fluvoxamine treatment in obsessive-compulsive disorder: a double-blind, placebo-controlled study. *Eur Neuropsychopharmacol* 2005;**15**:69–74.

92. Shapira NA, Ward HE, Mandoki M *et al.* A double-blind, placebo-controlled trial of olanzapine addition in fluoxetine-refractory obsessive-compulsive disorder. *Biol Psychiatry* 2004;**55**:553–555.

93. Bystritsky A, Ackerman DL, Rosen RM *et al.* Augmentation of serotonin reuptake inhibitors in refractory obsessive-compulsive disorder using adjunctive olanzapine: a placebo-controlled trial. *J Clin Psychiatry* 2004;**65**:565–568.

94. D'Amico G, Cedro C, Muscatello MR, *et al.* Olanzapine augmentation of paroxetine-refractory obsessive-compulsive disorder. *Prog Neuropsychopharmacol Biol Psychiatry* 2003;**27**:619–623.

95. Atmaca M, Kuloglu M, Tezcan E, Gecici O. Quetiapine augmentation in patients with treatment resistant obsessive-compulsive disorder: a single-blind, placebo-controlled study. *Int Clin Psychopharmacol* 2002;**17**:115–119.

96. Denys D, van Megen H, Westenberg H. Quetiapine addition to serotonin reuptake inhibitor treatment in patients with treatment-refractory obsessive-compulsive disorder: an open-label study. *J Clin Psychiatry* 2002;**63**:700–703.

97. Denys D, de Geus F, van Megen HJ, Westenberg HG. A double-blind, randomized, placebo-controlled trial of quetiapine addition in patients with obsessive-compulsive disorder refractory to serotonin reuptake inhibitors. *J Clin Psychiatry* 2004;**65**:1040–1048.

98. Carey PD, Vythilingum B, Seedat S, Muller JE, van Ameringen M, Stein DJ. Quetiapine augmentation of SRIs in treatment refractory obsessive-compulsive disorder: a double-blind, randomised, placebo-controlled study [ISRCTN83050762]. *BMC Psychiatry* 2005;**5**:5.

99. Vulink NC, Denys D, Fluitman SB, Meinardi JC, Westenberg HG. Quetiapine augments the effect of citalopram in non-refractory obsessive-compulsive disorder: a randomized, double-blind, placebo-controlled study of 76 patients. *J Clin Psychiatry* 2009;**70**:1001–1008.

100. McDougle CJ, Barr LC, Goodman WK *et al.* Lack of efficacy of clozapine monotherapy in refractory obsessive-compulsive disorder. *Am J Psychiatry* 1995;**152**:1812–1814.

101. Matsunaga H, Nagata T, Hayashida K, Ohya K, Kiriike N, Stein DJ. A long-term trial of the effectiveness and safety of atypical antipsychotic agents in augmenting SSRI-refractory obsessive-compulsive disorder. *J Clin Psychiatry* 2009;**70**:863–868.

102. Ipser JC, Carey P, Dhansay Y, Fakier N, Seedat S, Stein DJ. Pharmacotherapy augmentation strategies in treatment-resistant anxiety disorders. *Cochrane Database Syst Rev* 2006 Oct 18;(4):CD005473.

103. McDougle CJ, Price LH, Goodman WK, Charney DS, Heninger GR. A controlled trial of lithium augmentation in fluvoxamine-refractory obsessive-compulsive disorder: lack of efficacy. *J Clin Psychopharmacol* 1991;**11**:175–184.

104. McDougle CJ, Goodman WK, Leckman JF *et al.* Limited therapeutic effect of addition of buspirone in fluvoxamine-refractory obsessive-compulsive disorder. *Am J Psychiatry* 1993;**150**:647–649.

105. Barr LC, Goodman WK, Anand A, McDougle CJ, Price LH. Addition of desipramine to serotonin reuptake inhibitors in treatment-resistant obsessive-compulsive disorder. *Am J Psychiatry* 1997;**154**:1293–1295.

106. Seedat S, Stein DJ. Inositol augmentation of serotonin reuptake inhibitors in treatment-refractory obsessive-compulsive disorder: an open trial. *Int Clin Psychopharmacol* 1999;**14**:353–356.

107. Crockett BA, Churchill E, Davidson JR. A double-blind combination study of clonazepam with sertraline in obsessive-compulsive disorder. *Ann Clin Psychiatry* 2004;**16**:127–132.

108. Dannon PN, Sasson Y, Hirschmann S, Iancu I, Grunhaus LJ, Zohar J. Pindolol augmentation in treatment-resistant obsessive compulsive disorder: a double-blind placebo controlled trial. *Eur Neuropsychopharmacol* 2000;**10**:165–169.

109. Koran LM, Aboujaoude E, Bullock KD, Franz B, Gamel N, Elliott M. Double-blind treatment with oral morphine in treatment-resistant obsessive-compulsive disorder. *J Clin Psychiatry* 2005;**66**:353–359.

110. Mula M, Pini S, Cassano GB. The role of anticonvulsant drugs in anxiety disorders: a critical review of the evidence. *J Clin Psychopharmacol* 2007;**27**:263–272.

111. Hemeryck A, Belpaire FM. Selective serotonin reuptake inhibitors and cytochrome P-450 mediated drug–drug interactions: an update. *Curr Drug Metab* 2002;**3**:13.

112. Spina E, Santoro V, D'Arrigo C. Clinically relevant pharmacokinetic drug interactions with second-generation antidepressants: an update. *Clin Ther* 2008;**30**:1206–1227.

113. Gillman PK. Tricyclic antidepressant pharmacology and therapeutic drug interactions updated. *Br J Pharmacol* 2007;**151**:737–748.

114. Szegedi A, Wetzel H, Leal M, Hartter S, Hiemke C. Combination treatment with clomipramine and fluvoxamine: drug monitoring, safety, and tolerability data. *J Clin Psychiatry* 1996;**57**:257–264.

115. Koran LM, Sallee FR, Pallanti S. Rapid benefit of intravenous pulse loading of clomipramine in obsessive-compulsive disorder. *Am J Psychiatry* 1997;**154**:396–401.

116. Fallon BA, Liebowitz MR, Campeas R *et al.* Intravenous clomipramine for obsessive-compulsive disorder refractory to oral clomipramine: a placebo-controlled study. *Arch Gen Psychiatry* 1998;**55**:918–924.

117. Pallanti S, Quercioli L, Koran LM. Citalopram intravenous infusion in resistant obsessive-compulsive disorder: an open trial. *J Clin Psychiatry* 2002;**63**:796–801.

118. Figueroa Y, Rosenberg DR, Birmaher B, Keshavan MS. Combination treatment with clomipramine and selective serotonin reuptake inhibitors for obsessive-compulsive disorder in children and adolescents. *J Child Adolesc Psychopharmacol* 1998;**8**:61–67.

119. Denys D, van Megen HJ, van der Wee N, Westenberg HG. A double-blind switch study of paroxetine and venlafaxine in obsessive-compulsive disorder. *J Clin Psychiatry* 2004;**65**:37–43.

120. Simpson HB, Foa EB, Liebowitz MR *et al.* A randomized, controlled trial of cognitive-behavioral therapy for augmenting pharmacotherapy in obsessive-compulsive disorder. *Am J Psychiatry* 2008;**165**:621–630.

121. Wilhelm S, Buhlmann U, Tolin DF *et al.* Augmentation of behavior therapy with D-cycloserine for obsessive-compulsive disorder. *Am J Psychiatry* 2008;**165**:335–341; quiz 409.

122. Abramowitz JS, Taylor S, McKay D. Obsessive-compulsive disorder. *Lancet* 2009;**374**:491–499.

123. Kushner MG, Kim SW, Donahue C *et al.* D-cycloserine augmented exposure therapy for obsessive-compulsive disorder. *Biol Psychiatry* 2007;**62**:835–838.

124. Baxter LR Jr, Phelps ME, Mazziotta JC, Guze BH, Schwartz JM, Selin CE. Local cerebral glucose metabolic rates in obsessive-compulsive disorder. A comparison with rates in unipolar depression and in normal controls. *Arch Gen Psychiatry* 1987;**44**:211–218.

125. Saxena S, Brody AL, Ho ML *et al.* Differential cerebral metabolic changes with paroxetine treatment of obsessive-compulsive disorder vs major depression. *Arch Gen Psychiatry* 2002;**59**:250–261.

126. Saxena S, Brody AL, Ho ML, Zohrabi N, Maidment KM, Baxter LR Jr. Differential brain metabolic predictors of response to paroxetine in obsessive-compulsive disorder versus major depression. *Am J Psychiatry* 2003;**160**:522–532.

127. Saxena S, Brody AL, Schwartz JM, Baxter LR. Neuroimaging and frontal-subcortical circuitry in obsessive-compulsive disorder. *Br J Psychiatry Suppl* 1998;(35):26–37.

128. Adams BL, Warneke LB, McEwan AJ, Fraser BA. Single photon emission computerized tomography in obsessive compulsive disorder: a preliminary study. *J Psychiatry Neurosci* 1993;**18**:109–112.

129. Carlsson ML. On the role of prefrontal cortex glutamate for the antithetical phenomenology of obsessive compulsive disorder and attention deficit hyperactivity disorder. *Prog Neuropsychopharmacol Biol Psychiatry* 2001;**25**:5–26.

130. Carlsson ML. On the role of cortical glutamate in obsessive-compulsive disorder and attention-deficit hyperactivity disorder, two phenomenologically antithetical conditions. *Acta Psychiatr Scand* 2000;**102**:401–413.

131. Chakrabarty K, Bhattacharyya S, Christopher R, Khanna S. Glutamatergic dysfunction in OCD. *Neuropsychopharmacology* 2005;**30**:1735–1740.

132. Pittenger C, Kelmendi B, Wasylink S, Bloch MH, Coric V. Riluzole augmentation in treatment-refractory obsessive-compulsive disorder: a series of 13 cases, with long-term follow-up. *J Clin Psychopharmacol* 2008;**28**:363–367.

133. Tye SJ, Frye MA, Lee KH. Disrupting disordered neurocircuitry: treating refractory psychiatric illness with neuromodulation. *Mayo Clin Proc* 2009;**84**:522–532.

134. Dell'Osso B, Altamura AC, Allen A, Hollander E. Brain stimulation techniques in the treatment of obsessive-compulsive disorder: current and future directions. *CNS Spectrums* 2005;**10**:966–79, 983.
135. Martin JL, Barbanoj MJ, Perez V, Sacristan M. Transcranial magnetic stimulation for the treatment of obsessive-compulsive disorder. *Cochrane Database Syst Rev* 2003;(3):CD003387.
136. Denys D, Mantione M, Figee M *et al.* Deep brain stimulation of the nucleus accumbens for treatment-refractory obsessive-compulsive disorder. *Arch Gen Psychiatry* 2010;**67**:1061–1068.
137. Greist JH, Jefferson JW, Kobak KA, Katzelnick DJ, Serlin RC. Efficacy and tolerability of serotonin transport inhibitors in obsessive-compulsive disorder. A meta-analysis. *Arch Gen Psychiatry* 1995;**52**:53–60.
138. Piccinelli M, Pini S, Bellantuono C, Wilkinson G. Efficacy of drug treatment in obsessive-compulsive disorder. A meta-analytic review. *Br J Psychiatry* 1995;**166**:424–443.
139. Stein DJ, Spadaccini E, Hollander E. Meta-analysis of pharmacotherapy trials for obsessive-compulsive disorder. *Int Clin Psychopharmacol* 1995;**10**:11–18.
140. Abramowitz JS. Effectiveness of psychological and pharmacological treatments for obsessive-compulsive disorder: a quantitative review. *J Consult Clin Psychol* 1997;**65**:44–52.
141. Kobak KA, Greist JH, Jefferson JW, Katzelnick DJ, Henk HJ. Behavioral versus pharmacological treatments of obsessive compulsive disorder: a meta-analysis. *Psychopharmacology (Berl)* 1998;**136**:205–216.
142. Ackerman DL, Greenland S. Multivariate meta-analysis of controlled drug studies for obsessive-compulsive disorder. *J Clin Psychopharmacol* 2002;**22**:309–317.
143. Joel D, Stein DJ, Schreiber R. Animal models of obsessive-compulsive disorder: From bench to bedside via endophenotypes and biomarkers. In: McArthur RA, Borsini F (eds), *Animal and Translational Models for CNS Drug Discovery, Volume 1: Psychiatric Disorders*. Amsterdam: Elsevier, 2008.

CHAPTER 3

Cognitive Behavioural Therapy in Obsessive-Compulsive Disorder: State of the Art

Martin E. Franklin,[1] Addie Goss[2] and John S. March[3]

[1] *University of Pennsylvania School of Medicine;* [2] *Bryn Mawr College;*
[3] *Duke University Medical Center*

THEORETICAL MODELS

Several cognitive and behavioural theories have been put forward to explain the development and maintenance of obsessive-compulsive disorder (OCD) symptoms, yet the theory advanced by Mowrer [1,2] continues to be strongly influential in explaining the maintenance of OCD symptoms. Mowrer's two-stage theory [1,2] proposes that a neutral event first becomes associated with fear when it is paired with a stimulus that by nature provokes distress or pain. Through conditioning processes, objects, thoughts and images suggestive of the event acquire the ability to produce discomfort. The individual then develops escape or avoidance behaviours to reduce the distress evoked by the conditioned stimuli. In OCD, behavioural avoidance and escape take the form of rituals. They are maintained because they reduce the distress.

Adding a more integrated cognitive behavioural perspective, Foa and Kozak [3] proposed that OCD is characterized by erroneous cognitions: that, first, OCD sufferers assign a high probability of danger to situations that are relatively safe; and second, individuals with OCD exaggerate the cost of the bad things they

Obsessive-Compulsive Disorder: Current Science and Clinical Practice, First Edition. Edited by Joseph Zohar.
© 2012 John Wiley & Sons, Ltd. Published 2012 by John Wiley & Sons, Ltd.

believe can happen. Foa and Kozak further suggested that individuals with OCD conclude that, in the face of a lack of evidence that a situation or an object is safe, the situation or object is dangerous; therefore, OCD sufferers require constant evidence for safety, and compulsions are one means by which individuals with OCD attempt to restore this feeling of safety.

Salkovskis [4] offered a comprehensive cognitive account of OCD. He proposed that intrusive obsessional thoughts are stimuli that may provoke certain negative automatic thoughts. According to Salkovskis, an exaggerated sense of responsibility and self-blame are the central themes in the OCD sufferer's belief system (e.g. only bad people have sexual thoughts). Compulsions can be understood as 'neutralizations' – attempts to reduce this sense of responsibility and to prevent blame. Salkovskis outlined five dysfunctional assumptions typical of OCD:

1. Having a thought about an action is like performing the action.
2. Failing to prevent or to try to prevent harm is the same as having caused the harm.
3. Responsibility is not reduced by other factors, such as a low probability of occurrence.
4. Not neutralizing in response to an intrusion is similar or equivalent to wanting the intrusion to occur.
5. One can and should exercise control over one's thoughts [ref. 4, p. 579].

Each of the aforementioned models proposes a specific therapeutic emphasis. For example, Salkovskis's cognitive model suggests that OCD treatment should focus on identifying erroneous assumptions and modifying automatic thoughts. Theories that blend cognitive and behavioural elements, such as Foa and Kozak's Emotional Processing Theory [3], suggest cognitive and behavioural treatment strategies, with the aim of providing the patient with corrective information about the world and about his or her own fear responses. The treatments described below flow from these prevailing conceptual models. However, evidence for the efficacy of these interventions provides only partial support for the theoretical foundations upon which they were built.

A detailed discussion of the neurobiology of OCD and the specific unique role of selective serotonin reuptake inhibitors (SSRIs) in OCD can be found in Chapter 9. Studies collectively suggest that clinically significant residual impairment is the norm. Accordingly, treatment development work has moved in the past decade towards augmentation of partial response to SRIs; findings from two large studies indicate that adding CBT to the treatment regimen is associated with greater acute symptom reductions than stress management training in adults [5], and to medication maintenance alone in youth [6].

TREATMENT

Exposure plus response prevention (ERP)

Brief description of ERP procedures

The psychosocial intervention that has garnered the most empirical support is exposure plus response prevention (ERP). ERP has been studied around the world for the last 40 years and has proven to be both effective and durable for patients with OCD across the developmental spectrum [7–10]. The adult literature supporting the efficacy of ERP has been built over the course of decades, and there are now dozens of positive trials conducted across the world that attest to its efficacy. A number of randomized studies conducted recently also support the efficacy of ERP in children and adolescents with OCD [e.g. 11–16].

Current ERP treatments are based largely on the blended theoretical model proposed by Foa and Kozak [3]. ERP typically includes prolonged exposure to obsessional cues, procedures aimed at blocking rituals, and informal discussions of mistaken beliefs conducted in anticipation of exposure exercises. Exposures are most often done in real-life settings (*in vivo*) and involve prolonged contact with the feared external (e.g. contaminated surfaces) or internal (e.g. images of harming a family member) stimuli that the patient reports as distressing. For patients who fear specific consequences if they refrain from performing rituals, these fears can be addressed through 'imaginal exposure': creating very detailed image scripts and listening to or reading these scripts repeatedly until they are perceived as less anxiety-provoking. Following from Foa and Kozak's theory, *in vivo* and imaginal exposures are designed specifically to prompt obsessional distress. It is believed that repeated, prolonged exposure to feared thoughts and situations serves to disconfirm mistaken associations and evaluations held by the patient, thereby promoting habituation [3]. Exposures are typically done gradually, with situations provoking moderate distress confronted before more upsetting ones. Exposure 'homework' is routinely assigned between sessions, and patients are asked to refrain from rituals to the extent possible. The stated goal is complete abstinence from rituals, yet therapists must be cognizant of the need to encourage patients to achieve this goal over time rather than simply insisting upon it immediately. Patients are reminded throughout treatment that ritualizing maintains fear, whereas refraining from rituals promotes dissipation of fear; accordingly, they are given recommendations as to how best to refrain from rituals when the urges do arise.

Exposure versus response prevention versus ERP

An experiment by Foa *et al.* [17] highlighted the importance of combining exposure with response prevention in treatment of OCD. Patients with washing rituals were randomly assigned to treatment by exposure only, response prevention only, or their combination (EX/RP). Patients in each condition were found to have improved at both post-treatment and follow-up, but EX/RP was superior at both assessment points. These findings clearly suggest that exposure and ritual prevention should be implemented concurrently. It is also important to convey this information to patients, who may experience difficulty in refraining from rituals or engaging in exposure exercises. In our clinical work we will often cite the results of this study when patients are conducting exposures and yet ritualizing afterwards, thus minimizing the long-term benefits of their hard work.

Implementation of response prevention

ERP protocols emphasize that patients refrain consistently from ritualizing and avoidance; the success of these efforts is critical for symptom reduction [18]. The therapist can support the patient in doing so through encouragement, suggested alternatives to ritualizing, and involvement of family members to support the patient. Family members can be trained in how best to respond when the patient struggles with urges to ritualize, or when the patient is already in the midst of engaging in rituals.

Imaginal exposure

An early randomized study [19,20] found that treatment involving imaginal exposure plus *in vivo* ERP was superior at follow-up to *in vivo* ERP that did not include imaginal exposure; however, a later study [21] did not find an additive effect. The treatment programmes in these studies differed considerably, however, and thus the source of these inconsistencies cannot be identified.

Clinically, we have found that imaginal exposure is particularly helpful for patients who report that disastrous consequences will result if they refrain from rituals. Because many of these consequences cannot be readily translated into *in vivo* exposure exercises (e.g. burning in hell), imaginal exposure gives the patient an opportunity to confront these feared thoughts. Patients who suffer primarily from 'Not Just Right' OCD, which is more tic-like and less likely to be associated with specific feared consequences, typically benefit from exclusive focus on *in vivo* exposure plus resisting urges to ritualize; in such cases, imaginal exposure may well be superfluous.

Frequency of exposure sessions

ERP studies have been conducted using visit schedules ranging from weekly to intensive schedules, although only a few studies have directly examined the effects of session frequency. Intensive exposure therapy typically involves daily sessions over the course of approximately 1 month, but good outcomes have also been found with more widely spaced sessions [e.g. 21–23]. A recent randomized controlled trial (RCT) in paediatric OCD found no difference between intensive and weekly treatment [14]. Clinically, we suggest that therapists take motivational factors, developmental level of the patient, psychiatric comorbidity, clinical need for a faster response, and cost into account when determining session frequency. Less frequent sessions may be sufficient for highly motivated patients with mild to moderate OCD symptoms who readily understand the importance of daily exposure homework exercises, whereas patients with very severe symptoms or who are experiencing difficulty completing EX/RP tasks between sessions might benefit more from a more intensive visit schedule.

Gradual versus abrupt exposures

No differences in OCD symptom reduction have been detected between patients who confront the most distressing situations first versus those who work up to them [24]. However, given that patient motivation is critical to the success of EX/RP, situations that provoke low to moderate distress are usually confronted in treatment first, followed by several intermediate steps before the most distressing exposures are attempted. This may be especially important in the treatment of children, where positive initial experiences with lower level exposures may set the stage for greater cooperation and buy-in as the practices become more challenging.

Duration of exposure

Duration of exposure is thought to be an important factor in treatment outcomes: prolonged, continuous exposure has been found to be more effective than short, interrupted exposure [25]. Exposure may be extended beyond 90 minutes if the patient has not experienced anxiety reduction within that time; it may be terminated if the patient reports substantial reduction in obsessional distress sooner.

Family involvement

Family members affect and are affected by OCD, particularly when the patient is a child or adolescent. In paediatric OCD, families often accommodate to the child's symptoms [14,26]; family conflict and comorbid externalizing symptoms tend to be worse when families attempt to refrain from accommodation [26]. Studies of paediatric OCD have yet to indicate the optimal amount of family involvement necessary for robust and durable symptom reduction. However, our clinical observations suggest that some combination of family and individual sessions is best for most patients aged 9 years and older. In our protocol for paediatric OCD, we include several sessions that involve the whole family. Some investigators have emphasized family work even more in the development of their CBT protocols [e.g. 27] With younger patients, the role of the family in treatment is generally greater [28].

Cognitive therapies

Several treatment protocols, emerging from cognitive conceptualizations of OCD, emphasize that modifying maladaptive beliefs can serve to reduce OCD symptoms. Several recent studies [29–32] have found that cognitively oriented protocols, compared with EX/RP, achieved clinically significant and equivalent symptom reductions; however, procedural overlap in the form of behavioural experiments in the cognitive conditions make these findings somewhat difficult to interpret. Vogel and colleagues' randomized augmentation study [33] demonstrated that the addition of cognitive procedures following a course of EX/RP yielded further improvement, but this design did not address whether full integration of cognitive and behavioural techniques yields better outcomes than each technique alone. More recently, Whittal and colleagues [34] failed to find a difference between cognitive therapy that included behavioural elements and stress management training for individuals with obsessions not accompanied by overt compulsions; substantial and lasting benefits were observed in both groups at the end of the acute phase of the trial and at 12-month follow-up.

ERP plus medication

The issue of pharmacotherapy per se is covered in Chapters 2 and 5. With respect to the relative and combined efficacy of pharmacotherapy and ERP, the largest and perhaps most definitive placebo-controlled study was conducted by Foa and colleagues [35], who compared clomipramine (CMI) with intensive ERP and their combination in adults with OCD. Findings indicated that each of the active treatments was superior to placebo, EX/RP was superior to CMI, and the combination of the two treatments was not superior to EX/RP alone; relapse was more evident following treatment discontinuation in the CMI group than in either of the treatments that included intensive EX/RP [35]. However, the design used in this study may not have optimally allowed for an additive effect for CMI because the EX/RP programme was largely completed before patients reached their maximum dose of CMI. Experts have speculated that combined treatment effects may be more evident when intensive EX/RP is not used [18].

The Pediatric OCD Treatment Study (POTS) was the first randomized trial in paediatric OCD to directly compare the efficacy of an established medication (sertraline), OCD-specific CBT involving ERP, and their combination, with a control condition, pill placebo, in the acute treatment of paediatric OCD. Results showed a significant advantage for all three active treatments compared with placebo. Combined treatment proved superior to CBT and to sertraline, which did not differ from one another, although a site effect did emerge in which CBT monotherapy yielded a larger effect size at one site than it did at the other [36]. ERP was conducted weekly in POTS I, which may have permitted the emergence of the overall combined treatment effect.

Patients who respond to selective serotonin reuptake inhibitors (SSRIs) often experience residual OCD symptoms and associated impairment, which has promoted interest in developing augmentation strategies that would yield further symptom improvements. A recent randomized trial indicated that augmentation with twice-weekly CBT involving ERP yielded greater improvements and retention of gains than augmentation with stress management training for SSRI partial responders [5]. SRI partial response also appears to be common in youths with OCD, which led to an RCT examining the efficacy of ERP augmentation in children and adolescents who had experienced a partial response to an adequate medication trial (for details see [37]). Its findings are convergent with the adult trial in support of the efficacy of augmentation with ERP (Franklin *et al.*, submitted).

In OCD subspecialty clinical practices in the United States, it is quite common to encounter patients presenting for EX/RP treatment who are already receiving SSRIs. Concomitant pharmacotherapy is also used in clinical practice to manage comorbid symptoms known to negatively impact EX/RP outcomes, such as depression and attention-deficit hyperactivity disorder (ADHD), though optimal sequencing of these treatments has yet to be established empirically. From the data collected thus far on combined approaches, we can conclude that concomitant pharmacotherapy does not inhibit EX/RP treatment response, yet is not required for every patient to benefit substantially from EX/RP.

OCD PROTOCOLS

Assessment

Several instruments are available to quantify the severity of OCD symptoms. These instruments will assist the therapist in evaluating treatment progress for a given patient.

Yale–Brown Obsessive Compulsive Scale (Y–BOCS)

The Y–BOCS [38,39] is a standardized semi-structured interview that takes approximately 30 minutes to complete. The test's severity scale includes 10 items (five assess obsessions and five compulsions), each of which is rated on a five-point scale ranging from 0 (no symptoms) to 4 (severe symptoms). Assessors rate the time occupied by the obsessions and compulsions, the degree of interference with functioning, the level of distress, attempts to resist the symptoms, and the level of control over the symptoms. The Y–BOCS has shown adequate interrater agreement, internal consistency and validity [38,39]. A version of this instrument was also developed for use with children and adolescents, the Children's Yale–Brown Obsessive Compulsive Scale (CY–BOCS) [40]. The structure and content of the instrument are very similar to the adult version, although some of the language was adapted to make it more developmentally appropriate.

Self-report measures

Obsessive Compulsive Inventory – Revised (OCI-R)

The Obsessive Compulsive Inventory – Revised (OCI-R) [41] is an 18-item self-report measure that assesses the distress associated with obsessions and compulsions; total scores range from 0 to 72, with each subscale score ranging from 0 to 12. In addition to the total score, six separate subscale scores are calculated by adding the three items that comprise each subscale: Washing, Checking, Ordering, Obsessing, Hoarding and Neutralizing. Foa *et al.* [41] report good internal consistency and test-retest reliability, and good discriminant validity in clinical patients with OCD, post-traumatic stress disorder (PTSD), generalized social phobia (GSP) and non-anxious controls. A version of this instrument now exists for use with children and adolescents as well [42].

Other self-report measures

A few self-report instruments for assessing OCD symptoms are also available, such as the Leyton Obsessional Inventory [43] and the Lynfield Obsessional Compulsive Questionnaire [44]. These instruments are limited in that they assess only certain forms of obsessive-compulsive behaviour and/or they include items that are unrelated to OCD symptoms. More recently, Storch and colleagues have developed the Children's Florida Obsessive Compulsive Inventory [45], which is intended primarily for screening purposes rather than for tracking symptoms over the course of treatment.

Adult ERP protocol

The treatment programme typically consists of four phases: (i) psychoeducation; (ii) information gathering and hierarchy development; (iii) ERP; and (iv) a maintenance and relapse prevention phase. Once a patient is judged to be appropriate for treatment with ERP, the psychoeducation and information gathering phases can begin. These two phases typically consist of 4 to 6 hours of contact with the patient conducted over a period of two to three double sessions if possible; this permits completion of this phase quickly so that the core of the programme, ERP, can commence as soon as possible. During these initial phases, the therapist collects information about the patient's OCD, general history and the history of treatment for OCD. The theoretical model of OCD and the rationale for treatment that flows from this model is discussed in detail, the ERP programme as it would be applied to the patient specifically is described in detail, patients are taught to monitor their rituals, and OCD treatment hierarchies are developed according to each current obsessional theme.

The ERP treatment programme that we typically recommend for adults consists of 15 90-minute treatment sessions conducted twice per week for 8 weeks. Each session begins with a 10–15-minute discussion of homework assignments and ritual monitoring since the previous in-person session. The rest of the session is devoted to in-session exposure; depending on the patient's particular presentation of OCD, the session time can be allocated to *in vivo* exposure only or to *in vivo* and imaginal exposure. The final 10–15 minutes of the session are spent discussing homework assignments to be completed before the next in-person visit. This format should be adjusted when necessary. For example, if an *in vivo* exposure requires that the therapist and patient drive along city streets to provoke anxiety about having struck pedestrians, the entire session will be devoted to this activity and may even require a longer duration. Some patients with feared consequences have difficulty engaging emotionally in imaginal exposures (i.e. the images fail to elicit distress). In these cases, treatment should focus exclusively on *in vivo* exercises.

In the beginning of each session it is suggested that the therapist discusses the plan for that particular session. Barring any unusual circumstances, for example a patient's stated objection to proceeding with the planned exposure, it is important to keep these discussions brief, so as to leave sufficient time for exposure. OCD patients are often very fearful of engaging in exposure tasks, and elaborated discussion of the task at hand may serve as a form of avoidance from going ahead with the exposure. These pre-exposure discussions are also fertile ground for assurance seeking, that is, the patient asking the therapist if they are certain that the proposed exercise is safe. The therapist should answer such questions carefully, avoiding either extreme of providing compulsive reassurance or of conveying to the patient that the proposed exposure is objectively dangerous.

Once the core of ERP has been completed, the maintenance phase begins. During this phase, in addition to prescribing continued self-exposure tasks to help the patient maintain therapy gains, the therapist may also wish to ask the patient to generate more suggestions about what kinds of exposures need to be done and why. These maintenance sessions may be used to plan additional exposures, refine guidelines for normal behaviour, and address issues that arise as the patient adjusts to life without OCD. There is some evidence that OCD patients benefit from continued contact with the therapist following the acute treatment phase. In one study, 12 weekly booster sessions (no exposure exercises) appeared to reduce the number of relapses in a sample of individuals with OCD treated with 3 weeks of intensive exposure and response prevention [46]. In another study, following the intensive treatment with 1 week of daily cognitive behavioural sessions followed by eight brief (10-minute) weekly telephone contacts resulted in better long-term outcome than following intensive treatment with 1 week of treatment with free association [47].

Paediatric ERP protocol

Taking into account developmental and practical limitations that are inherent in treating youths, our clinical protocol for paediatric OCD involves 14 hour-long visits over 12 weeks spread across five phases. Psychoeducation (Phase 1), Cognitive Training (Phase 2) and Mapping OCD (Phase 3) take place during visits 1–4; Exposure and Response Prevention (Phase 4) takes place during visits 5–12; and Relapse Prevention and Generalization Training (Phase 5) occurs during visits 13–14. Each session includes a statement of goals, review of the previous week, provision of new information, therapist-assisted practice, homework for the coming week and monitoring procedures. Visits occur once per week, last 1 hour, and include between-visit 10-minute telephone contact scheduled in weeks 3 and 12.

Parents are centrally involved at sessions 1, 7 and 11, with the latter two sessions devoted to guiding the parent(s) through their role in helping the child with homework assignments. Parents are also significantly involved in the sessions devoted to preventing relapse. Cases in which the family is extensively involved in rituals may require that family members play a more central role in treatment. This is also the case in treatment with younger children [28] and with children with developmental disabilities.

The therapist must adjust the level of discourse to meet the child's developmental level. For example, younger patients require more redirection and activities to sustain attention; adolescents are less likely to appreciate giving OCD a 'nasty nickname' than younger children. Developmentally appropriate metaphors relevant to the child's areas of interest and knowledge are also used to promote active involvement in the treatment process.

DISSEMINATION

Much has been learned in the past several decades about the efficacy of treatments for OCD in adults and in youths, and this information now guides us in providing empirically informed treatment recommendations for OCD patients encountered in clinical practice. However, critics of the methods used to examine treatment efficacy have raised concerns about whether findings from RCTs designed specifically to emphasize internal validity have done so at the expense of generalizability to more typical clinical patients and psychotherapy practice settings (e.g. [48]). Many of these criticisms have been addressed in detail elsewhere (e.g. [49,50]), yet the prevailing question of how well these treatments hold up outside the academic research is an important and extremely relevant one. Thus far, at least with respect to ERP specifically, it appears that good outcomes are not limited to highly selected RCT samples [51], and can be achieved in OCD subspecialty private practice settings [52,53] and in community agencies by supervised therapists who are not themselves OCD experts (e.g. [54,55]).

The effectiveness studies conducted thus far in OCD may well serve as building blocks for the development of the infrastructure needed to disseminate ERP into the many communities where those with OCD cannot access it at present. The problem of limited access, however, is certainly not specific to ERP. In a particularly thoughtful and timely paper, Shafran and colleagues [56] noted that empirically supported treatments for many disorders are rarely available in community settings and, even when they are, they are often delivered suboptimally. In order to facilitate the use of empirically supported CBT protocols in routine practice, they suggest that:

1. Treatment developers should state explicitly how existing trials address comorbidity.
2. Clinicians should have easy access to training in diagnostic assessment and outcome measures.
3. Effectiveness studies should provide adequate training and supervision for therapists when studying how well treatments work in routine clinical populations.
4. CBT trials and effectiveness studies should examine therapist effects and establish the effects of levels of training on outcome.
5. Reliable assessment of competence should be conducted.
6. More research should be conducted on methods of disseminating treatment procedures.
7. Mechanisms of efficacious action should be studied more closely.
8. Methods should be established to examine which patients require more intensive contact.

We concur with their views, and remain hopeful that the next decade of clinical research in OCD will expand our understanding of ERP's efficacy and effectiveness, and the mechanisms that underlie its effects, which, in turn, will improve our precision about what specific elements of treatment are essential to produce the best and most lasting outcomes possible for this complex and sometimes vexing disorder.

FUTURE RESEARCH

Although we have witnessed in the past 20 years a period of almost unprecedented growth in our knowledge about OCD and its treatment across the developmental spectrum, there are several key issues that require further study. First, studies that have examined the relative versus combined efficacy of ERP and medications thus far have failed to clarify which patients actually need both treatments, nor have they shed sufficient light on the issue of optimal treatment sequencing for initial treatments. More research is also needed on the issue of managing partial and non-response to the available treatments: only one such study in adults has been published [5]. Findings anticipated soon from large studies examining ERP augmentation in paediatric partial responders to SRIs [6,37] and medication augmentation strategies for partial response to ERP will contribute to knowledge about how best to develop optimal treatment regimes. The relative efficacy of augmentation with ERP versus augmentation with an atypical neuroleptic is currently being examined in a multicenter trial (E. Foa & B. Simpson, PIs), which will provide patients and providers with more definitive information about the risk-to-benefit ratio of each approach.

There is also a need to look carefully at patient characteristics in order to develop ideal treatment approaches. For example, the effect of OCD subtype on treatment outcome needs to be examined in larger studies, as insufficient sample sizes and method variance across studies have resulted in inconsistent findings thus far. Further, it is high time to develop treatment innovations to target specific mediators known to affect ERP outcomes, such as family dysfunction and certain comorbidity patterns. Recent findings on the efficacy of Acceptance and Commitment Therapy for OCD [57] raise an even broader question about the mechanism that underlies effective treatment for OCD including ERP, in that a weekly treatment founded on the framework of relational frame theory that did not include any in-session exposure yielded substantial and clinically significant changes in OCD symptoms that were clearly superior to what was achieved with a psychosocial control condition (relaxation). No issue facing the field, however, is as critical to address as our dissemination crisis, since failure to improve access to care is a threat to the relevance of all of the psychological treatments of established efficacy for OCD including ERP.

SUMMARY

The extant literature reviewed above offers guidance for clinicians regarding the likelihood of patients' responsiveness to ERP and to other treatment approaches, and thus should be referenced and emphasized during the discussion of treatment alternatives with patients seeking professional assistance. At the same time, findings from studies that have examined the efficacy and effectiveness of treatments are based on aggregated data, and thus do not provide certainty for individual outcomes; this point must also be acknowledged openly. In adult OCD, where the literature is deeper, there is greater confidence regarding the expected responses to ERP and SRI pharmacotherapy, as dozens of studies conducted around the world have contributed to the knowledge base about these treatments. The treatment outcome literature in paediatric OCD has grown substantially over the past decade in particular, yet the number of studies, associated sample sizes and methodological quality of the studies published to date leave many important questions still unanswered. In the case of both the adult and paediatric literatures, however, the data on prediction of treatment response has generally yielded divergent and sometimes even inconsistent findings. Such investigations have generally been hampered by relatively small sample sizes within specific treatment conditions; these sample size issues may directly flow from the reality that OCD is a relatively low base rate disorder, which makes efficient collection of large samples impractical. Accordingly, it may be the case that efforts to identify predictors (factors that are generally associated with differential treatment response) and moderators (factors that are associated with differential response to specific treatments) will only advance if databases from sites conducting similar treatments on similar samples can be combined, since the current generation of treatment trials have typically been powered to examine outcome but not moderation. Such an undertaking poses many practical barriers given that the study assessment batteries may not overlap entirely, yet the potential yield from such cooperation may well provide the best opportunity to do so. Such steps may be necessary if we are ever to improve our precision in answering the most fundamental question still unanswered, namely, which treatments will work best for which patients with which characteristics? Child psychiatry has already made some positive steps in this direction (Child & Adolescent Psychiatry Trials Network, CAPTN [58]), although such efforts have not been attempted in OCD specifically as yet.

REFERENCES

1. Mowrer OH. A stimulus-response analysis of anxiety and its role as a reinforcing agent. *Psychol Rev* 1939;**46**:553–565.
2. Mowrer OH. *Learning Theory and Behavior*. New York: John Wiley & Sons, Ltd, 1960.
3. Foa EB, Kozak MJ. Emotional processing of fear: Exposure to corrective information. *Psychol Bull* 1986;**99**:20–35.
4. Salkovskis PM. Obsessional compulsive problems: A cognitive-behavioral analysis. *Behav Res Ther* 1985;**23**:571–583.
5. Simpson HB, Foa EB, Liebowitz MR *et al*. A randomized controlled trial of cognitive-behavioral therapy for augmenting pharmacotherapy in obsessive-compulsive disorder. *Am J Psychiat* 2008;**165**:621–630.

6. Franklin ME, Saptya J, Freeman JB et al. Cognitive-behavior therapy augmentation of pharmacotherapy in pediatric obsessive compulsive disorder: The Pediatric OCD Treatment Study II (POTS II) randomized, controlled trial. *JAMA* 2011; **306**(11):1224–1232.

7. Abramowitz JS. Variants of exposure and response prevention in the treatment of obsessive compulsive disorder: A meta-analysis. *Behav Ther* 1996;**27**:583–600.

8. Abramowitz JS, Whiteside SP, Deacon BJ. The effectiveness of treatment for pediatric obsessive-compulsive disorder: A meta-analysis. *Behav Ther* 2005;**36**:55–63.

9. National Institute for Health and Clinical Excellence. *Obsessive Compulsive Disorder: Core Interventions in the Treatment of Obsessive-Compulsive Disorder and Body Dysmorphic Disorder*. London: NICE, 2005.

10. Rosa-Alcázar AI, Sánchez-Meca J, Gómez-Conesa A, Marín-Martínez F. Psychological treatment of obsessive-compulsive disorder: A meta-analysis. *Clin Psychol Rev* 2008;**28**:1310–1325.

11. Barrett P, Healy-Farrell L, March JS. Cognitive-behavioral family treatment of childhood obsessive-compulsive disorder: A controlled trial. *J Am Acad Child Adolesc Psychiat* 2004;**43**:46–62.

12. Bolton D, Perrin S. Evaluation of exposure with response-prevention for obsessive compulsive disorder in childhood and adolescence. *J Behav Ther Exp Psychiat* 2008;**39**:11–22.

13. Freeman JB, Garcia AM, Coyne L *et al.* Early childhood OCD: Preliminary findings from a family-based cognitive-behavioral approach. *J Am Acad Child Adolesc Psychiat* 2008;**47**:593–602.

14. Storch EA, Geffken GR, Merlo LJ *et al.* Family-based cognitive-behavioral therapy for pediatric obsessive-compulsive disorder: Comparison of intensive and weekly approaches. *J Am Acad Child Adolesc Psychiat* 2007;**46**:469–78.

15. Watson HJ, Rees CS. Meta-analysis of randomized, controlled trials for pediatric obsessive-compulsive disorder. *J Child Psychol Psychiat* 2008;**49**:489–498.

16. Williams TI, Salkovskis PM, Forrester L, Turner S, White H, Allsopp MA. A randomised controlled trial of cognitive behavioural treatment for obsessive compulsive disorder in children and adolescents. *Eur Child Adolesc Psychiat* 2010;**19**:449–456.

17. Foa EB, Steketee G, Grayson JB, Turner RM, Latimer P. Deliberate exposure and blocking of obsessive-compulsive rituals: Immediate and long-term effects. *Behav Ther* 1984;**15**:450–472.

18. Foa EB, Franklin ME, Moser J. Context in the clinic: How well do CBT and medications work in combination? *Biol Psychiat* 2002;**51**:989–997.

19. Foa EB, Steketee G, Turner RM, Fischer SC. Effects of imaginal exposure to feared disasters in obsessive-compulsive checkers. *Behav Res Ther* 1980;**18**:449–455.

20. Steketee GS, Foa EB, Grayson JB. Recent advances in the behavioral treatment of obsessive-compulsives. *Arch Gen Psychiat* 1982;**39**:1365–1371.

21. DeAraujo LA, Ito LM, Marks IM, Deale A. Does imaginal exposure to the consequences of not ritualising enhance live exposure for OCD? A controlled study: I. Main outcome. *Brit J Psychiat* 1995;**167**:65–70.

22. Abramowitz JS, Foa EB, Franklin ME. Exposure and ritual prevention for obsessive compulsive disorder: Effects of intensive versus twice-weekly sessions. *J Consult Clin Psychol* 2003;**71**:394–399.

23. Franklin ME, Kozak MJ, Cashman L, Coles M, Rheingold A, Franklin ME. Cognitive behavioral treatment of pediatric obsessive compulsive disorder: An open clinical trial. *J Am Acad Child Adolesc Psychiat* 1998;**37**:412–419.

24. Hodgson RJ, Rachman S. The effects of contamination and washing in obsessional patients. *Behav Res Ther* 1972;**10**:111–117.

25. Rabavilas AD, Boulougouris JC, Stefanis C. Duration of flooding sessions in the treatment of obsessive-compulsive patients. *Behav Res Ther* 1976;**14**:349–355.

26. Peris TA, Bergman RL, Langley A, Chang S, McCracken JT, Piacentini J. Correlates of accommodation of pediatric obsessive-compulsive disorder: Parent, child and family characteristics. *J Am Acad Child Adolesc Psychiat* 2008;**47**:1173–1181.

27. Piacentini J, Bergman RL, Jacobs C, McCracken JT, Kretchman J. Open trial of cognitive behavior therapy for childhood obsessive-compulsive disorder. *J Anxiety Disord* 2002;**16**:207–219.

28. Freeman JB, Choate-Summers ML, Moore PS *et al.* Cognitive behavioral treatment for young children with obsessive compulsive-disorder. *Biol Psychiat* 2007;**61**:337–343.

29. Cottraux J, Note I, Yao SN. A randomized controlled trial of cognitive therapy versus intensive behavior therapy in obsessive compulsive disorder. *Psychother Psychosom* 2001;**70**:288–297.

30. McLean PL, Whittal ML, Thordarson DS. Cognitive versus behavior therapy in the group treatment of obsessive-compulsive disorder. *J Consult Clin Psychol* 2001;**69**:205–214.

31. Whittal ML, Thordarson DS, McLean PD. Treatment of obsessive-compulsive disorder: Cognitive behavior therapy vs. exposure and response prevention. *Behav Res Ther* 2005;**43**:1559–1576.

32. Whittal ML, Robichaud M, Thordarson DS, McLean PD. Group and individual treatment of obsessive-compulsive disorder using cognitive therapy and exposure plus response prevention: A 2-year follow-up of two randomized trials. *J Consult Clin Psychol* 2008;**76**:1003–1014.

33. Vogel PA, Stiles TC, Götestam KG. Adding cognitive therapy elements to exposure therapy for obsessive compulsive disorder: A controlled study. *Behav Cogn Psychother* 2004;**32**:275–290.

34. Whittal ML, Woody SR, McLean PD, Rachman S, Robichaud M. Treatment of obsessions: A randomized controlled trial. *Behav Res Ther* 2010;**48**:295–303.

35. Foa EB, Liebowitz MR, Kozak MJ *et al.* Treatment of obsessive compulsive disorder by exposure and ritual prevention, clomipramine, and their combination: A randomized, placebo-controlled trial. *Am J Psychiat* 2005;**162**:151–161.

36. Pediatric OCD Treatment Study Team. Cognitive-behavioral therapy, sertraline, and their combination for children and adolescents with obsessive-compulsive disorder: The Pediatric OCD Treatment Study randomized controlled trial. *JAMA* 2004;**292**:1969–1976.

37. Freeman JB, Choate-Summers ML, Garcia AM *et al.* The Pediatric Obsessive-Compulsive Disorder Treatment Study II: Rationale, design and methods. *Child Adolesc Psychiat Ment Hlth* 2009;**3**:1–15.

38. Goodman WK, Price LH, Rasmussen SA *et al.* The Yale-Brown Obsessive Compulsive Scale: II. Validity. *Arch Gen Psychiat* 1989;**46**:1012–1016.

39. Goodman WK, Price LH, Rasmussen SA *et al.* The Yale-Brown Obsessive Compulsive Scale: I. Development, use, and reliability. *Arch Gen Psychiat* 1989;**46**:1006–1011.

40. Scahill L, Riddle MA, McSwiggin-Hardin M *et al.* Children's Yale-Brown Obsessive Compulsive Scale: reliability and validity. *J Am Acad Child Adolesc Psychiat* 1997;**36**:844–52.

41. Foa EB, Huppert JD, Leiberg S *et al.* The Obsessive-Compulsive Inventory: Development and validation of a short version. *Psychol Assessment* 2002;**14**:485–495.

42. Foa EB, Coles M, Huppert JD, Pasupuleti RV, Franklin ME, March J. Development and validation of a child version of the Obsessive Compulsive Inventory. *Behav Ther* 2010;**41**:121–132.

43. Kazarian SS, Evans DL, Lefave K. Modification and factorial analysis of the Leyton obsessional inventory. *J Clin Psychol* 1977;**33**:422–425.

44. Allen JJ, Tune GS. The Lynfield obsessional/compulsive questionnaire. *Scot Med J* 1975;**20**:21–24.

45. Storch EA, Khanna M, Merlo LJ *et al.* Children's Florida Obsessive Compulsive Inventory: Psychometric properties and feasibility of a self-report measure of obsessive-compulsive symptoms in youth. *Child Psychiat Hum Dev* 2009;**40**:467–483.

46. Foa EB, Kozak MJ, Steketee G, McCarthy PR. Treatment of depressive and obsessive-compulsive symptoms in OCD by imipramine and behavior therapy. *Brit J Clin Psychol* 1992;**31**:279–292.

47. Hiss H, Foa FB, Kozak MJ. A relapse prevention program for treatment of obsessive compulsive disorder. *J Consult Clin Psychol* 1994;**62**:801–808.

48. Westen D, Novotny CM, Thompson-Brenner H. The empirical status of empirically supported psychotherapies: Assumptions, findings, and reporting in controlled clinical trials. *Psychol Bull* 2004;**130**:631–663.

49. Crits-Christoph P, Wilson GT, Hollon SD. Empirically supported psychotherapies: Comment on Westen, Novotny, and Thompson-Brenner (2004). *Psychol Bull* 2005;**131**:412–417.

50. Weisz JR, Weersing VR, Henggeler SW. Jousting with straw men: Comment on Westen, Novotny, and Thompson-Brenner, 2004. *Psychol Bull* 2005;**131**:418–426.

51. Franklin ME, Abramowitz JS, Kozak MJ, Levitt J, Foa EB. Effectiveness of exposure and ritual prevention for obsessive compulsive disorder: Randomized compared with non-randomized samples. *J Consult Clin Psychol* 2000;**68**:594–602.

52. Rothbaum BO, Shahar F. Behavioral treatment of obsessive-compulsive disorder in a naturalistic setting. *Cogn Behav Pract* 2000;**7**:262–270.

53. Warren R, Thomas JC. Cognitive-behavior therapy of obsessive-compulsive disorder in private practice: An effectiveness study. *J Anxiety Disord* 2001;**15**:277–85.

54. Nakatani E, Mataix-Cols D, Micali N, Turner C, Heyman I. Outcomes of cognitive behaviour therapy for obsessive compulsive disorder in a clinical setting: A 10-year experience from a specialist OCD service for children and adolescents. *Child Adolesc Psychiat Ment Hlth* 2009;**14**:133–139.

55. Valderhaug R, Larsson B, Götestam KG, Piacentini J. An open clinical trial of cognitive-behaviour therapy in children and adolescents with obsessive-compulsive disorder administered in regular outpatient clinics. *Behav Res Ther* 2007;**45**:577–89.

56. Shafran R, Clark DM, Fairburn CG *et al.* Mind the gap: Improving the dissemination of CBT. *Behav Res Ther* 2009;**47**:902–909.
57. Twohig MP, Hayes SC, Plumb JC *et al.* A randomized clinical trial of Acceptance and Commitment therapy versus progressive relaxation training for obsessive-compulsive disorder. *J Consult Clin Psychol* 2010;**78**:705–716.
58. Shapiro M, Silva SG, Compton S *et al.* The child and adolescent psychiatry trials network (CAPTN): Infrastructure development and lessons learned. *Child Adolesc Psychiat Ment Hlth* 2009;**3**:12.
59. Merlo, L.J., Lehmkuhl, H.D., Geffken, G.R., Storch, E.A. (2009). Decreased family accommodation associated with improved therapy outcome in pediatric obsessive–compulsive disorder. *Journal of Consulting and Clinical Psychology*, **77**(2): 355–360.
60. Storch, E.A., Geffken, G.R., Merlo, L.J., Jacob, M.L., Murphy, T.K Grabill, K. (2007b). Family accommodation in pediatric obsessive–compulsive disorder. *Journal of Clinical Child and Adolescent Psychology*, **36**(2):207–216.
61. Torres, A.R., Prince, M.J., Bebbington, P.E., Bhugra, D., Brugha, T.S Singleton, N. (2006). Obsessive–compulsive disorder: Prevalence, comorbidity, impact, and help–seeking in the British National Psychiatric Morbidity Survey of 2000. *American Journal of Psychiatry*, **163**, 1978–1985.
62. Wever, C. & Rey, J.M. (1997). Juvenile obsessive compulsive disorder. *Australian and New Zealand Journal of Psychiatry*, **31**, 105–113.

CHAPTER 4

Electroconvulsive Therapy, Transcranial Magnetic Stimulation and Deep Brain Stimulation in OCD

Rianne M. Blom,[1] **Martijn Figee,**[1] **Nienke Vulink**[1] **and Damiaan Denys**[1,2]

[1]*Department of Psychiatry, Academic Medical Center, University of Amsterdam, Amsterdam, The Netherlands;* [2]*The Netherlands Institute for Neuroscience, an institute of the Royal Netherlands Academy of Arts and Sciences, Amsterdam, The Netherlands*

INTRODUCTION

Patients with obsessive-compulsive disorder (OCD) are usually treated with antidepressants or cognitive behavioural therapies. Although three out of four patients experience an average symptom decrease of almost 40% with selective serotonin reuptake inhibitors (SSRIs) or behavioural therapy, eventually, 1 out of 10 patients cannot be helped with these regular treatments. In this case a physical intervention might be a solution. This chapter describes the physical interventions that have been used in (refractory) obsessive-compulsive disorder: electroconvulsive therapy (ECT), repetitive transcranial magnetic stimulation (rTMS), surgical lesioning and deep brain stimulation (DBS).

ELECTROCONVULSIVE THERAPY

Electroconvulsive therapy (ECT), in which seizures are electrically induced under narcosis, is regularly used in treatment-refractory major depression [1]. The literature of ECT in obsessive-compulsive disorder (OCD) is sparse, and most clinicians

Obsessive-Compulsive Disorder: Current Science and Clinical Practice, First Edition. Edited by Joseph Zohar.
© 2012 John Wiley & Sons, Ltd. Published 2012 by John Wiley & Sons, Ltd.

do not perceive ECT as a valid treatment option for OCD. Two reviews concluded that ECT is not efficacious in OCD [2,3]. One small open-label study from 1988 reported a short-term efficacy for ECT in refractory OCD; however, 6 months after initial treatment the symptoms returned to pre-ECT levels [2]. Since then, only isolated case reports have been published. Three cases report long-lasting diminished OCD symptoms in patients with OCD and comorbid major depression after single [3] or several ECT sessions [4,5]. One Japanese study describes the reduction of OCD symptoms in a 36-year-old pregnant OCD patient after two sessions of moderate ECT [6]. Furthermore, some single effective ECT cases have been reported in late-onset OCD (right unilateral) [7], schizophrenia with comorbid OCD (bitemporal) [4] and a case of comorbid Tourette syndrome and OCD (unilateral) [5]. None of the recent studies investigated ECT solely for OCD and none were designed as prospective double-blind controlled trials. In conclusion, case studies suggest ECT may be effective only for the comorbid affective or psychotic disorders of OCD cases.

TRANSCRANIAL MAGNETIC STIMULATION

With repetitive transcranial magnetic stimulation (rTMS) it has become possible to modulate local neural activity by inducing a depolarizing magnetic field pulse [8] (Figure 4.1). Since OCD may be related to increased neural activity in prefrontal-subcortical circuits [9], the inhibitory effect of rTMS was hypothesized to be beneficial in OCD treatment. In 1997, Greenberg *et al.* [10] introduced rTMS as a new treatment approach for OCD. Earlier, rTMS had been shown to have

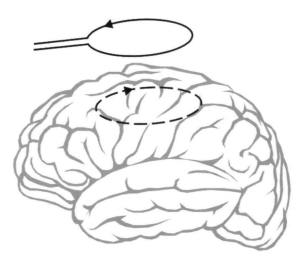

Figure 4.1 Transcranial magnetic stimulation (TMS) is a non-invasive technique that uses electromagnets to create localized electrical currents in the brain.

a modest positive effect on mood disorders, with stimulation of the prefrontal cortex [11]. Greenberg *et al.* [10] hypothesized that inhibition of the prefrontal activity with rTMS might reduce obsessive-compulsive symptoms. They applied rTMS (80% motor threshold, 20 Hz/2 seconds per minute) for 20 minutes to 12 patients with OCD and found significantly decreased compulsive urges for 8 hours after stimulation. Since then rTMS has been investigated in OCD, targeting several brain areas within the corticostriatal network. First, the mechanism of action will be discussed, then the efficacy and side effects of rTMS at various brain targets, and finally implications for the future.

Mechanism of action

In the early 1980s, the transcranial magnetic stimulation (TMS) device was developed by Barker and his colleagues [8]. The device stimulates the human cortex directly by a contactless and non-invasive method. It uses a strong pulse of electrical current, which is sent through a coil and induces a magnetic field pulse in the area under the coil. This pulse has the capacity to depolarize superficial local neurons [8]. To create a longer lasting effect of the depolarized neurons application of repetitive TMS is needed. The magnitude and direction of rTMS-induced neuronal modulation depends on extrinsic factors such as motor threshold, frequency and total number of stimuli, and intrinsic factors such as the functional state of the cortex [12]. For example, it appears that low-frequency rTMS (0–5 Hz) results in decreased neural excitability and regional cerebral blood flow as opposed to high-frequency rTMS (5–20 Hz), which increases both [13].

Since knowledge of involvement of specific brain circuits in OCD is advancing, rTMS has been applied to several brain targets (Table 4.1). The rationale for the first rTMS studies in OCD was based on functional neuroimaging studies of OCD that demonstrated abnormalities in the orbito-frontal-subcortical circuits, especially in the orbital frontal gyri and medial caudate nuclei [14]. This circuitry may be manipulated with rTMS by: (i) stimulation of the dorsolateral prefrontal cortex (DLPFC) [17]; (ii) by inhibition of the orbitofrontal cortex directly [15]; or (iii) by inhibition of the supplementary motor area (SMA). The SMA was chosen as a useful target for rTMS since it has extensive connections with regions implicated in cognitive processes and motor control [16,17].

Efficacy of rTMS in OCD

A total of 110 OCD patients in 10 studies have been treated with rTMS, targeting the dorsolateral prefrontal cortex (DLPFC), the orbitofrontal cortex (OFC) or the supplementary motor area (SMA). Four studies investigated the efficacy of rTMS in OCD in a double-blind, randomized, sham-controlled design [13,18–21], three

Table 4.1 Repetitive transcranial magnetic stimulation (rTMS) in obsessive-compulsive disorder (OCD).

	Year	Author	Target	Number	Diagnosis	Medication continuation	Intervention	Time	Mean (SD) Y–BOCS Pre-rTMS	Mean (SD) Y–BOCS Post-rTMS	Mean (SD) Moodscale Pre-rTMS	Mean (SD) Moodscale Post-rTMS
Intervention	1997	Greenberg	Right LPFC or Left LPFC	12	OCD	Yes, n = 8 (stable SRI treatment)	20 Hz/2 s/min 80% of motor threshold	1 session of 20 min; measurement after 8 h	–	Compulsions decreased rPFC $p = 0.02$ lPFC $p = 0.05$	–	No sig. positive mood increase
Control			Mid-occipital	12[a]	OCD		20 Hz/2 s/min 80% of motor threshold	1 session of 20 min; measurement after 8 h	–	Compulsions decreased Mid-occipital $p = 0.07$	–	No sig. positive mood increase
Intervention	2001	Sachdev	Right PFC	6	Treatment-resistant OCD	Yes, n = 10 (stable SRI, benzodiazepines, neuroleptics treatment)	10 Hz 110% motor threshold	10 sessions of 2,5 minutes in 2 weeks Measurement 4 weeks after last session	27.2 (9.0)	12.0 (3.9)	23.2 (12.5) BDI	11.6 (14.6) BDI
Control			Left PFC	6	Treatment-resistant OCD		10 Hz 110% motor threshold	10 sessions of 2,5 minutes in 2 weeks Measurement 4 weeks after last session	22.5 (6.3)	16.5 (8.3)	19.7 (12.5) BDI	10.8 (7.9) BDI

	Year	Author	Location	n	Condition	Medication	Stimulation	Sessions				
Intervention	2001	Alonso	Right DLPFC	10	OCD	Yes n = 7 (stable SRI, TCA treatment)	1 Hz 110% of motor threshold	18 sessions of 20 min in 10 weeks Measurement after 10 weeks	24.0 (5.3)	20.6 (9.1)	11.1 (5.1) HAM-D	10.8 (4.8) HAM-D
Control	—		Right DLPFC	8	OCD	Yes n = 6 (stable SRI, TCA treatment)	Sham condition	18 sessions of 20 min in 10 weeks Measurement after 10 weeks	25.6 (6.1)	25.3 (8.3)	11.7 (2.7) HAM-D	12.0 (3.0) HAM-D
Intervention	2006	Mantovani	SMA	10	OCD/TS	Yes n = 10 (stable SRI, benzodiazepines, neuroleptics treatment)	1 Hz 100% of motor threshold	10 sessions of 20 min in 2 weeks Measurement 2 weeks after last stimulation	36.4 (7.5)	26.0 (10.5)	20.7 (11.4) HAM-D	10.8 (10.7) HAM-D
Control	—	—	—	—	—	—	—	—	—	—	—	—
Intervention	2006	Prasko	Left DLPFC	15	SRI-resistant OCD	Yes n = 15 (stable SRI treatment)	1 Hz 110% of motor threshold	10 sessions of 30 min in 2 weeks Measurement 2 weeks after last stimulation	29.8 (5.8)	21.4 (9.2)	—	—
Control			Left DLPFC	15	SRI-resistant OCD	Yes n = 15 (stable SRI treatment)	Sham condition	10 sessions of 30 min in 2 weeks Measurement 2 weeks after last stimulation	23.4 (5.0)	16.9 (5.9)	—	—

(Continued)

Table 4.1 Repetitive transcranial magnetic stimulation (rTMS) in obsessive-compulsive disorder (OCD). (*Continued*)

	Year	Author	Target	Number	Diagnosis	Medication continuation	Intervention	Time	Mean (SD) Y-BOCS Pre-rTMS	Mean (SD) Y-BOCS Post-rTMS	Mean (SD) Moodscale Pre-rTMS	Mean (SD) Moodscale Post-rTMS
Intervention	2007	Sachdev	Left DLPFC	10	OCD	Yes n = 9 (unknown treatment)	10 Hz 110% motor threshold	2.5 min of 10 sessions in 2 weeks Measurement directly after last stimulation	26.0	20.0	–	Symptoms improved over time; but no difference between groups
Control			Left DLPFC	8	OCD	Yes n = 4 (unknown treatment)	Sham condition	2.5 min of 10 sessions in 2 weeks Measurement directly after last stimulation	24.0	19.0	–	Symptoms improved over time; but no difference between groups
Intervention	2009	Ruffini	Left OFC	16	Drug-resistant OCD	Yes n = 23 (stable SRI, neuroleptics, antiepileptics, benzodiazepines treatment)	1 Hz 80% of motor threshold	10 min of 15 sessions in 3 weeks Measurement 12 weeks after last session	32.1 (6.0)	27.3 (9.4)	–	No mood improvement over time
Control			Left OFC	7	Drug-resistant OCD		Sham condition	10 min of 15 sessions in 3 weeks Measurement 12 weeks after last session	31.4 (6.9)	29.6 (6.7)	–	No mood improvement over time
Intervention	2009	Kang	Right DLPFC and SMA	10	Treatment-resistant OCD	Yes n = 10 (stable SRI, benzodiazepines treatment)	1 Hz 110% of motor threshold	14 sessions of 10 min in 2 weeks Measurement 2 weeks after last	26.5 (5.6)	23.6 (7.4)	18.1 (6.6) BDI	17.2 (10.9) BDI

	Target	N	Diagnosis	Medication	Condition	Protocol				
Control	Right DLPFC and SMA	10	Treatment-resistant OCD	Yes n = 10 (stable SRI, benzodiazepines treatment)	Sham condition	14 sessions of 10 min in 2 weeks Measurement 2 weeks after last session	26.3 (4.1)	22.9 (6.2)	16.7 (10.0) BDI	15.8 (14.4) BDI
Intervention 2010 Mantovani	SMA	9	OCD	Yes n = 13 (stable SRI treatment)	1 Hz 100% of motor threshold	20 sessions of 20 min in 4 weeks Measurement direct after last stimulation	26.0 (5.4)	19.4 (5.6)	15.3 (10.6) HAM-D	12.1 (11.4) HAM-D
Control	SMA	9	OCD		Sham condition	20 sessions of 20 min in 4 weeks Measurement direct after last stimulation	26.7 (5.5)	23.5 (9.0)	14.8 (6.9) HAM-D	14.1 (8.8) HAM-D
Intervention 2010 Sarkhel	Right DLPFC	21	OCD	Yes n = 21 (TCA, SRI treatment)	10 Hz 110% motor threshold	10 sessions in 2 weeks, measurement 2 weeks after last session	25.7 (3.9)	Change in score 5.0 (2.3)	12.5 (2.2) HAM-D	Change in score 3.8 (1.6) HAM-D
Control	Right DLPFC	21	OCD	Yes n = 21 (TCA, SRI treatment)	Sham condition	10 sessions in 2 weeks, measurement 2 weeks after last session	23.6 (3.7)	Change in score 4.2 (1.8)	12.1 (2.7) HAM-D	Change in score 3.2 (1.0) HAM-D

aSame 12 subjects as investigated in the intervention group.
BDI, Beck Depression Inventory; DLPFC, dorsolateral prefrontal cortex; HAM-D, Hamilton Depression Rating Scale; LPFC, lateral prefrontal cortex; PFC, prefrontal cortex; OFC, orbito-frontal cortex; SD, standard deviation; SMA, supplementary motor area; SRI, serotonin reuptake inhibitors; TCA, Tricyclic Antidepressants; TS, Tourette syndrome; Y-BOCS, Yale–Brown Obsessive-Compulsive Scale.
Transcranial Magnetic Stimulation is a non-invasive technique that uses electromagnets to create localized electrical currents in the brain. Reproduced from Scholarpedia.

studies had a sham-controlled design, although not double-blind [20,22,23], and three case studies reported on rTMS in an open fashion [10,16,24]. The characteristics of each study are summarized in Table 4.1.

Dorsolateral prefrontal cortex (DLPFC)

The DLPFC has been the most investigated target for rTMS in OCD. In 1997, Greenberg *et al.* treated 12 OCD patients with rTMS to the right DLPFC, the left DLPFC, and lastly the mid-occipital cortex as a control condition [10]. Eight out of 12 patients were stable on SRI treatment. rTMS was randomly applied to these targets in an open fashion on separate days, at 80% threshold, 20 Hz/2 seconds per minute for 20 minutes. Compulsions decreased significantly by 34.8% immediately after right-DLPFC stimulation ($p < 0.01$) and remained significant 8 hours afterwards ($p < 0.02$), whereas obsessions did not decrease significantly. Depressive symptoms decreased significantly as well, although the effect did not last longer than 8 hours. Compulsions decreased instantly by 26.8% ($p < 0.03$) following left-DLPFC stimulation but, similar to depressive symptoms, they returned after 8 hours. Mid-occipital stimulation increased compulsions, albeit non-significantly ($p = 0.07$).

In 2001, Sachdev *et al.* tried to replicate this study in 12 patients with treatment-resistant OCD [16]. Right ($n = 6$) and left ($n = 6$) DLPFC stimulation was applied in an open fashion at 10 Hz, 100% motor threshold for 10 sessions of 2.5 minutes. At 4 weeks of follow-up rTMS led to a mean decrease on the Y–BOCS of 57% for the right DLPFC and a 27% reduction for the left DLPFC. All 12 subjects were analyzed together as there were no differences on any of the parameters measured; they showed a significant decrease of 42% on the Y–BOCS at 1 month follow-up ($p = 0.003$). However, after corrections for depression scores on the Montgomery Asberg Depression Rating Scale (MADRS) the significance disappeared ($p = 0.06$). In the same year, the first randomized sham-controlled double-blind rTMS OCD trial was completed. Alonso *et al.* randomly assigned 18 patients with OCD to real rTMS ($n = 10$) or sham rTMS ($n = 8$) at the right DLPFC [19]. The rTMS lasted 20 minutes at 1 Hz for both conditions, but the motor threshold was 110% for real rTMS and 20% for sham rTMS. This study failed to find significant improvement on the Y–BOCS and Hamilton Depression Rating Scale (HAM-D) after 18 sessions.

In 2006, this randomized sham-controlled double-blind design was repeated, stimulating the left instead of the right DLPFC in 30 treatment-resistant OCD patients [21]. Patients were given 10 daily sessions of sham or real rTMS (1 Hz, 110% motor threshold) in addition to ongoing SRI treatment. After 2 weeks of follow-up, obsessive-compulsive symptoms improved, with mean Y–BOCS reductions of 28%, but no differences between sham and real TMS were observed. The authors concluded that rTMS did not result in an effect in OCD by stimulating the left DLPFC. Similarly, in a study by Sachdev *et al.* [18], high-frequency (10 Hz, 110% motor threshold) rTMS of the left DLPFC demonstrated significant Y–BOCS decreases (6.0 points, 23.1%) over 2 weeks in 10 OCD patients, but the effects were similar after sham TMS in eight patients (5.0 points, 20.4%).

Last, in an Indian sham-controlled study, active rTMS at 10 Hz, 110% motor threshold ($n = 21$) and sham rTMS ($n = 21$) of the right DLPFC elicited similar improvement in obsessions and compulsions 2 weeks after the 10th session [17]. The Y–BOCS reduction for active rTMS was 5.0 points (19.5%), whereas for sham rTMS it was 4.2 points (17.7%). Interestingly, depressive scores, as measured by the HAM-D, reduced significantly over time in the real TMS group compared to the sham TMS group ($p > 0.04$). Of the subjects receiving real rTMS, 76.2% were partial responders (25% reduction in HAM-D scores from baseline) compared to 66.7% in the sham group. The authors concluded that right DLPFC rTMS has no effect on OCD but is modestly effective in the treatment of comorbid depressive symptoms.

In conclusion, in open-label studies, high-frequency rTMS of the right and/or left DLPFC appears to be effective in reducing obsessive-compulsive symptoms. However, this could not be replicated in double-blind sham-controlled studies. In those studies, neither low nor high-frequency rTMS, whether applied to the left or right DLPFC, appeared more effective than sham rTMS.

Orbitofrontal cortex (OFC)

In 2009, Ruffini and colleagues examined the orbitofrontal cortex as a new target for rTMS in drug-resistant OCD patients [15]. The subjects received 10 minutes of 1 Hz left-sided rTMS at 80% motor threshold for 15 sessions to the left OFC; the coil was placed parallel (active $n = 16$) or perpendicular (sham $n = 7$) to the scalp. They found a significant reduction of Y–BOCS scores comparing active versus sham treatment for 10 weeks after the end of rTMS ($p < 0.02$), with loss of significance after 12 weeks ($p < 0.06$). Y–BOCS reduction was 19.7% immediately after rTMS and 14.7% after 12 weeks of follow-up, compared with 6.7% and 5.7% respectively for the sham condition. There was also a benefit in terms of depressive and anxiety symptoms but not at a significant level in the two groups. Similar to findings for DLPFC TMS, this study suggests that low-frequency rTMS of the OFC may only acutely improve obsessive-compulsive symptoms.

Supplementary motor area (SMA)

Two groups investigated the efficacy of low-frequency rTMS to the SMA in addition to ongoing pharmacotherapy. In 2006, Mantovani *et al.* reported an open-label study of 10 subjects with OCD, Tourette syndrome or both [24]. Subjects were treated with active rTMS to the SMA for 10 daily sessions at 1 Hz, 100% motor threshold. After 2 weeks of daily rTMS, the Y–BOCS reduction (28.6%) and HAM-D reduction (47.8%) were both significant and remained stable after 3 months of follow-up in both the OCD and OCD/TS groups. In 2010, the same group examined rTMS (at 1 Hz and 100% motor threshold) to the SMA bilaterally in a randomized sham-controlled double-blind design [20]. After 4 weeks of stimulation the Y–BOCS decreased significantly ($p < 0.001$) in the active group (6 points, 25.4%) and in the sham group (3.2 points, 12.0%), without significant differences between treatment conditions.

Lastly, an open sham-controlled study investigated the possible therapeutic effects and safety of sequentially combined low-frequency (1 Hz, 110% threshold) rTMS to the right DLPFC and the SMA in 10 patients with treatment-resistant OCD [13]. Similar improvements of obsessive-compulsive and depressive symptoms were observed for both sham and real TMS at 2 weeks after the last of 14 sessions. The Y–BOCS reduction was 2.9 points (10.9%) and 3.4 points (12.9%) for real and sham rTMS respectively. rTMS was a safe method, and there was no significant change in cognitive functioning after stimulation. Similar to DLPFC and OFC stimulation, rTMS to the SMA was a safe method for immediately improving obsessive-compulsive symptoms; however, the improvement did not persist over time.

In conclusion, the efficacy of low- and high-frequency rTMS to the left or right DLPFC, the OFC or the SMA has been investigated in a total of 110 obsessive-compulsive patients over the last decade. Although open studies have initially demonstrated beneficial effects of rTMS on obsessive-compulsive and depressive symptoms during the first hours after stimulation, these effects disappeared during follow-up, and more importantly rTMS did not show any advantages over sham stimulation in double-blind sham-controlled studies.

Side effects and safety

Repetitive transcranial magnetic stimulation is generally regarded as a safe and non-invasive therapeutic technique. Although extremely rare, the most severe acute adverse effect for rTMS is the induction of epileptic seizures. The chance of getting a seizure during high-frequency rTMS is greater than that during low-frequency rTMS. Other reported side effects are induction of hypomania, local pain, headache, paraesthesia, hearing changes, and alterations in blood concentrations of thyroid stimulating hormone (TSH) and lactate. The two latter have only been reported in high-frequency rTMS [25].

In the studies of rTMS in OCD patients, low-frequency rTMS occasionally induced headache or localized scalp pain [13,19,24], whereas with high-frequency rTMS side effects were more often noted. The most common complaint in the latter studies was headache, followed by localized scalp pain, facial nerve stimulation, fainting and weepiness [16–18]. None of the side effects persisted for more than 4 weeks after stimulation and no serious adverse events (e.g. seizures) or memory or cognition problems were disclosed.

Conclusion and future directions

Since 1997, rTMS has been applied as an experimental treatment in refractory OCD. Local induction of a depolarizing magnetic field pulse may decrease obsessive-compulsive symptoms by normalizing hypermetabolism in orbitofrontal-striatal circuits. The technique is non-invasive and has no or only mild side effects, of which headache is the most common. Due to the lack of studies with comparable stimulation or treatment parameters and reliable designs, it is difficult to draw clear conclusions. Explorations of rTMS to the DLPFC, OFC or SMA in a total of 10 studies have demonstrated only acute effects of rTMS on obsessive-compulsive symptoms, and no differences from sham treatment.

The results of these studies show that further research is necessary. Careful consideration of target regions and stimulation parameters, longer follow-up times, and the use of a double-blind sham-controlled design, is needed to draw firm conclusions in the future. Besides, as the efficacy of rTMS is often time-limited, the need for futher rTMS after several weeks should be investigated. Moreover, functional MRI studies of rTMS in OCD are needed to clarify the specific stimulation region of rTMS. Nevertheless, rTMS may play an important role in research settings. For example, rTMS could be used to modulate obsessive-compulsive symptoms and brain activity in functional MRI and receptor binding studies. Also, as the improvement of symptoms is often present in the sham setting, it would be interesting to investigate the neural underpinnings of the placebo effect due to sham rTMS. Finally, recently novel stimulation paradigms have been designed, namely theta burst stimulation (TBS) and deep TMS. TBS is a low-intensity burst of rTMS at 50 Hz, considered to be a safer, more consistent and longer-lasting form of rTMS [22]. Deep TMS, using an H1 coil, can produce a larger and deeper spread of field than rTMS and has been shown to be effective in the treatment of depression [26–29]. The results of a first case study with the TBS paradigm in OCD and depression are promising and warrant further exploration [30]. Deep TMS still needs to be explored in OCD.

LESIONING

In the case of severe treatment-refractory OCD that is incapacitating in all aspects of daily life, an OCD patient might be a candidate for neurosurgical treatment. Surgery for OCD has a controversial history. Traditionally, procedures were undertaken to physically disconnect brain targets in the emotional system [31]. Nowadays, because the neural circuitries in OCD are better known and surgical techniques have been refined, functional neurosurgery is still performed [32]. The most common lesioning treatments for treatment-refractory OCD are anterior capsulotomy and anterior cingulotomy, performed using either traditional surgical techniques or with stereotactic radiosurgery (e.g. the 'gamma knife') [32,33]. Overall, lesioning procedures offer therapeutic benefit to 30–60% of patients with treatment-refractory OCD [33–37]. Cognitive deficits due to the lesioning and other serious adverse events, such as epileptic seizures and hallucinations, are reported in up to 20% of cases [32,34,36,37]. Due the high risk of these side effects and complications and due to its irreversible character, physicians remain cautious about performing lesion surgery.

DEEP BRAIN STIMULATION

During the past two decades, a shift has occurred in the field of stereotactic neuro-surgery since deep brain stimulation (DBS) became an established reversible and adjustable method for the alleviation of movement disorders (Figure 4.2). The first deep brain stimulation procedures were selective stimulation of the anterior limb of the internal capsule in order to imitate the effects of earlier capsulotomies. Since then more targets have been explored, and as OCD is one of the few diseases in psychiatry in which more functional data on neuroanatomical correlates are becoming available, linking specific brain areas to pathophysiology, DBS can nowadays be applied in OCD with a more rational approach.

Efficacy of DBS in OCD

Up to April 2011, approximately 100 patients with treatment-refractory OCD had received experimental DBS treatment. The efficacy of DBS has been reported in eight double-blind controlled studies [38–46] and six case studies [23,47–51]. Five targets have been used for DBS in OCD: the anterior limb of the internal capsule (ALIC), the ventral capsule/ventral striatum (VC/CS), the nucleus accumbens (NAcc), the subthalamic nucleus (STN) and the inferior thalamic peduncle (ITP) (Table 4.2).

Anterior limb of internal capsule (ALIC)

The use of DBS in OCD was initiated in 1998 at the Karolinska institute in Stockholm, where two patients received bilateral implantation in the ALIC, but the results were never published (S. Andreewitch, personal communication). In

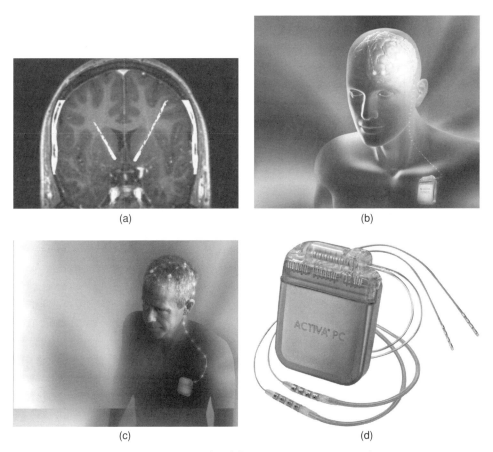

(a)   (b)

(c)   (d)

Figure 4.2 (a) Postoperative DBS lead locations superimposed on a preoperative magnetic resonance imaging scan. (b,c) In deep brain stimulation (DBS) a stimulator in the chest connects with the electrodes in the brain. (d) An implantable DBS device delivers carefully controlled electrical pulses to precisely targeted areas of the brain. Parts a–c reproduced by permission of Medtronic.

1999, the Leuven Group reported on bilateral ALIC DBS in four patients [38]. In a subsequent paper, these four patients and two others were followed-up for a period of 21 months [39]. Three out of four patients who completed the study experienced a $\geq$35% decrease in symptoms. An average symptom change of 40% was observed in the double-blind controlled part of the study in which the stimulator was switched on and off. In 2005, the Michigan Group reported another study of implantation of electrodes in the ALIC of four patients. Patients were stimulated in a double-blind way in a phase of four 3-week periods in which the stimulation was on or off, followed by an open phase [40]. Only one patient had a decrease of more than 35% in the double-blind phase. In the open phase, this patient progressed from severe disability to relatively normal life, with a 73% improvement over baseline in

Table 4.2 Deep brain stimulation (DBS) in obsessive-compulsive disorder (OCD).

Year	Author	Side	Target	Number	Diagnosis	Mean Y–BOCS preoperative	Mean Y–BOCS postoperative
1999	Nuttin et al.	Bilateral	Anterior limb of capsula interna	4	OCD	No Y–BOCS scores reported	In three of four patients effects were found
2003	Nuttin et al.	Bilateral	Anterior limb of capsula interna	6	OCD		*Cross-over phase:* Stimulation off: 32.3 ± 3.9 Stimulation on: 19.8 ± 8
2003	Anderson et al.	Bilateral	Anterior limb of capsula interna	1	OCD	34	7
2005	Abelson et al.	Bilateral	Anterior limb of capsula interna	4	OCD	32.8	*Open stimulation:* 23 *Double-blind phase:* 1 patient: at least 35% decrease 1 patient: 17% decrease 2 patients: non-responders
2006	Greenberg et al.	Bilateral	Anterior limb of capsula interna	10	OCD	34.6 ± 0.6	*Open stimulation:* After 3 months: 25 ± 1.6 After 36 months (8 patients): 22.3 ± 2.1
2008	Greenberg et al. (combined results)	Bilateral	Capsula interna/ventral striatum	26	OCD	34.0 ± 0.6	*Open stimulation:* After 3 months: 21.0 ± 1.8 After 36 months: 20.9 ± 2.4

Year	Author	Laterality	Target	n	Diagnosis	Y-BOCS baseline	Outcome
2010	Goodman et al.	Bilateral	Capsula interna/ventral striatum	6	OCD	33.7	After 12 months: 18 ± 4.1
2003	Sturm et al.	Unilateral	Nucleus accumbens (right)	4	OCD	No Y–BOCS scores reported.	Three of four patients almost complete remission of anxiety and OCD symptoms
2009	Hoff et al.	Unilateral	Nucleus accumbens (right)	10	OCD	32.2 ± 4	*Open stimulation:* After 12 months: 25.4 ± 6.7 *Cross-over phase:* Stimulation on: 27.9 ± 6.4 Stimulation off: 31.1 ± 5.0
2004	Aouizerate et al.	Bilateral	Nucleus accumbens + caudate nucleus	1	OCD + depressive disorder	25	*Open stimulation:* After 12 months : 10 After 15 months: 14 After 27 months: 12
2010	Franzini et al.	Bilateral	Nucleus accumbens	2	OCD	34	*Follow-up after 24–27 months:* 21
2002	Mallet et al.	Bilateral	Subthalamic nucleus	2	OCD + Parkinson disease	No Y–BOCS scores reported.	Patient 1: 58% improvement Patient 2: 64% improvement
2004	Fontaine et al.	Bilateral	Subthalamic nucleus	1	OCD + Parkinson disease	32	*Follow-up after 1 year:* 1

Y–BOCS, Yale–Brown Obsessive-Compulsive Scale.

8 months. Another patient who experienced only a 17% decline in the double-blind phase, showed improvement in the open phase, with a final reduction of 44% after completing an intensive behavioural treatment programme. In the two patients who were considered responders, positron emission tomography (PET) scans showed decreased activity of the orbitofrontal cortex. In another case study of ALIC DBS, a patient experienced a 79% reduction of symptoms at 3-month follow-up [47]. At 10-month follow-up the patient was able to return to work with compulsions in complete remission. These first studies show that the ALIC is a potential effective target for the treatment of therapy-refractory OCD. However, the effects are modest and subsequent targets were localized in a more ventral position.

Ventral capsule/ventral striatum (VC/VS)

In 2006, an American-Belgian group published the results of 10 patients who had undergone bilateral stimulation of the VC/VS [41]. Eight of them were followed over 3 years after bilateral implantation. Over these 3 years, OCD symptoms improved from severe to moderate, with a 30% decrease on average. Four of eight patients were considered responders with a symptom reduction of at least 35%. The Leuven Group, the American-Belgian Group and a group from the University of Florida published the combined results of VC/VS DBS in 26 patients [42]. During this period, targeting within the VC/VS evolved from anterior to a more posterior area. The percentage of responders was 62% at 36 months, with more effective stimulation at lower currents of the more posterior targets. A recent pilot study reported on VC/VS in six treatment-refractory OCD patients [43]. Patients were stimulated at either 30 or 60 days post-surgery under blinded conditions. Four of six patients (67%) were responders, with a decrease of at least 35% of symptoms. Interestingly, depressive symptoms improved significantly in all patients.

Nucleus accumbens (NAcc)

A German group aimed at the right NAcc as the stimulation target in four OCD patients [44]. In three out of four patients, open stimulation resulted in nearly total recovery from both anxiety and OCD symptoms at 24–30 months. The lack of effect in the fourth patient appeared to be caused by a displacement of the electrode in the caudoventral direction thereby missing the target area. The same group subsequently published a double-blind study on unilateral right-sided NAcc DBS in 10 OCD patients [45]. A modest improvement of just 10% was observed in the double-blind part of the study, which was initiated 6 months after the stimulator had been implanted. At 1-year follow-up, 5 out of 10 patients showed symptom decreases of more than 25%, and one patient more than 35%. Depression scores improved within 1 year, but anxiety failed to respond. A case study on one patient with OCD and depression reported a marked but delayed reduction of symptoms of up to 52% at 15 months follow-up [49]. An Italian group recently reported delayed effects of NAcc stimulation in two OCD patients [51]. On average, symptoms improved by 38% after 1 year of stimulation in the first patient and after 2 years in the second patient with depression scores improving concomitantly. In a recent Dutch study 16 treatment-resistant OCD patients were stimulated in an open 8-month treatment phase, followed by a double-blind crossover phase with randomly assigned 2-week periods of active or sham stimulation and ending with an open 12-month maintenance phase [46]. In the open phase, the mean (SD) Y–BOCS score decreased by 46%, from 33.7 (3.6) at baseline to 18.0 (11.4) after 8 months ($p < 0.001$). Nine of 16 patients were responders, with a mean (SD) Y–BOCS score decrease of 23.7 (7.0), or 72%. In the double-blind, sham-controlled phase ($n = 14$), the mean (SD) Y–BOCS score difference between active and sham stimulation was 8.3 (2.3), or 25% ($p = 0.004$). Depression and anxiety decreased significantly.

Subthalamic nucleus (STN)

The STN was long known as an effective target for DBS in treatment for Parkinson disease, and in some patients positive effects of STN stimulation on OCD symptoms were reported [23,48]. In 2008, the French group reported on the efficacy of bilateral STN stimulation in 18 OCD patients [52]. STN DBS resulted in positive effects on compulsive behaviour but appeared to have no effect on mood and global functioning within the first 6 months.

Thalamic peduncle

In 2004 and 2007, two case reports in patients with OCD and major depression were published, in which DBS targeted the ventral caudate nucleus/nucleus accumbens [49] and inferior thalamic peduncle [53]. In the first study, a marked but delayed reduction of symptoms of up to 52% was seen at 15 months follow-up. Likewise, in the second study, stimulation showed a significant reduction of obsessive and compulsive symptoms. The latter finding was substantiated by the same Mexican group that described a 49% reduction of symptoms following open stimulation of the bilateral inferior thalamic peduncle in five patients with OCD [54].

Efficacy: conclusions

In conclusion, DBS targeted to the ALIC, VC/VS, NAcc, STN and inferior thalamic peduncle has shown to be effective in therapy-refractory OCD. Fifty-eight of 94 reported patients experienced a $\geq 35\%$ reduction of obsessive-compulsive symptoms. Sixty-three percent of the patients are thus considered responders, making DBS a promising technique. However, efficacy varied strongly, not only between different brain targets but also among patients targeted at the same area. Moreover, DBS at different targets appears to modulate different symptoms of OCD: VC/VS DBS improved mood, obsessions and compulsions whereas STN DBS predominantly improved compulsions. Another significant difference was the time to response between the different studies. In the earlier studies, Mallet *et al.* [23] and Nuttin *et al.* [38,39] reported an acute relief of anxiety and obsessions whereas in the later studies of Nuttin *et al.*, reduction of obsessions and compulsions was not observed until a week of stimulation. Sturm *et al.* [44] reported the onset of clinical improvement a few days to several weeks after the beginning of the stimulation. In the study of Abelson *et al.* [40], beneficial effects were seen within the 3-week blinded study period, whereas Mallet *et al.* [52] reported improvement of symptoms after 3 months, Aouizerate *et al.* [49] after 9 months, and Franzini *et al.* [51] only after 1–2 years.

Mechanism of action of DBS in OCD

Since OCD has been associated with hyperactivity of the cortico-striato-thalamocortical (CSTC) network [55], the efficacy of DBS in OCD is most likely related to functional changes within this network. Electrical stimulation appears to be effective because it is assumed to induce a resetting of network oscillatory patterns across the CSTC network [56]. Studies in OCD combining DBS treatment with neuroimaging methods have confirmed changes within the CSTC network. A PET study in six OCD patients, which was carried out 2 weeks after implantation of electrodes in the VC/VS, demonstrated DBS-induced activation of the orbitofrontal cortex (OFC), anterior cingulate cortex, striatum, pallidus and thalamus [57]. However, no clinical effects of DBS had occurred at that point. Postoperative functional magnetic resonance imaging (fMRI) in an OCD patient with ALIC DBS showed increased activity in the frontal cortex and striatum compared to preoperative brain activity [39]. In the same study, clinical response after 3 months of continuous stimulation was related to a relative decrease of hyperactivity in the OFC. A study by Abelson *et al.* [40] showed decreased PET activity in the OFC after 3–6 weeks of ALIC DBS in two OCD responders, but not in the non-responders. In conclusion, sparse neuroimaging research suggests that DBS is effective in OCD because it induces functional changes, not limited to the target area but observable in the complete CSTC network, such as decreased activity in the OFC.

Side effects of DBS in OCD

Potential complications of DBS can arise (i) as a result of surgery ('procedure related'), (ii) due to the implanted device ('device related') or (iii) due to stimulation or cessation of stimulation. A potential risk of surgery is intracerebral haemorrhage. This was reported in 1 out of 10 patients by Greenberg *et al.* [41] and in one patient in the sample of Mallet *et al.* [52]. One patient had a single intraoperative generalized tonic-clonic seizure following electrode implantation [41]. Superficial surgical wound infection after implantation was reported in 1 of 10 patients by Greenberg *et al.* [41], and in 2 of 16 patients by Mallet *et al.* [52]. In the latter study, the implanted electrodes had to be removed. Other studies did not mention procedure-related complications. Device-related side effects were reported by Greenberg *et al.* [42], where a break in the electrode and subcutaneous extension cable required a replacement in one patient. Also, patients have reported that they disturbingly feel the material within their body, to the extent that some patients wanted it to be removed (one out of four patients: Nuttin *et al.* [39]).

The side effects of stimulation can be divided into acute effects and effects of chronic stimulation. The latter can be subdivided into effects on mood, cognition and personality. Stimulation may cause various acute physical and mental side effects, most of which are transitory and disappear after adaptation of stimulation parameters. Okun *et al.* [58] reported acute olfactory, gustatory and motor sensations that were strongly associated with the most ventral electrode positions, as well as physiological responses such as autonomic changes, increased breathing rate, sweating, nausea, cold sensation, heat sensation, fear and panic episodes. All effects reversed when DBS was stopped or parameters were changed. Acute mood changes during the first few days of stimulation of the ALIC and NAcc have been reported by Okun *et al.* [58], such as transient sadness, anxiety, euphoria or giddiness, sometimes to the extent of hypomanic symptoms (5 of 10 patients, Greenberg *et al.* [41]; 2 of 10 patients, Huff *et al.* [45]; four of six patients, Goodman *et al.* [43]). Chronic mood improvement is an unintended but favourable side effect of DBS since most treatment-refractory OCD patients suffer from comorbid major depression. Patients start to laugh, experience blissful feelings, and describe that they can see the world more brightly and clearly within seconds after stimulation. Abelson *et al.* [40] reported improvement of depression in one out of four patients while stimulating the ALIC. Decreased depression scores following VC/VS stimulation were found by Greenberg *et al.* [41]. Antidepressive effects seem to be especially related to DBS of the ventral striatum [40,41,44,49]. No improvement of depression was found following STN stimulation [44]. Apart from transient diminished concentration and verbal perseverations [42], DBS has not been associated with cognitive decline. Some patients did complain about memory and language problems but this has not been confirmed with neuropsychological tests. Gabriëls *et al.* [59], Abelson *et al.* [40], Aouizerate *et al.* [50], Goodman *et al.* [43] and Greenberg *et al.* [41] reported no decline in cognitive and executive functioning. On the contrary, in the latter study, a group analysis revealed significant improvements in memory recall. Using the Minnesota Multiphasic Personality Inventory (MMPI), Gabriëls *et al.* [59] reported no major adverse or harmful personality changes after 1 year of DBS. Neither patients nor family members reported changes in personality in the study of Abelson *et al*. [40]. Finally, remission of alcohol dependency [60] and unintended, effortless smoking cessation was observed following bilateral stimulation of the NAcc [61,62], supporting the idea of compulsivity with common circuitry in the processing of diverse rewards.

Follow-up treatment

Although studies indicate that DBS has the potential to significantly improve OCD symptoms in treatment-refractory patients, they also show that complete remission rarely is achieved. In addition, patients often continue to have problems in their daily life functioning after DBS, even when most OCD symptoms have disappeared. Compulsions and avoidance behaviour that have been almost lifelong in most therapy-refractory OCD patients may have become habitual. Therefore, follow-up treatment with behavioural therapy may be essential to motivate patients to implement the effects of DBS in their daily lives [46]. Studies are needed to investigate the additional efficacy of behavioural therapy following DBS.

Conclusions: DBS

Deep brain stimulation has been applied in therapy-refractory OCD in an experimental setting in approximately 100 patients over roughly a decade. Stimulation of five different targets has resulted in variable efficacy, ranging from no response to almost complete remission of symptoms. Overall, DBS in OCD may effect a decrease of 40–60% of symptoms in at least half of patients. Stimulating the VC/VS improves mood, obsessions and compulsions, whereas STN stimulation only improves compulsions. Most side effects are transitory and reverse after adaptation of stimulation parameters. The various stimulated brain areas, in many cases developed empirically, are consistent with recent theoretical findings on the neuroanatomy of OCD. DBS is probably effective in OCD because it modulates pathological activity within the CSTC network, resulting in a decrease of hyperactivity. DBS may be more effective when patients are followed up with behavioural therapy after surgery. DBS certainly has the potential to become the preferential treatment for a specific group of seriously ill, therapy-refractory OCD patients due to the low risk of the operation, the reversible nature of the technique, and the possibility to optimize treatment postoperatively.

CONCLUSION

Obsessive-compulsive disorder is a chronic and disabling disorder. Ten percent of patients remain treatment refractory despite several treatments. For these severe, treatment-refractory cases, physical interventions might be a treatment option. Of all physical interventions, DBS, as a replacement for the ablative neurosurgical therapies, seems to be the most promising. As yet, up to two-thirds of the treated patients experience more than 35% symptom reduction with mild to moderate adverse events. Currently, there is scant sound evidence supporting the use of rTMS and ECT as treatment options for OCD.

ACKNOWLEDGEMENTS

The authors thank Mariska Mantione MSc, Pepijn van den Munckhof MD and Rick Schuurman MD PhD, for their comments on the DBS section of the manuscript.

REFERENCES

1. Lisanby SH. Electroconvulsive therapy for depression. *N Engl J Med* 2007;**357**: 1939–1945.
2. Khanna S, Gangadhar BN, Sinha V, Rajendra PN, Channabasavanna SM. Electroconvulsive therapy in obsessive-compulsive disorder. *Convuls Ther* 1988;**4**:314–320.
3. Thomas SG, Kellner CH. Remission of major depression and obsessive-compulsive disorder after a single unilateral ECT. *J ECT* 2003;**19**:50–51.
4. Chaves MP, Crippa JA, Morais SL, Zuardi AW. Electroconvulsive therapy for coexistent schizophrenia and obsessive-compulsive disorder. *J Clin Psychiatry* 2005;**66**:542–543.
5. Strassnig M, Riedel M, Muller N. Electroconvulsive therapy in a patient with Tourette's syndrome and co-morbid Obsessive Compulsive Disorder. *World J Biol Psychiatry* 2004;**5**:164–166.
6. Fukuchi T, Okada Y, Katayama H *et al.* [A case of pregnant woman with severe obsessive-compulsive disorder successfully treated by modified-electroconvulsive therapy]. *Seishin Shinkeigaku Zasshi* 2003;**105**:927–932.
7. Loi S, Bonwick R. Electroconvulsive therapy for treatment of late-onset obsessive compulsive disorder. *Int Psychogeriatr* 2010;**22**:830–831.
8. Barker AT, Jalinous R, Freeston IL. Non-invasive magnetic stimulation of human motor cortex. *Lancet* 1985;**i**:1106–1107.
9. Whiteside SP, Port JD, Abramowitz JS. A meta-analysis of functional neuroimaging in obsessive-compulsive disorder. *Psychiatry Res* 2004;**132**:69–79.
10. Greenberg BD, George MS, Martin JD *et al.* Effect of prefrontal repetitive transcranial magnetic stimulation in obsessive-compulsive disorder: a preliminary study. *Am J Psychiatry* 1997;**154**:867–869.
11. George MS, Wassermann EM, Williams WA *et al.* Changes in mood and hormone levels after rapid-rate transcranial magnetic stimulation (rTMS) of the prefrontal cortex. *J Neuropsychiatry Clin Neurosci* 1996;**8**:172–180.
12. Siebner HR, Rothwell J. Transcranial magnetic stimulation: new insights into representational cortical plasticity. *Exp Brain Res* 2003;**148**:1–16.
13. Kang JI, Kim CH, Namkoong K, Lee CI, Kim SJ. A randomized controlled study of sequentially applied repetitive transcranial magnetic stimulation in obsessive-compulsive disorder. *J Clin Psychiatry* 2009;**70**:1645–1651.

14. Baxter LR Jr, Phelps ME, Mazziotta JC, Guze BH, Schwartz JM, Selin CE. Local cerebral glucose metabolic rates in obsessive-compulsive disorder. A comparison with rates in unipolar depression and in normal controls. *Arch Gen Psychiatry* 1987;**44**:211–218.
15. Ruffini C, Locatelli M, Lucca A, Benedetti F, Insacco C, Smeraldi E. Augmentation effect of repetitive transcranial magnetic stimulation over the orbitofrontal cortex in drug-resistant obsessive-compulsive disorder patients: a controlled investigation. *Prim Care Companion J Clin Psychiatry* 2009;**11**:226–230.
16. Sachdev PS, McBride R, Loo CK, Mitchell PB, Malhi GS, Croker VM. Right versus left prefrontal transcranial magnetic stimulation for obsessive-compulsive disorder: a preliminary investigation. *J Clin Psychiatry* 2001;**62**:981–984.
17. Sarkhel S, Sinha VK, Praharaj SK. Adjunctive high-frequency right prefrontal repetitive transcranial magnetic stimulation (rTMS) was not effective in obsessive-compulsive disorder but improved secondary depression. *J Anxiety Disord* 2010;**24**: 535–539.
18. Sachdev PS, Loo CK, Mitchell PB, McFarquhar TF, Malhi GS. Repetitive transcranial magnetic stimulation for the treatment of obsessive compulsive disorder: a double-blind controlled investigation. *Psychol Med* 2007;**37**:1645–1649.
19. Alonso P, Pujol J, Cardoner N *et al*. Right prefrontal repetitive transcranial magnetic stimulation in obsessive-compulsive disorder: a double-blind, placebo-controlled study. *Am J Psychiatry* 2001;**158**:1143–1145.
20. Mantovani A, Simpson HB, Fallon BA, Rossi S, Lisanby SH. Randomized sham-controlled trial of repetitive transcranial magnetic stimulation in treatment-resistant obsessive-compulsive disorder. *Int J Neuropsychopharmacol* 2010;**13**:217–227.
21. Prasko J, Paskova B, Zalesky R *et al*. The effect of repetitive transcranial magnetic stimulation (rTMS) on symptoms in obsessive compulsive disorder. A randomized, double blind, sham controlled study. *Neuro Endocrinol Lett* 2006;**27**:327–332.
22. Huang YZ, Edwards MJ, Rounis E, Bhatia KP, Rothwell JC. Theta burst stimulation of the human motor cortex. *Neuron* 2005;**45**:201–206.
23. Mallet L, Mesnage V, Houeto JL *et al*. Compulsions, Parkinson's disease, and stimulation. *Lancet* 2002;**360**:1302–1304.
24. Mantovani A, Lisanby SH, Pieraccini F, Ulivelli M, Castrogiovanni P, Rossi S. Repetitive transcranial magnetic stimulation (rTMS) in the treatment of obsessive-compulsive disorder (OCD) and Tourette's syndrome (TS). *Int J Neuropsychopharmacol* 2006;**9**:95–100.
25. Rossi S, Hallett M, Rossini PM, Pascual-Leone A. Safety, ethical considerations, and application guidelines for the use of transcranial magnetic stimulation in clinical practice and research. *Clin Neurophysiol* 2009;**120**:2008–2039.
26. Rosenberg O, Shoenfeld N, Zangen A, Kotler M, Dannon PN. Deep TMS in a resistant major depressive disorder: a brief report. *Depress Anxiety* 2010;**27**:465–469.
27. Rosenberg O, Zangen A, Stryjer R, Kotler M, Dannon PN. Response to deep TMS in depressive patients with previous electroconvulsive treatment. *Brain Stimul* 2010;**3**:211–217.
28. Levkovitz Y, Harel EV, Roth Y *et al*. Deep transcranial magnetic stimulation over the prefrontal cortex: evaluation of antidepressant and cognitive effects in depressive patients. *Brain Stimul* 2009;**2**:188–200.

29. Zangen A, Roth Y, Voller B, Hallett M. Transcranial magnetic stimulation of deep brain regions: evidence for efficacy of the H-coil. *Clin Neurophysiol* 2005;**116**:775–779.

30. Wu CC, Tsai CH, Lu MK, Chen CM, Shen WC, Su KP. Theta-burst repetitive transcranial magnetic stimulation for treatment-resistant obsessive-compulsive disorder with concomitant depression. *J Clin Psychiatry* 2010;**71**:504–506.

31. Moniz E. I succeeded in performing the prefrontal leukotomy. *J Clin Exp Psychopathol* 1954;**15**:373–379.

32. Bear RE, Fitzgerald P, Rosenfeld JV, Bittar RG. Neurosurgery for obsessive-compulsive disorder: contemporary approaches. *J Clin Neurosci* 2010;**17**:1–5.

33. Greenberg BD, Rauch SL, Haber SN. Invasive circuitry-based neurotherapeutics: stereotactic ablation and deep brain stimulation for OCD. *Neuropsychopharmacology* 2010;**35**:317–336.

34. Dougherty DD, Baer L, Cosgrove GR *et al.* Prospective long-term follow-up of 44 patients who received cingulotomy for treatment-refractory obsessive-compulsive disorder. *Am J Psychiatry* 2002;**159**:269–275.

35. Jung HH, Kim CH, Chang JH, Park YG, Chung SS, Chang JW. Bilateral anterior cingulotomy for refractory obsessive-compulsive disorder: Long-term follow-up results. *Stereotact Funct Neurosurg* 2006;**84**:184–189.

36. Kim CH, Chang JW, Koo MS *et al.* Anterior cingulotomy for refractory obsessive-compulsive disorder. *Acta Psychiatr Scand* 2003;**107**:283–290.

37. Oliver B, Gascon J, Aparicio A *et al.* Bilateral anterior capsulotomy for refractory obsessive-compulsive disorders. *Stereotact Funct Neurosurg* 2003;**81**:90–95.

38. Nuttin B, Cosyns P, Demeulemeester H, Gybels J, Meyerson B. Electrical stimulation in anterior limbs of internal capsules in patients with obsessive-compulsive disorder. *Lancet* 1999;**354**:1526.

39. Nuttin BJ, Gabriels LA, Cosyns PR *et al.* Long-term electrical capsular stimulation in patients with obsessive-compulsive disorder. *Neurosurgery* 2003;**52**:1263–1272.

40. Abelson JL, Curtis GC, Sagher O *et al.* Deep brain stimulation for refractory obsessive-compulsive disorder. *Biol Psychiatry* 2005;**57**:510–516.

41. Greenberg BD, Malone DA, Friehs GM *et al.* Three-year outcomes in deep brain stimulation for highly resistant obsessive-compulsive disorder. *Neuropsychopharmacology* 2006;**31**:2384–2393.

42. Greenberg BD, Gabriels LA, Malone DA Jr *et al.* Deep brain stimulation of the ventral internal capsule/ventral striatum for obsessive-compulsive disorder: worldwide experience. *Mol Psychiatry* 2010;**15**:64–79.

43. Goodman WK, Foote KD, Greenberg BD *et al.* Deep brain stimulation for intractable obsessive compulsive disorder: pilot study using a blinded, staggered-onset design. *Biol Psychiatry* 2010;**67**:535–542.

44. Sturm V, Lenartz D, Koulousakis A *et al.* The nucleus accumbens: a target for deep brain stimulation in obsessive-compulsive- and anxiety-disorders. *J Chem Neuroanat* 2003;**26**:293–299.

45. Huff W, Lenartz D, Schormann M *et al.* Unilateral deep brain stimulation of the nucleus accumbens in patients with treatment-resistant obsessive-compulsive disorder: Outcomes after one year. *Clin Neurol Neurosurg* 2010;**112**:137–143.

46. Denys D, Mantione M, Figee M *et al*. Deep brain stimulation of the nucleus accumbens for treatment-refractory obsessive-compulsive disorder. *Arch Gen Psychiatry* 2010;**67**:1061–1068.

47. Anderson D, Ahmed A. Treatment of patients with intractable obsessive-compulsive disorder with anterior capsular stimulation. Case report. *J Neurosurg* 2003;**98**:1104–1108.

48. Fontaine D, Mattei V, Borg M *et al*. Effect of subthalamic nucleus stimulation on obsessive-compulsive disorder in a patient with Parkinson disease. Case report. *J Neurosurg* 2004;**100**:1084–1086.

49. Aouizerate B, Cuny E, Martin-Guehl C *et al*. Deep brain stimulation of the ventral caudate nucleus in the treatment of obsessive-compulsive disorder and major depression. Case report. *J Neurosurg* 2004;**101**:682–686.

50. Aouizerate B, Martin-Guehl C, Cuny E *et al*. Deep brain stimulation for OCD and major depression. *Am J Psychiatry* 2005;**162**:2192.

51. Franzini A, Messina G, Gambini O *et al*. Deep-brain stimulation of the nucleus accumbens in obsessive compulsive disorder: clinical, surgical and electrophysiological considerations in two consecutive patients. *Neurol Sci* 2010;**31**:353–359.

52. Mallet L, Polosan M, Jaafari N *et al*. Subthalamic nucleus stimulation in severe obsessive-compulsive disorder. *N Engl J Med* 2008;**359**:2121–2134.

53. Jimenez F, Velasco F, Salin-Pascual R *et al*. Neuromodulation of the inferior thalamic peduncle for major depression and obsessive compulsive disorder. *Acta Neurochir Suppl* 2007;**97**:393–398.

54. Jimenez-Ponce F, Velasco-Campos F, Castro-Farfan G *et al*. Preliminary study in patients with obsessive-compulsive disorder treated with electrical stimulation in the inferior thalamic peduncle. *Neurosurgery* 2009;**65**:203–209.

55. Whiteside SP, Port JD, Abramowitz JS. A meta-analysis of functional neuroimaging in obsessive-compulsive disorder. *Psychiatry Res* 2004;**132**:69–79.

56. McIntyre CC, Hahn PJ. Network perspectives on the mechanisms of deep brain stimulation. *Neurobiol Dis* 2010;**38**:329–337.

57. Rauch SL, Dougherty DD, Malone D *et al*. A functional neuroimaging investigation of deep brain stimulation in patients with obsessive-compulsive disorder. *J Neurosurg* 2006;**104**:558–565.

58. Okun MS, Mann G, Foote KD *et al*. Deep brain stimulation in the internal capsule and nucleus accumbens region: responses observed during active and sham programming. *J Neurol Neurosurg Psychiatry* 2007;**78**:310–314.

59. Gabriëls L, Cosyns P, Nuttin B, Demeulemeester H, Gybels J. Deep brain stimulation for treatment-refractory obsessive-compulsive disorder: psychopathological and neuropsychological outcome in three cases. *Acta Psychiatr Scand* 2003;**107**:275–282.

60. Kuhn J, Lenartz D, Huff W *et al*. Remission of alcohol dependency following deep brain stimulation of the nucleus accumbens: valuable therapeutic implications? *J Neurol Neurosurg Psychiatry* 2007;**78**:1152–1153.

61. Kuhn J, Bauer R, Pohl S *et al*. Observations on unaided smoking cessation after deep brain stimulation of the nucleus accumbens. *Eur Addict Res* 2009;**15**:196–201.

62. Mantione M, van de Brink W, Schuurman PR, Denys D. Smoking cessation and weight loss after chronic deep brain stimulation of the nucleus accumbens: therapeutic and research implications: case report. *Neurosurgery* 2010;**66**:E218.

CHAPTER 5

Approaches to Treatment Resistance

Stefano Pallanti,[1,2,3] Giacomo Grassi[2] and Andrea Cantisani[2]

[1]*Department of Psychiatry, Mount Sinai School of Medicine, New York;*
[2]*Department of Psychiatry, University of Florence, Italy;* [3]*Institute of*
Neuroscience, Florence, Italy

Treatment resistance is a frequent situation in obsessive-compulsive disorder (OCD), which may occur at different stages throughout the course of the illness, having a strong impact on the long-term prognosis of the disease.

Although epidemiological studies indicate a prevalence of treatment-resistant patients of around 40–60% [1–7], treatment response is actually a symptom reduction of 35% (or more) of the initial Yale–Brown Obsessive-Compulsive Scale (Y–BOCS) score [8]. With other psychiatric disorders, patients with this slight degree of clinical improvement might still be regarded as non-responders. Considering these issues, even if in recent years some important progress has been made, many questions still remain open and represent notable obstacles for optimal intervention. Firstly, treatment for non-responders is largely not evidence-based; secondly, the research on predictors of response has not provided clear treatment recommendations for resistant patients, even if some elements (early onset, poor insight, hoarding symptom dimension) [9] have been individuated.

The difficulty in choosing the best therapeutic algorithm in a case of resistant-OCD is related to a remarkable lack of homogeneity of the disorder [10]. For example, the patient who responds to a selective serotonin reuptake inhibitor (SSRI) + dopamine antagonist combination could very likely be different from the one who responds to a SSRI + dopaminergic agent (such as dexamfetamine or caffeine), not only from a therapeutic point of view but also on a neurobiological and neurofunctional level. With regard to these issues, research into OCD endophenotypes and current animal models have yet to produce concrete strategies (see Chapters 9 and 12).

Obsessive-Compulsive Disorder: Current Science and Clinical Practice, First Edition. Edited by Joseph Zohar.
© 2012 John Wiley & Sons, Ltd. Published 2012 by John Wiley & Sons, Ltd.

TERMINOLOGICAL PROBLEMS AND OPERATIONAL DEFINITIONS

Despite the improvement that SSRIs have brought to the clinical condition of many patients affected by OCD (see Chapter 2), clinical evidence suggests that a high percentage of patients, ranging from 40% to 60%, do not obtain satisfactory symptom amelioration and do not adequately 'respond' to therapy [1–7], with a consequent strong impact on their quality of life, both in terms of disability and morbidity [11].

To describe the phenomenon of non-response several definitions, such as 'non-responder', 'treatment-resistant' and 'treatment refractory', are used with a significant lack of specificity. Although 'next step' treatment strategies have been used in recent years [7,12–19], due to the terminological issue it has not been possible to correctly interpret the collected data and to design new research studies on a reasonably homogeneous sample of so-called 'non-responsive' patients. This fact highlights the importance of this terminological and methodological problem.

Despite the terminological heterogeneity, there is substantial agreement on the instruments that have to be used to evaluate the individual's response to treatment. Validated and standardized clinical rating scales should be utilized both in clinical and research settings, and the response to treatment should be qualitatively assessed with periodic clinical interviews and the constant use of these scales.

The most frequently used is the Yale–Brown Obsessive-Compulsive Scale (Y–BOCS) [20,21]; initially developed for research purposes, it has quickly become a point of reference with regard to the clinical evaluation of the severity of obsessive-compulsive symptoms. Several studies have shown that approximately 60% of patients being treated with SSRIs obtained a reduction of 25–35% of their pre-treatment Y–BOCS score [22]: this value is now used globally as a cut-off point in the evaluation of the treatment response. Thereby a reduction of 35% of the Y–BOCS score after an adequate treatment is usually defined as a response, whereas a reduction of between 25% and 35% is considered a 'partial response'.

Even if these rates may seem slight, several trials show that the use of placebo usually causes a symptom improvement equivalent to a reduction in the range of only 3–5% of the Y–BOCS score [23]; besides, it is relevant to emphasize that in OCD there is no direct proportionality between the objective severity of the symptoms and the disability that they may cause in a patient's everyday life [24]: a reduction of 35% of the Y–BOCS score, although apparently small, may produce a major improvement in a patient's functionality.

Notwithstanding the specificity of it, this instrument has a relevant lack of sensitivity, in particular for severe and chronic cases, in detecting more subtle modifications in the psychopathological status of the patient, as for example a reduction from 5 to 3 hours per day of obsessive rituals. Instead, the Clinical Global

Impression (CGI) scale, although less specific, is considered to be sufficiently sensitive to capture this kind of modification and allows the clinician to estimate it and rate it in a more precise way. Patients with a CGI score of 1 (very much improved) and 2 (very improved) are usually considered as responders. The integrated use of these instruments may offer a standardized portrait of the treatment response of a patient.

Furthermore, in Y–BOCS-II (second edition, recently published by Storch *et al.* [25]), more attention was given to the sensitivity in detecting more subtle changes in symptom severity and to rate ritualistic avoidance (for more details, see Chapter 1).

However, these scales do not accurately evaluate an important dimension of the illness, namely subjective well-being. In recent years quality of life has gained increasing attention as an aspect of OCD research – one that was previously neglected; using standardized rating scales such as the Health Related Quality of Life (HRQL), the dimensional assessment of a patient's suffering should be included in the comprehensive evaluation of the patient and in particular with regard to non-responsive cases [26].

We proposed the introduction of operational criteria for the assessment of the 'stages of response' to help the clinician in planning the best treatment strategy [8] (Table 5.1). The response to treatment is seen as a continuum of stages ranging from refractoriness to all types of therapies, to 'remission'.

'Resistant' and 'refractory' are often used as synonyms, but the former term should be used in case of failure of one trial of therapy with a first-choice treatment (at least 10–12 weeks with full dose of an SRI), and the latter term after at least three trials with SRI agents (one of them with clomipramine), two augmentation

Table 5.1 Operational criteria for the assessment of stages of response to treatment in obsessive-compulsive disorder.

Stage of response	Stage	Description
I	Recovery	Not at all ill; less than 8 on Y–BOCS
II	Remission	Less than 16 on Y–BOCS
III	Full response	35% or greater reduction of Y–BOCS and CGI 1 or 2
IV	Partial response	Greater than 25% but less than 35% Y–BOCS reduction
V	Non-response	Less than 25% Y–BOCS reduction, CGI 4
VI	Relapse	Symptoms return (CGI 6 or 25% increase in Y–BOCS from remission score) after 3+ months of 'adequate' treatment
VII	Refractory	No change or worsening with all available therapies

CGI, Clinical Global Impression scale; Y–BOCS, Yale–Brown Obsessive-Compulsive Scale.

trials with atypical antipsychotics, and at least 20–30 hours of cognitive behavioural therapy.

Also the concept of 'recovery' should be differentiated from that of 'remission', as long-term studies suggest a range of outcomes from chronic refractory to complete remission. An episodic course has also been described in adults [27,28], and because of this the introduction of 'remission' and 'recovery' definitions in the staging of illness seems to be rational and practical, as proposed by Frank *et al.* [29] for depression.

'Recovery' represents an almost total absence of symptoms after treatment, basically a state that is indistinguishable from a healthy control, which corresponds to a Y–BOCS score of less than 8. Full recovery is a very uncommon clinical event that occurs in the 5% of patients with an episodic course of OCD [30]. Instead, the most probable result in cases of a non-episodic course is 'remission', a term that indicates a reduction of symptoms after treatment to a lower limit, associated with a Y–BOCS score of 16 or less (below the minimum threshold value needed to be included in a clinical trial).

Unfortunately, these results are uncommon in clinical practice, and very often there is a lower grade response that can be identified with the already mentioned stages of 'full response' or 'partial response': below that threshold (25% reduction of the Y–BOCS score) we propose to use the term 'non-response'.

A 25% increase in Y–BOCS score from the patient's score during response, or a CGI improvement score of 6 ('much worse') we consider a 'relapse', a definition that indicates a re-emergence of the symptoms during an ongoing but subclinical course of disease. As for the term 'recurrence', we propose to use this in the case of a new episode during a recovery phase and therefore it is applied only in case of an episodic course of the disorder [8].

Some studies [31–34] show that relapse is a very frequent phenomenon (65–90% of cases) after an acute discontinuation of SRI therapy, and that a lower level of response (to the same treatment that was effective during the previous episode) is often achieved [35]. The high prevalence of partial responses and this relapse pattern (after acute drug discontinuation) make the OCD course comparable to that of psychotic disorders [36]. An accurate evaluation of the timing of the return of symptoms, and whether they manifested during treatment or after discontinuation, is therefore necessary in determining whether a new episode or a relapse has occurred. Actually, it is still unclear whether a patient who has a relapse, which does not respond to a treatment that had previously been successful, should be labelled a non-responder [8]. A differentiation between episodic non-response and chronic non-response could be also useful [37]. A further question is defining the role of tachyphylaxis in determining resistance to treatment.

Another issue in determining non-response to treatment involves comorbid conditions. Non-responsive patients are more likely to meet criteria for comorbid axis I or axis II disorders, and the presence of a specific comorbid condition could be a distinguishing feature in OCD, with influence on the treatment adequacy and outcome [37]. Particularly, comorbid conditions such as bipolar disorder and ADHD (attention-deficit hyperactivity disorder) are common in treatment-resistant patients, but there are few studies investigating their impact on treatment resistance [38,39].

PHARMACOLOGICAL STRATEGIES IN RESISTANT OCD

Switching

Switching consists in replacing a serotoninergic agent with another one, or with an agent belonging to another class of drugs. Some studies suggest success in switching between SRIs in resistant patients [40–45], but there is no strong evidence supporting the possibility of predicting the response of the patient to another drug. Clinical experience indicates that the response rate to a successive treatment is around 50%, but also that it declines with an inverse relationship to the number of failed trials [46].

The majority of authors suggest switching from a SSRI to clomipramine (CMI) or vice versa, depending on which was the agent first used; the advantages of a shift from a SSRI to another one remain unclear [46,47]. The unique data available are those from an open-label trial showing that a non-response to a SSRI does not imply non-response to other molecules of the same class: 18 patients showing non-response to at least two SSRI trials were treated with citalopram 40 mg/day, with a response rate of 77% [48]. As for switching across classes, some trials have been performed with venlafaxine and mirtazapine. The switch from venlafaxine to paroxetine showed an improvement in 56% of cases after treatment, but when switching from paroxetine to venlafaxine the rate was only 19% [44]. The switch to mirtazapine is supported by one open pilot study and a double-blind discontinuation trial [49]. Moreover, in a case series, switching from a SSRI to the serotonin and noradrenaline reuptake inhibitor (SNRI) duloxetine was successful in a number of treatment-resistant patients [50].

So, although there are no double-blind studies that confirm the efficacy of switching from one SSRI to another, the rationale of this strategy derives from pharmacokinetic and side-effect issues. Citalopram and sertraline are, for example, poor inhibitors of cyt P450 (which is involved in the metabolism of many prescribed drugs), and could therefore be used in cases of complex pharmacological interactions. In contrast, fluoxetine and paroxetine significantly inhibit the CYP2D6 enzymes that metabolize tricyclic antidepressants, antipsychotics, antiarrhythmics and β-blockers. Fluoxetine has a long half-life and an active metabolite, which reduces the effects of abstinence, and this could be useful in patients with a low compliance [51]. Fluvoxamine inhibits CYP1A2 and CYP3A4, which are implicated respectively in the elimination of warfarin and tricyclics, benzodi-azepines and antiarrhythmics.

Infusion therapy

Some reports indicate that infusion therapy can be considered as a valid therapeutic strategy for treatment-resistant cases. Two agents are currently available for this kind of treatment of OCD, clomipramine and citalopram.

The rationale for using this route of administration is provided by both phar-macokinetic and clinical considerations. On the one hand, the absorption of an intravenously administered drug is rapid, constant, complete and not affected by malabsorption, gastric pH changes, intestinal motility, simultaneous administration of other drugs, or other factors. Moreover, intravenous administration allows by-passing of the liver on first pass, which considerably influences the biodispersibility of the drug (in other words, the amount of active drug that reaches the systemic circulation). On the other hand, from a clinical point of view infusion therapy may improve treatment compliance, reinforce the therapeutic alliance and reduce the frequency of adverse events.

Clomipramine is partially converted by first-pass metabolism into the metabo-lite desmethylclomipramine, which has a weaker serotoninergic effect. In-travenous administration may therefore increase the plasma clomipramine/desmethylclomipramine ratio and enhance the therapeutic effect. Fallon et al. [52] conducted a double-blind placebo-controlled study on 54 non-responder patients (following an 8-week trial with clomipramine per os) and reported a greater efficacy of clomipramine i.v. versus placebo.

Clomipramine can be administered with a gradual increase of the dose or with a 'pulse loading' strategy (150 mg i.v. on the first day, 200 mg i.v. on the second day, no administration for four consecutive days and then oral administration). Koran et al. [53] compared these two administration strategies in OCD-resistant patients and observed that a faster response was obtained with pulse loading administration.

Citalopram is the only SSRI available for infusion therapy. Pallanti et al. [54] administered intravenous citalopram for 3 weeks (followed by oral administra-tion for 9 weeks) to treatment-resistant OCD patients who were non-responders following at least two adequate trials with an SSRI but not citalopram: 59% of the patients showed a reduction of at least 25% of the initial Y–BOCS score after the first 3 weeks of therapy, and improved further at the end of the 12 weeks [54].

Ross et al. [55] conducted a follow-up study examining a sample of treatment-resistant patients with OCD 4 to 11 years after they were treated with intravenous clomipramine. This study revealed that almost half of these patients reported feeling much improved or very much improved compared to their state prior to treatment with intravenous clomipramine, and nearly one-third no longer met criteria for

OCD. These results suggest that a substantial percentage of treatment-resistant OCD patients improve symptomatically with time [55].

Cognitive behavioural therapy

Current research and clinical knowledge considers cognitive behavioural therapy (CBT) the most successful type of psychotherapy in the treatment of OCD. The most effective technique seems to be the exposure and response prevention (ERP) strategy [56–58]; this therapy essentially exposes OCD patients to feared stimuli and acts in order to prevent the following response. Currently, results of comparing CBT with pharmacological treatment are not conclusive [59]. However, CBT/ERP can be considered an effective first-choice treatment, as are SRIs; experts agree on the clinical utility of this kind of psychotherapy and on the fact that CBT should be considered as soon as resistance to SRIs appears [37].

In recent years, two studies have been published that investigated the efficacy of CBT as an augmentation strategy in treatment-resistant OCD patients, and provided similar results. Tundo and colleagues [60] treated 36 resistant patients with an ERP strategy, together with ongoing pharmacological treatment: at follow-up the 21 patients completing CBT showed statistically significant improvements on the outcome measures (Y–BOCS and CGI); at the end of the trial 15 patients of the 36 (42%) who were initially recruited had a CGI evaluation of 'much improved' or 'very much improved'.

Simpson *et al.* [61] recruited 107 patients who did not respond to at least a 12-week trial with a SRI and treated them with an ERP strategy or with stress management training (SMT) (pharmacological treatment underwent no changes during the trial period): 74% of the patients who received ERP responded to the treatment and had a decrease in symptom severity of at least 25%, versus 22% of those who received SMT.

Some interesting studies investigated the role of D-cycloserine as an augmentation agent in CBT. D-cycloserine (DCS) is a partial agonist of the neuronal N-methyl-D-aspartic acid (NMDA) receptor for glutamate and seems to improve the learning of fear extinction in animals exposed to fear stimuli. Storch and colleagues administered to their patients 250 mg of DCS or placebo 4 hours prior to the beginning of each ERP therapy (for 12 weeks). Although at the beginning of the trial an amelioration trend was noticed in the DCS group, in later stages of the trial there were no significant differences between the DCS and placebo groups [62]. Similar results came from a double-blind placebo-controlled study in which 125 mg of DCS or placebo were administered 2 hours before the exposure sessions: during the initial phase of the trial augmentation with DCS was successful in reducing the distress caused by obsessive symptoms compared to placebo, but the differences between the two groups were inconsistent by the end of the study [63]. These results were confirmed by another placebo-controlled trial in which

100 mg of DCS was administered 1 hour before exposure [64]. All these findings suggest that although DCS may accelerate the response to exposure therapy, it does not modify the final Y–BOCS score of the patients. Indeed, a recent meta-analysis confirmed these observations, yet this meta-analysis pointed out that the impact of DCS augmentation is related to the timing of its administration: being greater when administered a limited number of times and when given immediately before or after exposure therapy [65].

Serotoninergic agents

SRIs

This augmentation strategy consists of the combination of two serotoninergic drugs, usually clomipramine or an SSRI, depending on which was the initial agent. As already mentioned, sertraline and citalopram represent first-choice SSRI augmentation agents for clomipramine, due to their minor inhibitory effect on cyt P450 [47]. The efficacy of clomipramine as an augmentation agent for SSRIs is supported by several studies [66–68] and by an expert consensus [45]. In double-blind studies, intravenous clomipramine was more effective than oral clomipramine [52,59,69]; however, the experts recommend checking the plasma concentration of clomipramine and of its metabolite desmethylclomipramine during any augmentation therapy to maintain it below 500 ng/mL, because of cardiac and CNS toxic side effects. Fluvoxamine seems to be the SSRI that primarily has such an increasing effect [46].

Studies of the efficacy of SSRI augmentation during clomipramine treatment have focused on fluoxetine and sertraline. In a small open trial a 20–40 mg dose of fluoxetine was effective in clomipramine-resistant patients [70], and sertraline augmentation was more effective when compared to the dosage increase of the first-choice treatment [68].

Other serotoninergic agents

Besides SSRIs, the usefulness of other serotoninergic drugs has been investigated in a number of studies in recent years.

Buspirone

There have been some case reports of good results with the use of buspirone (a partial 5-HT$_{1A}$ agonist and D$_2$, α_1 and α_2 antagonist), but a subsequent double-blind placebo-controlled study did not replicate the positive results [71].

Pindolol

Augmentation with pindolol, a β-antagonist that probably has a blocking effect on 5-HT_{1A} presynaptic receptors, was moderately positive in one double-blind placebo-controlled study of patients treated with paroxetine [72], but it did not positively impact when added to fluvoxamine [73].

Lithium

Lithium is thought to increase the presynaptic release of serotonin, and on this basis it has been tested also in OCD cases; a double-blind placebo-controlled trial had negative results [74].

Clonazepam

Due to its serotoninergic effect, which differentiates it from the other benzodiazepines, clonazepam has been thought to be beneficial in the treatment of OCD. In the first study, results were encouraging [75], yet a recent controlled trial found this approach to be ineffective [76].

Trazodone

Trazodone was found to be scarcely useful as an augmentation strategy in a placebo-controlled trial [77].

Ondansetron

5-HT_3 receptor antagonists such as ondansetron have shown some interesting features, which may turn out to be useful in the treatment of OCD. A possible mechanism of its anti-obsessional efficacy involves dopaminergic inhibition by 5-HT_3 receptor blockade. In fact serotonin 5-HT_3 receptors are co-localized with GABA (gamma-aminobutyric acid) interneurons in the ventral tegmental area, and they act indirectly by inhibiting cortico-mesolimbic dopamine release [78]. It is of theoretical interest, with regard to OCD treatment, that 5-HT_3 receptor antagonists like ondansetron were shown to reduce the reinforcing effects of a variety of abused drugs, including alcohol and amphetamines [79]. This phenomenon was presumably explained by the attenuation of suprabasal cortico-mesolimbic dopamine release following withdrawal from cocaine use [80,81]. Furthermore, in humans ondansetron was also shown to inhibit increased right orbitofrontal cortex neuronal activation and cerebral blood flow in recently withdrawn cocaine addicts [82]. An increased neural activation of this region has been consistently reported in OCD [83].

The first study of 5-HT$_3$ antagonists in OCD patients was an open-label uncontrolled ondansetron monotherapy study [84]. This study reported a Y–BOCS score reduction of 28% in a small sample (eight patients) of non-treatment-resistant OCD patients [84]. In a recent single-blind trial our group administered augmentation therapy with ondansetron to treatment-resistant patients (receiving a stable therapy with SSRIs and antipsychotics). The drug was initiated at a dosage of 0.25 mg twice daily for 6 weeks and was then titrated to 0.5 mg twice daily for 6 weeks. At the endpoint, 9 of 14 enrolled patients (64.3%) reached the criteria for 'treatment response' (Y–BOCS score decrease of (25% and a CGI-I score of 1 or 2 – very much or much improved), while the average Y–BOCS reduction was around 23.2%, suggesting that low-dose ondansetron may have a role as an augmentation strategy for resistant patients [85]. Recently, Soltani *et al.* [86] conducted an 8-week pilot double-blind placebo-controlled trial of ondansetron augmentation of SSRI. In this study the patients were randomly assigned to receive either ondansetron (4 mg) plus fluoxetine or fluoxetine (20 mg/day) plus placebo. The ondansetron-treated group showed a statistically significant difference in the reduction of the Y–BOCS scores with respect to the placebo group, supporting the hypothesis that ondansetron may be a beneficial agent in treating OCD patients [86].

Dopaminergic agents

Rationale for the use of dopaminergic agents

Both preclinical and clinical evidence supports the relevance of the dopaminergic system in the pathophysiology of OCD. Experimental studies in animals, utilizing dopaminergic drugs (amphetamine, bromocriptine, apomorphine and L-dopa), have provided evidence for the involvement of dopamine in compulsive behaviours such as grooming and repetitive checking behaviours, which are commonly considered animal models of OCD [87–89]. Several findings of dopamine dysregulation in OCD in humans have also been reported. Neurological diseases associated with dopaminergic dysfunction such as Tourette syndrome, Sydenham chorea and Parkinson disease, often show obsessive-compulsive symptoms in their clinical presentation, providing indirect strong evidence of the role of dopamine in OCD [90–92]; in addition, the comorbidity of Tourette syndrome and OCD, mainly in the childhood-onset forms, suggests possible common neurobiological underpinnings and genetic factors for the two disorders [93]. Moreover, several drugs that increase synaptic dopamine levels such as cocaine and amphetamine, have been reported to exacerbate or induce as well as to improve OCD symptoms

[94]. Finally, interesting data about dopamine involvement in OCD come from neuroimaging studies. Perani *et al.* [93] conducted a PET (positron emission tomography) study in drug-naive OCD patients, measuring *in vivo* both serotonin ($5\text{-}HT_{2A}$) and dopamine (D2) receptor distributions. These authors found a reduction in D2 receptor binding potential suggesting a dopaminergic dysfunction, probably an endogenous dopaminergic hyperactivity, particularly in the ventral portion of the striatum.

Antipsychotic augmentation

Overview of effectiveness and long-term safety

Many studies have assessed the effectiveness of antipsychotic augmentation in OCD treatment-resistant patients. Available data show that antipsychotics used as an augmentation therapy are effective in one-third of SRI-treatment-resistant patients. Data from randomized double-blind placebo-controlled studies provide strong evidence of the efficacy of haloperidol and risperidone; however, evidence regarding the efficacy of quetiapine and olanzapine is inconclusive [95]. The reason for the greater effectiveness of haloperidol and risperidone is probably that they have a greater D2 dopamine receptor affinity. Augmentation with newer agents such as aripiprazole has not yet established sufficient basis for their wide use in OCD, but preliminary data reveal interesting perspectives. Since only one-third of the resistant patients appear to respond to the antipsychotics, it is desirable to identify predictors of antipsychotic response, but current evidence for these is limited. Several studies show that the subgroup of OCD patients with comorbid tics have a particularly beneficial response to this intervention (especially to haloperidol) as well as those with poor insight [96] and co-occurring schizotypical personality disorder [97,98]. Antipsychotic augmentation has a relatively rapid effect in the treatment of OCD, and patients are unlikely to improve if they have not responded after 3 months of intervention [95].

Until recently, all studies of atypical antipsychotic augmentation in OCD investigated only short-term responses. The only available data concerning the effectiveness and safety of long-term atypical antipsychotic augmentation in SRI-resistant patients come from a 1-year trial by Matsunaga *et al.* [99]. The main finding of this study was that although SRI-resistant patients responded to augmentation with atypical antipsychotics, they showed a significantly higher body mass index, as well as a significantly higher level of fasting blood sugar, compared to SRI-responders. Additionally, the SSRI + atypical antipsychotic group was relatively more likely to show elevated levels of triglycerides and total cholesterol. These data are consistent with previous findings from short-term clinical trials and emphasize the importance of assessing metabolic and nutritional factors in the management of OCD treatment-resistant patients.

Typical antipsychotics

- *Haloperidol.* In a double-blind placebo-controlled study, the addition of haloperidol to fluvoxamine [100] was effective particularly in patients with tic disorder. The mean dose of haloperidol was 6.2 mg/day. The response rate in patients with comorbid tics was 100%. The authors suggest beginning augmentation treatment with haloperidol at 0.25–0.5 mg/day, with subsequent increases every 4–7 days to a maximum of 2–4 mg/day, as clinically indicated. The authors also found that when this treatment strategy is effective, response will usually occur within 2–4 weeks of addition to the SRI [100].
- *Pimozide.* In an open-label case series, pimozide (6.5 mg/day), added to ongoing SRI treatment, was found to be effective in 9 of 17 OCD treatment-resistant patients. Seven of eight patients with comorbid chronic tic disorder or schizotypal personality disorder were responders compared with only two of nine patients without this comorbidity [98].

Atypical antipsychotics

- *Risperidone.* It has been demonstrated [101] in a double-blind placebo-controlled trial that risperidone at an average dose of 2.2 mg/day led to a significant improvement in Y–BOCS scores when compared to the addition of placebo. Hollander *et al.* [96] demonstrated similar findings in a double-blind placebo-controlled trial using risperidone augmentation of SRI at a mean dose of 2.5 mg/day with a maximum of 3 mg/day. Erzegovesi *et al.* [102] found that 5 of 10 fluvoxamine-resistant patients had a significant response when randomized to risperidone augmentation, while only two of nine patients improved after being randomized to placebo; notably, in this study the authors used a very low dosage of risperidone (equal to 0.5 mg/day). In a double-blind cross-over study, both haloperidol and risperidone were effective when added to an SSRI [103]. Interestingly, in a PET study of risperidone augmentation conducted by Hollander *et al.* [96], response to risperidone treatment was associated with significant increases in relative metabolic rate in the cingulate gyrus, the striatum, the prefrontal cortex, especially in the orbital region, and the thalamus. Patients with low relative metabolic rates in the striatum and high relative metabolic rates in the anterior cingulate gyrus were more likely to show a clinical response [96,104]. Interestingly, a recent study compared the efficacy of aripiprazole and risperidone augmentation in a single-blind randomized design. The study consisted of two different periods of treatment: a 12-week prospective period to determine resistance to SSRI treatment and an 8-week single-blind addition period for resistant patients only. At the end of the first period 59.4% of patients were considered treatment-resistant and were randomized to receive either risperidone (3 mg/day; $n = 20$) or aripiprazole (15 mg/day; $n = 21$) as augmentation of SSRI treatment.

At the end of this period 50% in the aripiprazole and 72.2% in the risperidone group met the response criterion of a Y–BOCS decrease $\geq 35\%$, suggesting, albeit in a small sample, that risperidone may be more effective than aripiprazole as augmentation therapy in treatment-resistant OCD [105].

- *Olanzapine.* Results of placebo-controlled studies with olanzapine are inconclusive. On the one hand, in a double-blind placebo-controlled trial, Shapira *et al.* [106] found no additional advantage of adding olanzapine in OCD patients resistant to fluoxetine, compared with extending the monotherapy trial. On the other hand, Bystritsky *et al.* [107], in a placebo-controlled trial, concluded that adding olanzapine to SSRIs is potentially efficacious in the short-term treatment of patients with resistant OCD. Finally, an 8-week, single-blind, randomized trial comparing risperidone with olanzapine augmentation of an SRI, revealed no difference between the two drugs [108].

- *Quetiapine.* To date, four double-blind placebo-controlled trials have compared quetiapine versus placebo augmentation of SRIs in OCD-resistant patients without conclusive results. In a large study (40 patients) by Denys *et al.* [109], quetiapine augmentation appeared to be more effective than placebo. In a smaller study, Fineberg *et al.* [110] found that quetiapine was more effective than placebo when added to SRIs; however, the difference did not reach statistical significance. Nevertheless, Carey *et al.* [111] found that quetiapine augmentation was no more effective than placebo in the augmentation of SRIs, but pointed out that their results might be influenced by the shorter duration of the SRI therapy before the addition of quetiapine, in comparison with that of other trials. Moreover, a recent study failed to find an additional effect of quetiapine augmentation versus placebo in patients with severe OCD [112]. Finally, a randomized open-label trial comparing quetiapine versus clomipramine in the augmentation of SSRI, corroborated quetiapine efficacy for treatment-resistant OCD and found that clomipramine did not produce a significant reduction in Y–BOCS scores [113].

- *Aripiprazole.* Aripiprazole augmentation in resistant patients has not yet a sufficient evidential basis for its wide use in OCD, but preliminary data highlight interesting possibilities. Aripiprazole is chemically different from other atypical agents. It is a quinolinone derivative with a high affinity for dopamine D2 and D3 receptors, as well as serotonin $5\text{-}HT_{1A}$, $5\text{-}HT_{2A}$ and $5\text{-}HT_{2B}$ receptors. Its pharmacological profile is characterized by a partial agonism at the dopamine D2 and serotonin $5\text{-}HT_{1A}$ receptors, whereas it works as an antagonist at serotonin $5\text{-}HT_{2A}$ receptors [114]. Aripiprazole was found to be effective in augmentation of SRI-resistant patients in several case reports [115–117], and as monotherapy in an 8-week, open-label, flexible dose (10–30 mg/day) pilot trial [118]. The first systematic study of aripiprazole augmentation was a 12-week, open-label, flexible-dose trial of aripiprazole addition to SRIs in treatment-resistant patients [119]. In this study aripiprazole was started at 5 mg/day and increased up to a maximum of 20 mg/day. At the end of the study, three patients (33.3%) met response criteria of ≥25% improvement in Y–BOCS total score versus baseline. Two of them had a reduction ≥35% in Y–BOCS total score. One patient reached response at week 8, and two patients at week 10. In this trial the most common adverse event reported was inner unrest. A recent double-blind placebo-controlled trial of aripiprazole augmentation of SRI therapy provided evidence of its efficacy in treatment-resistant OCD. In this study the patients treated with aripiprazole also showed an improvement in some cognitive functions, such as attentional resistance to interference (measured by the Stroop test) and executive functioning [120].

- *Ziprasidone.* To date there is insufficient evidence to support the use of ziprasidone in OCD. In a case report by Iglesias Garcia *et al.* [121] a severe OCD patient had a clinically significant improvement after switching from clozapine to ziprasidone, but in a retrospective comparative study of quetiapine and ziprasidone as adjuncts in treatment-resistant OCD, ziprasidone was found to be less effective than quetiapine.
- *Clozapine.* Clozapine was the first atypical antipsychotic agent to be systematically evaluated in OCD. In an open-label trial of clozapine monotherapy, none of the patients showed any statistically significant improvement in OC symptoms and none of the patients met criteria for treatment response [122].

Atypical antipsychotic-induced obsessive-compulsive symptoms

Since the introduction of atypical antipsychotics (AAP), both case reports [123–128] and clinical studies [129–131] have described either a *de novo* onset or exacerbation of existing subthreshold OC symptoms during treatment with these drugs. Conventional neuroleptics with high D2-blocking potency, such as haloperidol and pimozide, are not reported to worsen OCD whereas the lower potency conventional neuroleptic chlorpromazine was reported to induce OCS in two patients [132]. Most reports of APP-induced OC symptoms in schizophrenic patients relate to clozapine, olanzapine, risperidone and quetiapine [133–137]. Possible explanations include 5-HT$_{2A}$ receptor involvement, derived from the fact that serotonin and dopamine closely interact within the cortico-striato-thalamocortical loops [138]. Data from animal studies show that SSRIs and 5-HT$_{2A}$ receptor agonists inhibit dopamine release in the basal ganglia. Moreover, 5-HT$_{2A}$ antagonists stimulate dopamine release in the prefrontal cortex and the basal ganglia. Accordingly OC symptoms may derive from dopaminergic disinhibition in the 'wrong' cortico-striato-thalamocortical loops, especially the one involving the orbitofrontal cortex [137]. However, data from a genetic association study suggested a glutamate involvement in APP-induced OC symptoms [139]. In this study the authors found an association between sequence variations in the glutamate transporter gene *SLC1A1* and susceptibility to APP-induced OC symptoms in schizophrenic patients.

Dexamfetamine (dextroamphetamine) and caffeine augmentation

In two small, double-blind, placebo-controlled studies conducted before the introduction of SSRIs for OCD treatment [140,141], a single dose of dexamfetamine (D-amphetamine, or dextroamphetamine) 30 mg was found to be superior to placebo in immediately relieving OC symptoms. In addition, the combination of dexamfetamine and amphetamine salts (Adderall 30 mg) was found to be effective when administered as monotherapy in one case report [142] or as SSRI augmentation in a case series of childhood-onset OCD [143]. In an open-label, single-dose study methylphenidate (40 mg) had no significant effect on OCD symptoms [144]. However, methylphenidate monotherapy was found to be effective in two cases of co-morbid ADHD and OCD [145]. Recently Koran *et al.* [146] conducted a 5-week, double-blind, caffeine-controlled study of dexamfetamine in treatment-resistant OCD. In this study half of the subjects receiving dexamfetamine experienced an immediate marked reduction in OC symptoms severity, as did somewhat more than half of those receiving caffeine; the OC symptom improvement associated with both drugs was maintained or increased over the 5 weeks of the study. Caffeine appeared to be slightly more effective, in terms of both the number of responders (33% for dexamfetamine and 50% for caffeine) and the degree of response (mean Y–BOCS score decrease was 48% for dexamfetamine and 55% for caffeine). The authors argued that a possible explanation for the mechanism of this therapeutic effect could be that the increased release of dopamine induced by both drugs may increase D1 receptor stimulation in the prefrontal cortex; this enhancement is associated with improved attention regulation and working memory in patients with ADHD [147]. These functional improvements could lead to fewer obsessive intrusions, increased ability to shift attention away from them, and thus decreased urges to perform compulsions [146].

Glutamatergic agents

Rationale for the use of glutamatergic agents

Recent data support the notion that the excitatory neurotransmitter glutamate seems to play a role in the pathophysiology of OCD, suggesting the existence of a hyperglutamatergic state. A neuroimaging study used proton magnetic resonance spectroscopy to compare drug-naive paediatric OCD patients with healthy controls and found significantly higher caudate nucleus concentrations of GLX (glutamate plus glutamine) in the OCD group [148]. Furthermore, the enhanced glutamate activity normalized after paroxetine treatment [148–150]. Other neuroimaging studies showed similar results [148–152], and glutamate concentration in the cerebrospinal fluid was found to be significantly higher in OCD drug-naive patients compared with healthy controls [153].

The therapeutic action of neurosurgical lesion of part of the anterior limb of the internal capsule also supports the hypothesis of hyperglutamatergic activity in OCD. Because selective damage to this area interrupts the projections of the orbito-frontal cortex (OFC) to the caudate nucleus, and since the efferent axons of the OFC are glutamatergic neurons, it is thus likely that the neurochemical effect of capsulotomies might also be associated with interrupting the presumed increased glutamatergic transmission between the OFC and the caudate nucleus [154]. Genetic studies also highlight the possible implication of glutamate in the pathophysiology of OCD; in particular, a family study that found an association between the NMDA glutamate receptor subunit GRIN2B (glutamate receptor, ionotropic, N-methyl-D-aspartate 2B) and OCD [155]. Another study found an association between OCD and a locus on chromosome 9p24 that codes for the amino acid transporter SLC1A1 (solute carrier family 1, member 1), which is considered to play an important role in extinguishing the action of glutamate and in maintaining the extracellular glutamate concentrations within the reference range [156,157].

Finally, research in animal models also supports an OCD-glutamate association. Welch *et al.* [158] conducted a genetic study on SAPAP3-mutant mice; SAPAP3 (SAP90/PSD95-associated protein 3) is a postsynaptic scaffolding protein in excitatory (glutamatergic) synapses, which is highly expressed in the striatum. In this study the authors showed that mice with a genetic deletion of SAPAP3 exhibit increased anxiety and compulsive grooming behaviour leading to facial hair loss and skin lesions; both behaviours were alleviated by a 6-day fluoxetine treatment [158].

Given the hypothesis of glutamatergic hyperactivity, several researchers are exploring the potential efficacy of glutamate receptor antagonists in order to (theoretically) obtain normalization of glutamate activity.

Glutamatergic agent augmentation

- *Memantine.* This is a non-competitive NMDA receptor antagonist that has been approved by the US Food and Drug Administration for the treatment of Alzheimer disease. Case series [159–161] and several systematic studies [162–164] found memantine to be effective in treatment-resistant OCD. In an open-label trial of memantine augmentation in 14 resistant patients, after 12 weeks of treatment (with a target dose of 20 mg/day), 42.9% of the patients responded to therapy [162]. In a recent single-blinded case-control study memantine showed its efficacy in a case of severe OCD [163]. Finally, in an open-label trial comparing the efficacy of memantine in the treatment of OCD versus GAD (generalized anxiety disorder), it appeared to be preferentially useful in treating OCD symptoms [164].
- *Riluzole.* This is a potent antiglutamatergic agent that reduces glutamatergic neurotransmission in several ways, such as by inhibiting glutamate release, inactivating voltage-dependent sodium channels in cortical neurons, and blocking

of GABA reuptake [165]. In an open-label trial of riluzole (50 mg twice a day) in treatment-resistant OCD patients, 54% of them became full responders (>35% reduction in Y–BOCS scores) and 39% responders [165]. In an open-label pae-diatric study of six OCD-resistant patients, four subjects responded to riluzole treatment [166].

- *Topiramate.* The role of topiramate (an anticonvulsant with glutamatergic prop-erties) in OCD treatment is still unclear. Topiramate in treatment-resistant OCD was found to be an effective approach in a retrospective, open-label case-series [167] and in one case report [168]. Berlin *et al.* [169] conducted the first double-blind, placebo-controlled trial of topiramate augmentation in OCD-resistant pa-tients; in this study, compared to the placebo group, the topiramate augmentation group exhibited a significantly greater decrease in Y–BOCS compulsions but did not differ on Y–BOCS obsessions or total scores. Thus the authors suggest that topiramate may be beneficial for compulsions, but not obsessions [169].
- *N-acetylcysteine (NAC).* This amino acid derivative, thought to attenuate gluta-matergic neurotransmission, was found to be effective as fluvoxamine augmen-tation in a case report of a treatment-resistant patient [170].

Opioids

The opioid system probably seems to be involved in the pathophysiology of OCD, as suggested by various preclinical and clinical evidence [49,171–175]. Although clinical trials have been performed to test the efficacy of opioid agents as augmen-tation in treatment-resistant cases, the results are controversial and currently there is insufficient evidence to support their use. Koran *et al.* [49] compared morphine, lorazepam and placebo in a double-blind study but only one patient had a sufficient response to morphine. In a double-blind trial the opioid antagonist naltrexone did not improve OCD symptomatology and instead caused a worsening of anxiety and depression [171]. However, Shapira and colleagues reported the efficacy of the opioid agonist tramadol (26% reduction of the Y–BOCS score after 2 weeks of treatment) [176].

PHYSICAL THERAPIES

Electroconvulsive therapy (ECT)

Although some case reports suggest the efficacy of ECT in refractory OCD [177, 178], the expert consensus is that it has a very limited role in OCD treatment, as it does not appear to control the core symptoms of OCD [59]. Anyway, it may represent a useful tool in the therapy of OCD comorbidities, such as depression and catatonia [179,180].

Repetitive transcranial magnetic stimulation (rTMS)

There is no clear evidence regarding the use of rTMS in the treatment of OCD. The studies are few and the collected data are inconclusive, due partly to the fact that the study designs differed in many important aspects such as site of stimulation, stimulation parameters, and treatment duration. In double-blind studies with sham rTMS as control, rTMS over the left dorsolateral prefrontal cortex was ineffective [181,182], as it was over the right prefrontal cortex too [183]. More recently, stimulation of the orbitofrontal cortex [184] and of the supplementary motor area [185], considered to be more specific targets on the basis of functional neuroimaging [186–190] and neurophysiological data [191,192], showed a significant reduction of Y–BOCS score when compared to sham stimulation, suggesting that future studies in this direction may lead to interesting results.

Finally, the use of a neuronavigational system, using the patient's brain magnetic resonance imaging (MRI) to position the magnetic coil above the selected cerebral region, could help to individualize and improve the effectiveness of this treatment procedure.

Deep brain stimulation (DBS)

Deep brain stimulation is still an experimental technique and a last resort for the treatment of OCD, but it has recently become a valid alternative to the neurosurgical interventions performed in treatment-resistant patients with extremely disabling symptoms. In DBS procedures, stimulating electrodes are implanted into specific brain regions and a continuous high-frequency electrical stimulus is delivered from an implanted, externally programmable pulse generator. DBS is reversible in that the stimulator can be turned on or off, and the output of the device and degree of stimulation can be controlled at the discretion of the clinician. The stimulation target that has been most widely investigated and has been shown to provide the best results is the anterior limb of the internal capsule (ALIC), the same site that is lesioned in capsulotomy. The stimulation of this area is believed to disrupt the activity in the loop fibres that connect the cortex with the thalamus, theoretically resulting in the interruption of that pathological circuit [193]. DBS in this site was successful in several case series [194–199]. In an open study, DBS was still effective 3 years after implantation [200]. Other targets have been tested with good results, even if on a smaller number of patients. One of the most effective was the nucleus accumbens (NAcc). Part of the ventral striatum, the NAcc is located where the head of the caudate and the anterior portion of the putamen meet, just beneath the ALIC, and is involved in functions ranging from reward processing to motivation and addiction. The NAcc is considered a promising target for DBS because there is evidence of dysfunction of the reward system in OCD. In a study by Figee et al. [201] using a monetary incentive delay task and functional MRI, OCD patients showed attenuated reward anticipation activity in the NAcc compared with healthy controls. In 2003 Sturm *et al.* showed efficacy of right nucleus accumbens stimulation: three of the four patients had total remission over 24–30 months [202]. Recently, Denys *et al.* [203] published a study of 16 patients with NAcc DBS for OCD. This study consisted of an open 8-month treatment phase, followed by a double-blind crossover phase with randomly assigned 2-week periods of active or sham stimulation. It ended with an open 12-month maintenance phase. This resulted in an average 46% symptom decrease after 8 months. Nine of 16 patients were responders during follow-up. These nine individuals had a mean Y–BOCS score decrease of 72% (23.7 points). In the double-blind, sham-controlled phase ($n = 14$), the mean Y–BOCS difference between active and sham stimulation was 25% (8.3 points). Several other studies have shown good efficacy of NAcc stimulation after 1 year of follow-up [204,205].

Very good results were obtained also during a multicentre study based on stimulation of the subthalamic nucleus in 16 patients with severe OCD [206]. In this study the authors used a randomized crossover design with 10 months of active or sham subthalamic stimulation. With active stimulation 10 patients had significant improvement of their symptoms and four recovered (Y–BOCS of 6 or less). However, the good results of this study are limited by the onset of some major adverse events (including a brain haemorrhage) and several minor adverse events. Finally, another case report suggests the efficacy of targeting the inferior thalamic peduncle [207].

FAMILY INTERVENTION

Another important aspect that has to be included in the global evaluation of an OCD patient, particularly a treatment-resistant one, is the impact of the disorder on the family. Patients' families are often involved to a large extent, and the caregiver burden in OCD is similar to that found for other important mental disorders such as schizophrenia [208]. In order to create the optimum therapeutic setting, the clinician has to include the family in the process, to carefully analyze the role of the relationships between the patient and the family, and to suggest the relevant strategy for effective intervention.

CONCLUSIONS AND FUTURE PERSPECTIVES

In conclusion, the therapeutic options for treatment-resistant patients are numerous, ranging from dopaminergic drugs (both agonists and antagonists) to glutamatergic agents, and a number of them seem to have some efficacy. Faced with all these possibilities how can the clinician choose the best one for any individual patient? Current research on animal and human models suggests that the discovery

Table 5.2

Drug	Anatomical and neurofunctional targets	Subjective sensations
Risperidone	ACC (anterior cingulate cortex) → DECISION-MAKING → EXECUTIVE PLANNING	Improvement in pathological doubt, executive planning
Ondansetron	mPFC (medial prefrontal cortex) → PRE-PULSE INHIBITION → STARTLE REFLEX	Negative feelings related to pre-pulse inhibition (PPI) reduced control
Dexamfetamine Caffeine	PFC (prefrontal cortex) → WORKING MEMORY → ATTENTION REGULATION	Increased ability to shift attention away from obsessions
SSRIs	Amygdala → FEAR AND ANXIETY LOOPS	Improvement in anxiety symptoms

of more precise and distinct neurofunctional targets is possible and that it may successfully lead to a patient-tailored treatment algorithm. For example, a treatment based on atypical antipsychotics could in the future be reserved for patients with dysfunction of the anterior cingulate networks [37], as well as ondansetron for those with impairment of the pre-pulse inhibition startle reflex [209,210] and dextroamphetamine for those with deficits in working memory functioning [146] (see Table 5.2). Categorizing patients and basing their treatment on reliable and easily detectable neurodysfunctional targets, in order to offer an evidence-based highly specific therapy, is one of the most desirable and exciting goals that may be achieved in the near future.

REFERENCES

1. CMI group. Clomipramine in the treatment of patients with obsessive-compulsive disorder. The clomipramine collaborative study group. *Arch Gen Psychiatry* 1991;**48**:730–738.
2. Goodman WK, Price LK. Assessment of severity and change in obsessive-compulsive disorder. *Psychiatr Clin N Am* 1992;**15**:861–869.
3. Jenike MA, Rauch SL. Managing the patients with treatment-resistant obsessive compulsive disorder: current strategies. *J Clin Psychiatry* 1994;**55**:11–17.
4. McDougle CJ, Goodman WK, Leckman JF, Price LH. The psychopharmacology of obsessive-compulsive disorder. Implications for treatment and pathogenesis. *Psychiatr Clin N Am* 1993;**15**:749–766.
5. Piccinelli M, Pini S, Bellantonio C, Wilkinson G. Efficacy of drug treatment in obsessive-compulsive disorder: a meta-analytic review. *Br J Psychiatry* 1995;**166**:242–243.

6. Pigott TA, Seay SM. A review of the efficacy of selective serotonin reuptake inhibitors in obsessive-compulsive disorder. *J Clin Psychiatry* 1999;**60**:101–106.

7. Rasmussen SA, Eisen JL, Pato MT. Current issues in the pharmacological management of obsessive-compulsive disorder. *J Clin Psichiatry* 1993;**54**:4–9.

8. Pallanti S, Hollander E, Bienstock C *et al*. Treatment non-response in OCD: methodological issues and operational definitions. *Int J Neuropsychopharmacol* 2002;**5**:181–191.

9. Erzegovesi S, Cavallini MC, Cavedini P, Diaferia G, Locatelli M, Bellodi L. Clinical predictors of drug response in obsessive-compulsive disorder. *J Clin Psychopharmacol* 2001;**21**:488–492.

10. Mataix-Cols D. Deconstructing obsessive-compulsive disorder: a multidimensional perspective. *Curr Opin Psychiatry* 2006;**19**:84–89.

11. Hollander E, Kwon JH, Stein DJ, Broatch J, Rowland CT, Himelein CA. Obsessive-compulsive and spectrum disorders: overview and quality of life issues. *J Clin Psychiatry* 1996;**57**(Suppl. 8):3–6.

12. Dominguez RA, Mestre SM. Management of treatment-refractory obsessive compulsive disorder patients. *J Clin Psychiatry* 1994;**55**:86–92.

13. Dominguez RA. Serotonergic antidepressants and their efficacy in obsessive compulsive disorder. *J Clin Psychiatry* 1992;**52**:56–59.

14. Goodman WK, McDougle CJ, Barr LC, Aronson SC, Price LH. Biological approach to treatment-resistant obsessive-compulsive disorder. *J Clin Psychiatry* 1993;**54**(6 Suppl.):16–26.

15. Pallanti S, Hollander E, Goodman WK. A qualitative analysis of nonresponse: management of treatment-refractory obsessive-compulsive disorder. *J Clin Psychiatry* 2004;**65**(Suppl. 14):6–10.

16. Jefferson JW, Altemus M, Jenike MA, Pigott TA, Stein DJ, Greist JH. Algorithm for treatment of obsessive-compulsive disorder. *Psychopharmacol Bull* 1995;**31**:487–490.

17. Jenike MA. Pharmacologic treatment of obsessive compulsive disorders. *Psychiatr Clin N Am* 1992;**15**:895–919.

18. March JS, Frances A, Kahn DA, Carpenter D. The expert consensus guideline series: treatment of obsessive-compulsive disorder. *J Clin Psychiatry* 1997;**58**(Suppl. 4):3–72.

19. Rasmussen S, Eisen JL. Treatment strategies for chronic and refractory obsessive-compulsive disorder. *J Clin Psychiatry* 1997;**58**(Suppl. 13):9–13.

20. Goodman W, Price L, Rasmussen S *et al*. The Yale-Brown Obsessive-Compulsive Scale (Y-BOCS), part I: development, use, and reliability. *Arch Gen Psychiatry* 1989;**46**:1006–1011.

21. Goodman W, Price L, Rasmussen S *et al*. The Yale-Brown Obsessive-Compulsive Scale (Y-BOCS), part II: validity. *Arch Gen Psychiatry* 1989;**46**:1012–1016.

22. Goodman W, McDougle C, Price L. Pharmacotherapy of obsessive-compulsive disorder. *J Clin Psychiatry* 1992;**43**:29–37.

23. Mavissalakian M, Turner SM, Michelson L, Jacob R. Tricyclic antidepressants in obsessive-compulsive disorder: antiobsessional or antidepressant agents? *Am J Psychiatry* 1985;**142**:572–576.

24. Apter A, Fallon T, King R *et al*. Obsessive-compulsive characteristics: from symptoms to syndrome. *J Am Acad Child Adolesc Psychiatry* 1996;**35**:907–912.

25. Storch EA, Rasmussen SA, Price LH, Larson MJ, Murphy TK, Goodman WK. Development and psychometric evaluation of the Yale–Brown Obsessive-Compulsive Scale – Second Edition. *Psychol Assess* 2010;**22**:223–232.

26. Koran LM. Quality of life in obsessive-compulsive disorder. *Psychiatr Clin N Am* 2000;**23**:509–517.

27. Perugi G, Akiskal HS, Gemingnani A *et al.* Episodic course in obsessive-compulsive disorder. *Eur Arch Psychiatry Clin Neurosci* 1998;**248**:240–244.

28. Ravizza L, Maina G, Bogetto F. Episodic and chronic obsessive-compulsive disorder. *Depress Anxiety* 1997;**6**:154–158.

29. Frank E, Prien R, Jarret R *et al.* Conceptualization and rationale for consensus definitions of terms in major depressive disorder. Remission, recovery, relapse, and recurrence. *Arch Gen Psychiatry* 1991;**48**:851–855.

30. Rasmussen SA, Eisen JL. Treatment strategies for chronic and refractory obsessive-compulsive disorder. *J Clin Psychiatry* 1997;**58**(Suppl. 13):9–13.

31. Pato M, Zohar-Kadouch R, Zohar J, Murphy DL. Return of symptom after discontinuation of clomipramine in patients with obsessive-compulsive disorder. *Am J Psychiatry* 1988;**145**:1521–1525.

32. Pato MT, Hill JL, Murphy DL. A clomipramine dosage reduction study in the course of long-term treatment of obsessive-compulsive disorder patients. *Psychopharmacol Bull* 1990;**26**:211–214.

33. Leonard HL, Swedo SE, Lenane MC *et al.* A double-blind desipramine substitution during long-term clomipramine treatment in children and adolescents with obsessive-compulsive disorder. *Arch Gen Psychiatry* 1991;**48**:922–927.

34. Mundo E, Bareggi S, Pirola R, Bellodi L, Smeraldi E. Long-term pharmacotherapy of obsessive-compulsive disorder: a double-blind controlled study. *J Clin Psychopharmacol* 1997;**17**:4–10.

35. Maina G, Albert U, Bogetto F. Relapses after discontinuation of drug associated with increased resistance to treatment in obsessive-compulsive disorder. *Int Clin Psychopharmacol* 2001;**16**:33–38.

36. Emsley RA. Partial response to antipsychotic treatment: the patient with enduring symptoms. *J Clin Psychiatry* 1999;**60**(Suppl. 23):10–13.

37. Pallanti S, Quercioli L. Treatment-refractory obsessive-compulsive disorder: methodological issues, operational definitions and therapeutic lines. *Prog Neuropsychopharmacol Biol Psychiat* 2006;**30**:400–412.

38. Sheppard BA, Chavira D, Azzam A *et al.* ADHD prevalence and association with hoarding behaviors in childhood-onset OCD. *Depress Anxiety* 2010;**27**:667–674.

39. Magalhães PV, Kapczinski NS, Kapczinski F. Correlates and impact of obsessive-compulsive comorbidity in bipolar disorder. *Compr Psychiatry* 2010;**51**:353–356.

40. Goodman WK, Ward H, Kablinger A, Murphy T. Fluvoxamine in the treatment of obsessive compulsive disorder and related conditions. *J Clin Psychiatry* 1997;**58**(Suppl. 5):32–49.

41. Rasmussen S, Baer L, Eisen J, Shera D. Previous SRI treatment and efficacy of sertraline for OCD: combined analysis of four multicenter trials. Poster presented at the 150th Annual Meeting of the American Psychiatry Association, San Diego, CA, 1997; pp. 17–22.

42. Ackerman D, Grennland S, Bystritsky A. Clinical characteristics of response to fluoxetine treatment of obsessive-compulsive disorder. *J Clin Psychopharmacol* 1998;**18**:185–192.

43. Hollander E, Bienstock C, Koran L *et al.* Refractory obsessive compulsive disorder: state-of-the-art treatment. *J Clin Psychiatry* 2002;**63**(Suppl. 6):20–29.

44. Denys D, van Megen H, van der Wee N, Westenberg H. A double-blind switch study of paroxetine and venlafaxine in obsessive compulsive disorder. *J Clin Psychiatry* 2004;**65**:37–43.

45. Koran L, Aboujaoude E, Ward H *et al.* Pulse-loaded intravenous clomipramine in treatment-resistant obsessive compulsive disorder. *J Clin Psychopharmacol* 2006;**26**:79–83.

46. Koran L, Hanna G, Hollander E *et al.* Practice guideline for the treatment of patients with obsessive-compulsive disorder. *Am J Psychiatry* 2007;**164**(7 Suppl.):1–56.

47. Bogetto F, Maina G, Locatelli M, Lucca A. Terapie biologiche nel DOC. In: Smeraldi E (ed) *Il Disturbo Ossessivo-Compulsivo e Il Suo Spettro*, 3rd edn. Milan: Masson, 2003; pp. 336–366.

48. Marazziti D, Dell'Osso L, Gemignani A *et al.* Citalopram in refractory obsessive-compulsive disorder: an open study. *Int Clin Psychopharmacol* 2001;**16**:215–219.

49. Koran LM, Aboujaoude E, Bullok KD, Franz B, Gamel N, Elliott M. Double-blind treatment with oral morphine in treatment resistant obsessive-compulsive disorder. *J Clin Psychiatry* 2005;**66**:353–359.

50. Dell'Osso B, Mundo E, Marazziti D, Altamura A. Switching from serotonin reuptake inhibitors to duloxetine in patients with resistant obsessive compulsive disorder: a case series. *J Psychopharmacol* 2008;**22**:210–213.

51. Pallanti S, Koran LM. *La Cura del Paziente con Disturbo Ossessivo Compulsivo Resistente*. Milan: Airon Edizione, 2003.

52. Fallon B, Liebowitz M, Campeas R *et al.* Intravenous clomipramine for obsessive-compulsive disorder refractory to oral clomipramine: a placebo-controlled study. *Arch Gen Psychiatry* 1998;**55**:918–924.

53. Koran L, Pallanti S, Quercioli L, Paiva R. Pulse loading versus gradual dosing of intravenous clomipramine in obsessive-compulsive disorder. *Eur Neuropsychopharmacol* 1998;**8**:121–126.

54. Pallanti S, Quercioli L, Koran LM. Citalopram intravenous infusion in resistant obsessive-compulsive disorder: an open trial. *J Clin Psychiatry* 2002;**63**:796–801.

55. Ross S, Fallon BA, Petkova E, Feinstein S, Liebowitz MR. Long-term follow-up study of patients with refractory obsessive-compulsive disorder. *J Neuropsychiatry Clin Neurosci* 2008;**20**:450–457.

56. Abramowitz JS. Does cognitive-behavioral therapy cure obsessive-compulsive disorder? A meta-analytic evaluation of clinical significance. *Behav Ther* 1998;**29**:339–355.

57. Eddy KT, Dutra L, Bradley R, Westen D. A multidimensional meta-analysis of psychotherapy and pharmacotherapy for obsessive-compulsive disorder. *Clin Psychol Rev* 2004;**24**:1011–1030.

58. Fisher PL, Wells A. How effective are cognitive and behavioral treatments for obsessive-compulsive disorder? A clinical significance analysis. *Behav Res Ther* 2005;**43**:1543–1558.

59. Bandelow B, Zohar J, Hollander E, *et al*. World Federation of Societies of Biological Psychiatry (WFSBP) guidelines for the pharmacological treatment of anxiety, obsessive-compulsive and post-traumatic stress disorders – first revision. *World J Biol Psychiatry* 2008;**9**:248–312.

60. Tundo A, Salvati L, Busto G, Spigno D, Falcini R. Addition of cognitive-behavioral therapy for nonresponders to medication for obsessive-compulsive disorders: a naturalistic study. *J Clin Psychiatry* 2007;**68**:1552–1556.

61. Simpson HB, Foa EB, Liebowitz MR. A randomized, controlled trial of cognitive-behavioral therapy for augmentation pharmacotherapy in obsessive-compulsive disorder. *Am J Psychiatry* 2008;**165**:621–630.

62. Storch E, Merlo L, Bengtson M *et al*. D-cycloserine does not enhance exposure-response prevention therapy in obsessive-compulsive disorder. *Int J Psychopharmacol* 2007;**22**:230–237.

63. Kushner MG, Kim SW, Donahue C *et al*. D-cycloserine augmented exposure therapy for obsessive compulsive. *Biol Psychiatry* 2007;**62**:835–838.

64. Wilhelm S, Buhlmann U, Tolin D *et al*. Augmentation of behavior therapy with d-cycloserine for obsessive compulsive disorder. *Am J Psychiatry* 2008;**165**:335–341.

65. Norberg M, Krystal J, Tolin D. A meta-analysis of D-cycloserine and the facilitation of fear extinction and exposure therapy. *Biol Psychiatry* 2008;**63**:1118–1126.

66. Pallanti S, Quercioli L, Paiva R. Citalopram for treatment-resistant obsessive-compulsive disorder. *Eur Psychiatry* 1999;**14**:101–106.

67. Szegedi A, Wetzel H, Leal M, Hartter S, Hiemke C. Combination treatment with clomipramine and fluvoxamine: drug monitoring, safety and tolerability data. *J Clin Psychiatry* 1996;**57**:257–264.

68. Ravizza L, Barzega G, Bellino S, Bogetto F, Maina G. Drug treatment of obsessive-compulsive disorder: long-term trial with clomipramine and selective serotonin reuptake inhibitors (SSRIs). *Psychopharmacol Bull* 1996;**32**:167–173.

69. Koran LM, Sallee FR, Pallanti S. Rapid benefit of intravenous pulse loading of clomipramine in obsessive-compulsive disorder. *Am J Psychiatry* 1997;**154**:396–401.

70. Simeon J, Thatte S, Wiggins D. Treatment of adolescent obsessive-compulsive disorder with a clomipramine-fluoxetine combination. *Psychopharmacol Bull* 1990;**26**:285–290.

71. Pigott TA, L'Heureux F, Hill JL, Bihari K, Bernstein SE, Murphy DL. A double-blind study of adjuvant buspirone hydrochloride in clomipramine-treated patients with obsessive-compulsive disorder. *J Clin Psychopharmacol* 1992;**12**:11–18.

72. Dannon PN, Sasson Y, Hirschmann S, Iancu I, Grunhaus LJ, Zohar J. Pindolol augmentation in treatment-resistant obsessive compulsive disorder: a double-blind placebo controlled trial. *Eur Neuropsychopharmacol* 2000;**10**:165–169.

73. Mundo E, Guglielmo E, Bellodi L. Effect of adjuvant pindolol on the antiobsessional response to fluvoxamine: a double blind placebo-controlled study. *J Clin Psychopharmacol* 1998;**13**:219–224.

74. McDougle C, Price L, Goodman W, Charney D, Heninger GR. A controlled trial of lithium augmentation in fluvoxamine-refractory obsessive-compulsive disorder: lack of efficacy. *J Clin Psychopharmacol* 1991;**11**:175–184.

75. Hewlett WA, Vinogradov S, Agras WS. Clomipramine, clonazepam, and clonidine treatment of obsessive-compulsive disorder. *J Clin Psychopharmacol* 1992;**12**:420–430.

76. Choi YJ. Efficacy of treatment for patients with obsessive-compulsive disorder: a systematic review. *J Am Acad Nurse Pract* 2009;**21**:207–213.

77. Pigott TA, L'Heureux F, Rubenstein CS, Bernstein SE, Hill JL, Murphy DL. A double-blind, placebo controlled study of trazodone in patients with obsessive-compulsive disorder. *J Clin Psychopharmacol* 1992;**12**:156–162.

78. Bloom FE, Morales M. The central 5-HT$_3$ receptor in CNS disorders. *Neurochem Res* 1998;**23**:653–659.

79. Dawes MA, Johnson BA, Ma JZ, Ait-Daoud N, Thomas SE, Cornelius JR. Reductions in and relations between "craving" and drinking in a prospective, open-label trial of ondansetron in adolescents with alcohol dependence. *Addict Behav* 2005;**30**:1630–1637.

80. Costall B, Domeney AM, Naylor RJ, Tyers MB. Effects of the 5-HT3 receptor antagonist, GR38032F, on raised dopaminergic activity in the mesolimbic system of the rat and marmoset brain. *Br J Pharmacol* 1987;**92**:881–894.

81. Di Chiara G, Imperato A. Drugs abused by humans preferentially increase synaptic dopamine concentrations in the mesolimbic system of freely moving rats. *Proc Natl Acad Sci U S A* 1988;**85**:5274–5278.

82. Adinoff B. Neurobiologic processes in drug reward and addiction. *Harv Rev Psychiatry* 2004;**12**:305–320.

83. Chamberlain SR, Menzies L, Hampshire A *et al.* Orbitofrontal dysfunction in patients with obsessive-compulsive disorder and their unaffected relatives. *Science* 2008;**321**:421–422.

84. Hewlett WA, Schmid SP, Salomon RM. Pilot trial of ondansetron in the treatment of 8 patients with obsessive-compulsive disorder. *J Clin Psychiatry* 2003;**64**:1025–1030.

85. Pallanti S, Bernardi S, Antonini S, Singh N, Hollander E. Ondansetron augmentation in treatment-resistant obsessive-compulsive disorder: a preliminary, single-blind, prospective study. *CNS Drugs* 2009;**23**:1047–1055.

86. Soltani F, Sayyah M, Feizy F, Malayeri A, Siahpoosh A, Motlagh I. A double-blind, placebo-controlled study of ondansetron for patients with obsessive-compulsive disorder. *Hum Psychopharmacol* 2010;**25**:509–513.

87. Denys D, Zohar J, Westenberg HG. The role of dopamine in obsessive-compulsive disorder: preclinical and clinical evidence. *J Clin Psychiatry* 2004;**65**(Suppl. 14): 11–17.

88. Pitman RK. Animal models of compulsive behavior. *Biol Psychiatry* 1989;**26**: 189–198.

89. Tizabi Y, Louis VA, Taylor CT, Waxman D, Culver KE, Szechtman H. Effect of nicotine on quinpirole-induced checking behavior in rats: implications for obsessive-compulsive disorder. *Biol Psychiatry* 2002;**51**:164–171.

90. Lochner C, Hemmings SM, Kinnear CJ *et al.* Cluster analysis of obsessive-compulsive spectrum disorders in patients with obsessive-compulsive disorder: clinical and genetic correlates. *Compr Psychiatry* 2005;**46**:14–19.

91. Pauls DL, Towbin KE, Leckman JF, Zahner GE, Cohen DJ. Gilles de la Tourette's syndrome and obsessive-compulsive disorder. Evidence supporting a genetic relationship. *Arch Gen Psychiatry* 1986;**43**:1180–1182.

92. Pauls DL, Alsobrook II JP, Goodman W, Rasmussen S, Leckman JF. A family study of obsessive-compulsive disorder. *Am J Psychiatry* 1995;**152**:76–84.
93. Perani D, Garibotto V, Gorini A *et al*. In vivo PET study of 5HT2A serotonin and D2 dopamine dysfunction in drug naive obsessive-compulsive disorder. *Neuroimage* 2008;**42**:306–314.
94. Westemberg HGM, Fineberg NA, Denys D. Neurobiology of obsessive-compulsive disorder: serotonin and beyond. *CNS Spectr* 2007;**12**:14–27.
95. Bloch MH, Landeros-Weisenberger A, Kelmendi B, Coric V, Bracken MB, Leckman JF. A systematic review: antipsychotic augmentation with treatment refractory obsessive-compulsive disorder. *Mol Psychiatry* 2006;**11**:622–632.
96. Hollander E, Baldini Rossi N, Sood E, Pallanti S. Risperidone augmentation in treatment-resistant obsessive-compulsive disorder: a double-blind, placebo-controlled study. *Int J Neuropsychopharmacol* 2003;**6**:397–401.
97. Bogetto F, Bellino S, Vaschetto P, Ziero S. Olanzapine augmentation of fluvoxamine-refractory obsessive-compulsive disorder (OCD): a 12-week open trial. *Psychiatry Res* 2000;**96**:91–98.
98. McDougle CJ, Goodman WK, Price LH *et al*. Neuroleptic addition in fluvoxamine-refractory obsessive-compulsive disorder. *Am J Psychiatry* 1990;**147**:652–654.
99. Matsunaga H, Nakata T, Hayashida K, Ohya K, Kiriike N, Stein DJ. A long term trial of effectiveness and safety of atypical antipsychotic agents in augmenting SSRI-refractory obsessive-compulsive disorder. *J Clin Psychiatry* 2009;**70**:863–868.
100. McDougle CJ, Goodman WK, Leckman JF, Lee NC, Heninger GR, Price LH. Haloperidol addition in fluvoxamine-refractory obsessive-compulsive disorder: a double-blind, placebo controlled study in patients with and without tics. *Arch Gen Psychiatry* 1994;**51**:302–308.
101. McDougle CJ, Epperson CN, Pelton GH, Wasylink S, Price LH. A double-blind, placebo-controlled study of risperidone addition in serotonin reuptake inhibitor-refractory obsessive-compulsive disorder. *Arch Gen Psychiatry* 2000;**57**:794–801.
102. Erzegovesi S, Guglielmo E, Siliprandi F, Bellodi L. Low dose risperidone augmentation of fluvoxamine treatment in obsessive-compulsive disorder: a double-blind, placebo-controlled study. *Eur Neuropsychopharmacol* 2005;**15**:69–74.
103. Li X, May RS, Tolbert LC, Jackson WT, Flournoy JM, Baxter LR. Risperidone and haloperidol augmentation of serotonin reuptake inhibitors in refractory obsessive-compulsive disorder: a crossover study. *J Clin Psychiatry* 2005;**66**:736–743.
104. Pallanti S, Buchsbaum M, Hollander E. Neuroleptic augmentation in OCD: clinical and neuroimaging of risperidone. Presented at the 13th AEP Congress, Munich, 2–6 April, 2005.
105. Selvi Y, Atli A, Aydin A, Besiroglu L, Ozdemir P, Ozdemir O. The comparison of aripiprazole and risperidone augmentation in selective serotonin reuptake inhibitor-refractory obsessive-compulsive disorder: a single-blind, randomized study. *Hum Psychopharmacol* 2011;**26**:51–57.
106. Shapira NA, Ward HE, Mandoki M *et al*. A double-blind, placebo-controlled trial of olanzapine addition in fluoxetine-refractory obsessive-compulsive disorder. *Biol Psychiatry* 2004;**55**:553–555.

107. Bystritsky A, Ackerman DL, Rosen RM *et al*. Augmentation of serotonin reuptake inhibitors in refractory obsessive-compulsive disorder using adjunctive olanzapine: a placebo-controlled trial. *J Clin Psychiatry* 2004;**65**:565–568.

108. Maina G, Pessina E, Albert U, Bogetto F. 8-week, single-blind, randomized trial comparing risperidone versus olanzapine augmentation of serotonin reuptake inhibitors in treatment-resistant obsessive-compulsive disorder. *Eur Neuropsychopharmacol* 2008;**18**:364–372.

109. Denys D, De Geus F, Van Megen HJ, Westenberg HG. A double-blind, randomized, placebo-controlled trial of quetiapine addition in patients with obsessive-compulsive disorder refractory to serotonin reuptake inhibitors. *J Clin Psychiatry* 2004;**65**:1040–1048.

110. Fineberg NA, Sivakumaran T, Roberts A, Gale T. Adding quetiapine to SRI in treatment-resistant obsessive-compulsive disorder: a randomized controlled treatment study. *Int Clin Psychopharmacol* 2005;**20**:223–226.

111. Carey PD, Vythilingum B, Seedat S, Muller JE, van Ameringen M, Stein DJ. Quetiapine augmentation of SRIs in treatment refractory obsessive-compulsive disorder: a double-blind, randomised, placebo-controlled study [ISRCTN83050762]. *BMC Psychiatry* 2005;**5**:44.

112. Kordon A, Wahl K, Koch N *et al*. Quetiapine addition to serotonin reuptake inhibitors in patients with severe obsessive-compulsive disorder: a double-blind, randomized, placebo-controlled study. *J Clin Psychopharmacol* 2008;**28**:550–554.

113. Diniz JB, Shavitt RG, Pererira CA *et al*. Quetiapine versus clomipramine in the augmentation of selective serotonin reuptake inhibitors for the treatment of obsessive-compulsive disorder: a randomized, open label trial. *J Psychopharmacol* 2010;**24**:297–307.

114. Shapiro DA, Renock S, Arrington E *et al*. Aripiprazole, a novel atypical antipsychotic drug with a unique and robust pharmacology. *Neuropsychopharmacology* 2003;**28**:1400–1411.

115. Da Rocha FF, Correa H. Successful augmentation with aripiprazole in clomipramine-refractory obsessive-compulsive disorder. *Prog Neuropsychopharmacol Biol Psychiatry* 2007;**31**:1550–1551.

116. Sarkar R, Klein J, Kruger S. Aripiprazole augmentation in treatment refractory obsessive-compulsive disorder. *Psychopharmacology (Berl)* 2008;**197**:687–688.

117. Storch EA, Lehmkuhl H, Geffken GR, Touchton A, Murphy TK. Aripiprazole augmentation of incomplete treatment response in an adolescent male with obsessive-compulsive disorder. *Depress Anxiety* 2008;**25**:172–174.

118. Connor KM, Payne VM, Gadde KM, Zhang W, Davidson JRT. The use of aripiprazole in obsessive-compulsive disorder: preliminary observations in 8 patients. *J Clin Psychiatr* 2005;**66**:49–51.

119. Pessina E, Albert U, Bogetto F, Maina G. Aripiprazole augmentation of serotonin reuptake inhibitors in treatment-resistant obsessive-compulsive disorder: a 12-week open-label preliminary study. *Int Clin Psychopharmacol* 2009;**24**:265–269.

120. Muscatello MR, Bruno A, Pandolfo G *et al*. Effect of aripiprazole augmentation of serotonin reuptake inhibitors or clomipramine in treatment-resistant obsessive-compulsive disorder: a double-blind placebo-controlled study. *J Clin Psychopharmacol* 2011;**31**:174–179.

121. Iglesias Garcia C, Santamarina Montila S, Alonso Villa MJ. Ziprasidone as coadjuvant treatment in resistant obsessive-compulsive disorder treatment. *Actas Esp Psiquiatr* 2006;**34**:277–279.

122. McDougle CJ, Barr LC, Goodman WK *et al*. Lack of efficacy of clozapine monotherapy in refractory obsessive-compulsive disorder. *Am J Psychiatry* 1995;**152**:1812–1814.

123. Lykouras L, Alevizos B, Michalopoulou P, Rabavilas A. Obsessive-compulsive symptoms induced by atypical antipsychotics: a review of the reported cases. *Prog Neuropsychopharmacol Biol Psychiatry* 2003;**27**:333–346.

124. Alevizos B, Papageorgiou C, Christodoulou GN. Obsessive-compulsive symptoms with olanzapine. *Int J Neuropsychopharmacol* 2004;**7**:375–377.

125. Diler RS, Yolga A, Avci A, Scahill L. Risperidone–induced obsessive–compulsive symptoms in two children. *J Child Adolesc Psychopharmacol* 2003;**13**(Suppl. 1):89–92.

126. Ke CL, Yen CF, Chen CC, Yang SJ, Chung W, Yang MJ. Obsessive-compulsive symptoms associated with clozapine and risperidone treatment: three case reports and review of the literature. *Kaohsiung J Med Sci* 2004;**20**:295–301.

127. Ozer S, Arsava M, Ertugrul A, Demir B. Obsessive compulsive symptoms associated with quetiapine treatment in a schizophrenic patient: a case report. *Prog Neuropsychopharmacol Biol Psychiatry* 2006;**30**:724–727.

128. Stamouli S, Lykouras L. Quetiapine-induced obsessive-compulsive symptoms: a series of five cases. *J Clin Psychopharmacol* 2006;**26**:396–400.

129. Baker RW, Chengappa KN, Baird JW, Steingard S, Christ MA, Schooler NR. Emergence of obsessive compulsive symptoms during treatment with clozapine. *J Clin Psychiatry* 1992;**53**:439–442.

130. de Haan L, Linszen DH, Gorsira R. Clozapine and obsessions in patients with recent onset schizophrenia and other psychotic disorders. *J Clin Psychiatry* 1999;**60**:364–365.

131. Ertugrul A, Anil Yagcioglu AE, Eni N, Yazici KM. Obsessive-compulsive symptoms in clozapine-treated schizophrenic patients. *Psychiatry Clin Neurosci* 2005;**59**:219–222.

132. Howland RH. Chlorpromazine and obsessive-compulsive symptoms. *Am J Psychiatry* 1996;**153**:1503.

133. Baker RW, Ames D, Umbricht DS *et al*. Obsessive-compulsive symptoms in schizophrenia: a comparison of olanzapine and placebo. *Psychopharmacol Bull* 1996;**32**:89–93.

134. Reznik I, Yavin I, Stryjer R *et al*. Clozapine in the treatment of obsessive-compulsive symptoms in schizophrenia patients: a case series study. *Pharmacopsychiatry* 2004;**37**:52–56.

135. Ghaemi SN, Zarate CA Jr, Popli AP, Pillay SS, Cole JO. Is there a relationship between clozapine and obsessive compulsive disorder? A retrospective chart review. *Compr Psychiatry* 1995;**36**:267–270.

136. Khullar A, Chue P, Tibbo P. Quetiapine and obsessive-compulsive symptoms (OCS): case report and review of atypical antipsychotic-induced OCS. *J Psychiatry Neurosci* 2001;**26**:55–59.

137. Tranulis C, Potvin S, Gourgue M, Leblanc G, Mancini-Marie A, Stip E. The paradox of quetiapine in obsessive-compulsive disorder. *CNS Spectr* 2005;**10**:356–361.

138. Kapur S, Remington G. Serotonin-dopamine interaction and its relevance to schizophrenia. *Am J Psychiatry* 1996;**153**:466–476.

139. Kwon JS, Joo YH, Nam HJ *et al*. Association of the glutamate transporter gene SLC1A1 with atypical antipsychotics-induced obsessive-compulsive symptoms. *Arch Gen Psychiatry* 2009;**66**:1233–1241.

140. Insel TR, Hamilton JA, Guttmacher LB. D-amphetamine in obsessive-compulsive disorder. *Psychopharmacology (Berl)* 1983;**80**:231–235.

141. Joffe RT, Swinson RP, Levitt AJ. Acute psychostimulant challenge in primary obsessive-compulsive disorder. *J Clin Psychopharmacol* 1991;**11**:237–241.

142. Albucher RC Curtis CG. Adderall for obsessive-compulsive disorder. *Am J Psychiatry* 2001;**158**:818–819.

143. Owley T, Owley S, Leventhal B, Cook EH Jr. Case series: Adderall augmentation of serotonin reuptake inhibitors in childhood-onset obsessive-compulsive disorder. *J Child Adolesc Psychopharmacol* 2002;**12**:165–171.

144. Joffe RT, Swinson RP. Methylphenidate in primary obsessive-compulsive disorder. *J Clin Psychopharmacol* 1987;**7**:420–422.

145. Van der Feltz-Cornelis CM. Intractable obsessive-compulsive disorder: comorbidity with unrecognized adult attention-deficit hyperactivity disorder? *J Nerv Ment Dis* 1999;**187**:243–245.

146. Koran LM, Aboujaoude E, Gamel NN. Double-blind study of dextroamphetamine versus caffeine augmentation for treatment-resistant obsessive-compulsive disorder. *J Clin Psychiatry* 2009;**70**:1530–1535.

147. Arnsten AFT. Fundamentals of attention-deficit/hyperactivity disorder: circuits and pathways. *J Clin Psychiatry* 2006;**67**:7–12.

148. Rosenberg DR, MacMaster FP, Keshavan MS, Fitzgerald KD, Stewart CM, Moore GJ. Decrease in caudate glutamatergic concentrations in pediatric obsessive-compulsive disorder patients taking paroxetine. *J Am Acad Child Adolesc Psychiatry* 2000;**39**:1096–1103.

149. Rosenberg DR, MacMillan SN, Moore GJ. Brain anatomy and chemistry may predict treatment response in pediatric obsessive-compulsive disorder. *Int J Neuropsychopharmacol* 2001;**4**:179–190.

150. Bolton J, Moore GJ, MacMillan S, Stewart CM, Rosenberg DR. Case study: caudate glutamatergic changes with paroxetine persist after medication discontinuation in pediatric OCD. *J Am Acad Child Adolesc Psychiatry* 2001;**40**:903–906.

151. Moore GJ, MacMaster FP, Stewart C, Rosenberg DR. Case study: caudate glutamatergic changes with paroxetine therapy for pediatric obsessive-compulsive disorder. *J Am Acad Child Adolesc Psychiatry* 1998;**37**:663–667.

152. Carlsson ML. On the role of cortical glutamate in obsessive-compulsive disorder and attention-deficit hyperactivity disorder, two phenomenologically antithetical conditions. *Acta Psychiatr Scand* 2000;**102**:401–413.

153. Chakrabarty K, Bhattacharyya S, Christopher R, Khanna S. Glutamatergic dysfunction in OCD. *Neuropsychopharmacology* 2005;**30**:1735–1740.

154. El Mansari M, Blier P. Mechanism of action of current and potential pharmacotherapies of obsessive-compulsive disorder. *Prog Neuropsychopharmacol Biol Psychiatry* 2006;**30**:362–373.

155. Arnold PD, Rosenberg DR, Mundo E, Tharmalingam S, Kennedy JL, Richter MA. Association of a glutamate (NMDA) subunit receptor gene (GRIN2B) with

obsessive-compulsive disorder: a preliminary study. *Psychopharmacology (Berl)* 2004;**174**:530–538.

156. Arnold PD, Sicard T, Burroughs E, Richter MA, Kennedy JL. Glutamate transporter gene SLC1A1 associated with obsessive-compulsive disorder. *Arch Gen Psychiatry* 2006;**63**:769–776.

157. Dickel DE, Veenstra-VanderWeele J, Cox NJ *et al*. Association testing of the positional and functional candidate gene SLC1A1/EAAC1 in early-onset obsessive-compulsive disorder. *Arch Gen Psychiatry* 2006;**63**:778–785.

158. Welch JM, Lu J, Rodriguiz RM *et al*. Cortico-striatal synaptic defects and OCD-like behavior in SAPAP3 mutant mice. *Nature* 2007;**448**:894–900.

159. Poyurovsky M, Weizman R, Weizman A, Koran L. Memantine for treatment-resistant OCD. *Am J Psychiatry* 2005;**162**:2191–2192.

160. Pasquini M, Biondi M. Memantine augmentation for refractory obsessive-compulsive disorder. *Prog Neuropsychopharmacol Biol Psychiatry* 2006;**30**:1173–1175.

161. Hezel DM, Beattie K, Stewart SE. Memantine as augmenting agent for severe pediatric OCD. *Am J Psychiatry* 2009;**166**:237.

162. Aboujaoude E, Barry JJ, Gamel N. Memantine augmentation in treatment-resistant obsessive-compulsive disorder. *J Clin Psychopharmacol* 2009;**29**:51–55.

163. Stewart SE, Jenike EA, Hezel DM *et al*. A single-blinded case-control study of memantine in severe obsessive-compulsive disorder. *J Clin Psychopharmacol* 2010;**30**:34–39.

164. Feusner JD, Kerwin L, Saxena S, Bystritsky A. Differential efficacy of memantine for obsessive-compulsive disorder vs. generalized anxiety disorder: an open label trial. *Psychopharmacol Bull* 2009;**42**:81–93.

165. Coric V, Taskiran S, Pittenger C *et al*. Riluzole augmentation in treatment-resistant obsessive-compulsive disorder: an open-label trial. *Biol Psychiatry* 2005;**58**:424–428.

166. Grant P, Lougee L, Hirschtritt M, Swedo SE. An open-label trial of riluzole, a glutamate antagonist, in children with treatment resistant obsessive-compulsive disorder. *J Clin Adolesc Psychopharmacol* 2007;**17**:761–767.

167. Van Ameringen M, Mancini C, Patterson B, Bennet M. Topiramate augmentation in treatment-resistant obsessive-compulsive disorder: a retrospective, open-label case series. *Depress Anxiety* 2006;**23**:1–5.

168. Hollander E, Dell'Osso B. Topiramate plus paroxetine in treatment-resistant obsessive-compulsive disorder. *Int Clin Psychopharmacol* 2006;**21**:189–191.

169. Berlin HA, Koran ML, Jenike MA *et al*. Double-blind, placebo-controled trial of topiramate augmentation in treatment-resistant obsessive-compulsive disorder. *J Clin Psychiatry* 2010;**72**:716–721.

170. Lefleur DL, Pittenger C, Kelmendi B *et al*. N-acetylcysteine augmentation in serotonin reuptake inhibitor refractory obsessive-compulsive disorder. *Psychopharmacology (Berl)* 2006;**184**:254–256.

171. Amiaz R, Fostick L, Gershon A, Zohar J. Naltrexone augmentation in OCD: a double-blind placebo-controlled cross-over study. *Eur Neuropsychopharmacol* 2008;**18**:455–461.

172. McDougle C, Barr L, Goodman W, Price L. Possible role of neuropeptides in obsessive compulsive disorder. *Psychoneuroendocrinology* 1999;**24**:1–24.

173. Roy B, Benkelfalt C, Hill J *et al*. Serum antibody for somatostatin-14 and prodynorphine in patients with obsessive-compulsive disorder, schizophrenia, Alzheimer's desease, multiple sclerosis, and advanced HIV infection. *Biol Psychiatry* 1994;**35**:335–344.

174. Urraca N, Camarena B, Gomez-Caudillo L, Esmer MC, Nicolini H. Mu opioid receptor gene as a candidate for the study of obsessive compulsive disorder with and without tics. *Am J Med Genet B Neuropsychiatr Genet* 2004;**127B**:94–96.

175. Warneke L. A possible new treatment approach to obsessive compulsive disorder. *Can J Psychiatry* 1997;**42**; 667–668.

176. Shapira N, Keck P, Goldsmith T, McConville BJ, Eis M, McElroy SL. Open-label pilot study of tramadol hydrochloride in treatment-refractory obsessive-compulsive disorder. *Depress Anxiety* 1997;**6**:170–173.

177. Strassnig M, Riedel M, Miller N. Electroconvulsive therapy in a patient with Tourette's syndrome and co-morbid Obsessive Compulsive Disorder. *World J Biol Psychiatry* 2004;**5**:164–166.

178. Fukuschi T, Okada Y, Katayama H *et al*. [A case of pregnant woman with severe obsessive-compulsive disorder successfully treated by modified electroconvulsive therapy]. *Seishin Shinkeigaku Zasshi* 2003;**105**:927–932.

179. Hanish F, Friedmann J, Piro J, Gutmann P. Maintenance electroconvulsive therapy for comorbid pharmacotherapy-refractory obsessive-compulsive and schizoaffective disorder. *Eur J Med Res* 2009;**14**:367–368.

180. Casey DA, Davis MH. Obsessive-compulsive disorder responsive to electroconvulsive therapy in an elderly woman. *South Med J* 1994;**87**:862–864.

181. Prasko J, Paskova B, Zalesky R *et al*. The effect of repetitive transcranial magnetic stimulation (rTMS) on symptoms in obsessive compulsive disorder. A randomized, double blind, sham controlled study. *NeuroEndocrinol Lett* 2006;**27**:327–332.

182. Sachdev PS, Loo CK, Mitchell PB, McFarguhar TF, Malhi GS. Repetitive transcranial magnetic stimulation for the treatment of obsessive-compulsive disorder: a double-blind controlled investigation. *Psychol Med* 2007;**37**:1645–1649.

183. Alonso P, Pujol J, Cardoner N *et al*. Right prefrontal repetitive transcranial magnetic stimulation in obsessive-compulsive disorder: a double-blind, placebo-controlled study. *Am J Psychiatry* 2001;**158**:1143–1145.

184. Ruffini C, Locatelli M, Lucca A, Benedetti F, Insacco C, Smeraldi E. Augmentation effect of repetitive transcranial magnetic stimulation over the orbitofrontal cortex in drug-resistant obsessive-compulsive disorder patients: a controlled investigation. *J Clin Psychiatry* 2009;**11**:226–230.

185. Mantovani A, Simpson HB, Fallon BA, Rossi S, Lisanby SH. Randomized sham-controlled trial of repetitive transcranial magnetic stimulation in treatment-resistant obsessive-compulsive disorder. *Int J Neuropsychopharmacol* 2010;**13**:217–227.

186. Baxter LR, Schwartz JM, Mazziotta JC *et al*. Cerebral glucose metabolic rates in nondepressed patients with obsessive-compulsive disorder. *Am J Psychiatry* 1988;**145**:1560–1563.

187. Rubin RT, Villanueva-Meyer J, Ananth J, Trajmar PG, Mena I. Regional xenon 133 cerebral blood flow and cerebral technetium 99m HMPAO uptake in unmedicated patients with obsessive-compulsive disorder and matched normal control subjects:

determination by high-resolution single-photon emission computed tomography. *Arch Gen Psychiatry* 1992;**49**:695–702.

188. Molina V, Montz R, Martin-Loeches M, Jimenez-Viciozo A, Carreras JL, Rubia FJ. Drug therapy and cerebral perfusion in obsessive-compulsive disorder. *J Nucl Med* 1995;**36**:2234–2238.

189. Alptekin K, Degermenci B, Kivircik B *et al.* Tc-99m HMPAO brain perfusion SPECT in drug-free obsessive-compulsive patients without depression. *Psychiatry Res* 2001;**107**:51–56.

190. Yùcel M, Harrison BJ, Wood SJ *et al.* Functional and biochemical alterations of the medial frontal cortex in OCD. *Arch Gen Psychiatry* 2007;**64**:946–955.

191. Greenberg BD, Ziemann U, Harmon A, Murphy DL, Wassermann EM. Decreased neuronal inhibition in cerebral cortex in obsessive-compulsive disorder on transcranial magnetic stimulation. *Lancet* 1998;**352**:881–882.

192. Greenberg BD, Ziemann U, Cora-Locatelli G *et al.* Altered cortical excitability in obsessive-compulsive disorder. *Neurology* 2000;**54**:142–147.

193. Shah DB, Pesiridou A, Baltuch GH, Malone DA, O'Reardon JP. Functional neurosurgery in the treatment of severe obsessive compulsive disorder and major depression: overview of disease circuits and therapeutic targeting for the clinician. *Psychiatry (Edgmont)* 2008;**5**:24–33.

194. Abelson JL, Curtis GC, Sagher O *et al.* Deep brain stimulation for refractory obsessive-compulsive disorder. *Biol Psychiatry* 2005;**57**:510–516.

195. Anderson D, Ahmed A. Treatment of patients with intractable obsessive-compulsive disorder with anterior capsular stimulation. Case report. *J Neurosurg* 2003;**98**:1104–1108.

196. Gabriels L, Cosyns P, Nuttin B, Demeulemeester H, Gybels J. Deep brain stimulation for treatment-refractory obsessive-compulsive disorder: psychopathological and neuropsychological outcome in three cases. *Acta Psychiatr Scand* 2003;**107**:275–282.

197. Nuttin B, Cosyns P, Demeulemeester H, Gybels J, Meyerson B. Electrical stimulation in anterior limbs of internal capsules in patients with obsessive-compulsive disorder. *Lancet* 1999;**354**:1526.

198. Nuttin BJ, Gabriels LA, Cosyns PR *et al.* Long-term electrical capsular stimulation in patients with obsessive-compulsive disorder. *Neurosurgery* 2003;**52**:1263–1272.

199. Nuttin BJ, Gabriels LA, Cosyns PR *et al.* Long-term electrical capsular stimulation in patients with obsessive-compulsive disorder. *Neurosurgery* 2008;**62**:966–977.

200. Greenberg BD, Malone DA, Friehs GM *et al.* Three-year outcomes in deep brain stimulation for highly resistant obsessive-compulsive disorder. *Neuropsychopharmacology* 2006;**31**:2384–2393.

201. Figee M, Vink M, de Geus F *et al.* Dysfunctional reward circuitry in obsessive-compulsive disorder. *Biol Psychiatry* 2011 May 1;**69**(9):867–874. Epub 2011 Jan 26.

202. Sturm V, Lenartz D, Koulousakis A *et al.* The nucleus accumbens: a target for deep brain stimulation in obsessive-compulsive and anxiety disorders. *J Chem Neuroanat* 2003;**26**:293–299.

203. Denys D, Mantione M, Figee M *et al.* Deep brain stimulation of the nucleus accumbens for treatment-refractory obsessive-compulsive disorder. *Arch Gen Psychiatry* 2010;**67**:1061–1068.

204. Huff W, Lenarz D, Schormann M *et al.* Unilateral deep brain stimulation of the nucleus accumbens in patients with treatment-resistant obsessive-compulsive disorder: outcomes after one year. *Clin Neurol Neurosurg* 2010;**112**:137–143.

205. Aouizerate B, Cuny E, Martin-Guehl C *et al.* Deep brain stimulation of the ventral caudate nucleus in the treatment of obsessive-compulsive disorder and major depression. Case report. *J Neurosurg* 2004;**101**:682–686.

206. Mallet L, Polosan M, Jaafari N *et al.* Subthalamic nucleus stimulation in severe obsessive-compulsive disorder. *N Engl J Med* 2008;**359**:2121–2134.

207. Jimenez F, Velasco F, Salin-Pascual R *et al.* Neuromodulation of the inferior thalamic peduncle for major depression and obsessive compulsive disorder. *Acta Neurochir Suppl* 2007;**97**:393–398.

208. Karla H, Kamath P, Trivedi JK, Janca A. Caregiver burden in anxiety disorders. *Curr Opin Psychiatry* 2008;**21**:70–73.

209. Hoenig K, Hochrein A, Quednow BB, Maier W, Wagner M. Impaired prepulse inhibition of acoustic startle in obsessive-compulsive disorder. *Biol Psychiatry* 2005;**57**:1153–1158.

210. Harmer CJ, Reid CB, Ray MK, Goodwin GM, Cowen PJ. 5HT(3) antagonism abolishes the emotion potentiated startle effect in humans. *Psychopharmacology (Berl)* 2006;**186**:18–24.

Clinical Spotlights

CHAPTER 6

Subtypes and Spectrum Issues

Eric Hollander, Steven Poskar and Adriel Gerard

Albert Einstein College of Medicine, Montefiore Medical Center

THE OBSESSIVE-COMPULSIVE SPECTRUM

Introduction

The concept of a spectrum of obsessive-compulsive related disorders has gained prominence in the last 25 years [1–5]. This formulation was developed in response to observations that a number of disparate disorders, including body dysmorphic disorder (BDD), hypochondriasis, and several eating and impulse control disorders (ICDs), all share obsessive thinking and/or compulsive behaviour, the hallmark symptoms of obsessive-compulsive disorder (OCD). Although the content of the obsessions in these obsessive-compulsive spectrum disorders (OCSDs) can differ from those found in OCD [1], they are often significantly similar (e.g. symmetry, illness fears and need for reassurance). That these OCSDs share similar patient characteristics, course, comorbidity, neurobiology and treatment response further justifies that they should be considered as part of a spectrum of related disorders.

Cluster approach

The putative OSCDs can be conceptually divided into three distinct clusters: (i) body image/body sensitization/body weight concern disorders; (ii) ICDs; and (iii) neurological disorders with repetitive behaviours [2] (Figure 6.1). Cognitive preoccupation with the body is the defining characteristic of the first cluster disorders, which include hypochondriasis, body dysmorphic disorder, anorexia nervosa, binge eating disorder and depersonalization disorder. As Hollander [1] notes, these disorders share many structural similarities with OCD, including intense

Obsessive-Compulsive Disorder: Current Science and Clinical Practice, First Edition. Edited by Joseph Zohar.
© 2012 John Wiley & Sons, Ltd. Published 2012 by John Wiley & Sons, Ltd.

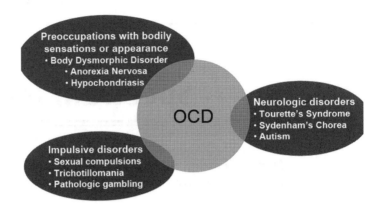

Figure 6.1   Reproduced from Hollander E, Friedberg JP, Wasserman S *et al*. The case for the OCD spectrum. In: Abramowitz JS, Houts AC (eds), *Concepts and Controversies in Obsessive-Compulsive Disorder*. Springer Science + Business Media B.V., 2005. With kind permission from Springer Science + Business Media B.V.

preoccupations that are often experienced as intrusive and anxiety-provoking, as well as engagement in repetitive behaviours, which are performed to reduce the distress caused by the obsessions (e.g. repeated visits to the doctor, requests for reassurance, mirror-checking, repeated cosmetic surgeries). Furthermore, the content of the preoccupations in the first cluster disorders frequently resembles that in OCD (e.g. health issues or symmetry preoccupations). The first cluster disorders and OCD also both involve overvalued ideas and ritualistic behaviours, indicating further overlap.

The second cluster, which is composed of ICDs, is characterized by impulsivity, in particular aggressive behaviours or behaviours that have negative consequences. Similar to those with OCD, individuals with these disorders often experience increased arousal and tension in relation to their impulsive behaviours. However, unlike those with OCD, these individuals typically derive some degree of pleasure from engaging in their impulsive behaviour [4]. In addition to pathological gambling, various sexual disorders, and trichotillomania (TTM), this cluster may be expanded to encompass three new disorders, which are currently being considered for inclusion in the forthcoming fifth edition of the *Diagnostic and Statistical Manual of Mental Disorders* (DSM-5), although they have not been fully validated: compulsive shopping disorder, internet usage disorder, and pathological excoriation (i.e. excessive skin-picking). In addition to their impulsive quality, the second cluster disorders also contain a compulsive element as their impulsive behaviour functions to reduce anxiety [6]. Obsessions are also prominent in many of these disorders; for example, pathological gamblers often have obsessive thoughts about gambling and demonstrate higher levels of obsessionality in comparison to controls [7].

The third cluster contains autism, Sydenham chorea, and Tourette syndrome (TS), disorders that share repetitive motor behaviours and in which obsessions are a less common feature compared to disorders of the first two clusters. A further distinction is evidence suggesting underlying neurological dysfunction in the third cluster disorders. The stereotyped, repetitive behaviours that mark these disorders have been attributed to functional disturbances in the basal ganglia, which have been found in individuals with these disorders [8–10]. The obsessions and compulsions seen in the third cluster disorders differ significantly from those found in OCD. TS, for example, has the distinct characteristics of mental play, echophenomena, touching and self-injurious behaviour [11]. Similarly, autism is distinguished by repetitive ordering, hoarding, telling/asking and touching; concerns about sexuality, religion, contamination and symmetry are less common as are checking, cleaning and counting compulsions, which are commonly seen in OCD [12].

Compulsivity and impulsivity

Initially, the OCSDs were conceptualized as lying along a compulsivity–impulsivity dimension [13–15] (Figure 6.2). Risk aversive/harm avoidant disorders, in which compulsions are performed in an effort to reduce anxiety or perceived threat, were placed at one end of this dimension. These disorders included conditions such as OCD, BDD and anorexia nervosa. At the other extreme of the dimension lay the impulsive/risk-taking disorders, such as sexual compulsions, compulsive shopping, pathological gambling, binge eating and kleptomania. A common characteristic of these disorders is that the individual fails to appreciate future negative

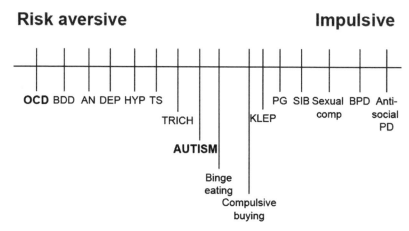

Figure 6.2 Reproduced from Hollander E, Friedberg JP, Wasserman S *et al*. The case for the OCD spectrum. In: Abramowitz JS, Houts AC (eds), *Concepts and Controversies in Obsessive-Compulsive Disorder*. Springer Science + Business Media B.V., 2005. With kind permission from Springer Science + Business Media B.V.

consequences, instead focusing on immediate gratification. However, it has now become evident that many of the OCSDs have both compulsive and impulsive features. As mentioned previously, disorders such as compulsive shopping, sexual compulsions, compulsive internet use and skin picking have both compulsive and impulsive qualities, and are relatively complex. Patients with autism who have many rigid routines and rituals coupled with impulsive-aggressive behaviour can also be included in this group, as can patients with TS who have compulsive rituals and impulsive-aggressive behaviour. So how can this be if compulsivity and impulsivity are diametric opposites? Currently it has been postulated that 'rather than polar opposites, compulsivity and impulsivity may represent key orthogonal factors that each contribute to varying degrees across these disorders' [16].

Repetitive behaviour domain

While initially these disorders were grouped together because they were all perceived to have obsessive-compulsive features, in fact there is more complexity to such a description. First, several of these disorders appear more impulsive than compulsive. Secondly, several of these disorders lack true obsessions. The one unifying feature of OCSDs seems to be that they all involve 'a decreased capacity to extinguish motor responses to affective states' [17]. These motor responses, driven by striatal hyperactivity, are the repetitive thoughts and behaviours seen throughout the obsessive-compulsive spectrum. In this way, all of the OCSDs can be said to be linked by a shared repetitive behaviour domain.

Previously, we have described one way of dividing the OCSDs using three distinct clusters. Alternatively, OCSDs can be subdivided into categories based on the different subtypes of repetitive behaviours displayed in each disorder. Repetitive behaviours can be subdivided into four distinct subtypes, which include: lower-order or motoric repetitive behaviours; higher-order or cognitive repetitive behaviours; reward seeking repetitive behaviours; and hoarding behaviour.

Lower-order repetitive behaviours comprise repetitive sensory and motoric behaviours and are believed to involve the more primitive brain. Examples of lower-order repetitive behaviour include the human stereotypies such as those demonstrated in pervasive developmental disorders and the tics exhibited in tic disorders [18]. The hair pulling seen in TTM and other body-focused repetitive symptoms (e.g. compulsive skin picking) seem to have some relation to these lower-order behaviours, which may serve to modulate self-arousal [19].

Higher-order repetitive behaviours are more cognitively mediated. These include the repetitive thoughts (obsessions) and repetitive behaviours (compulsions) that typify OCD, the recurrent and intrusive preoccupation with imagined ugliness and the compulsive behaviours (e.g. mirror-checking, camouflaging, requests for reassurance) present in BDD, and the preoccupation with illness and reassurance-seeking and body checking seen in hypochondriasis. Higher-order repetitive

behaviours also include the more complex cognitively mediated repetitive behaviours in autism spectrum disorders, such as ritualistic behaviours, preoccupations, desire to maintain sameness, circumscribed interests, repetitive language
and object attachments. Obsessive-compulsive personality disorder (OCPD) also
has what may be termed higher-order repetitive behaviours such as preoccupation
with organization, excessive devotion to work, and inflexible adherence to stan-
dards/rigidity. Compulsions and other higher-order repetitive behaviours may be
seen as a means of reducing anxiety.

In addition to higher-order and lower-order behaviours, a third group of repetitive behaviours have been classified in DSM-IV as ICDs not otherwise specified
or ICDs not otherwise classified and have been termed 'behavioural addictions'
[20,21]. These include pathological gambling, kleptomania, pyromania, impulsive-
compulsive buying disorder, impulsive-compulsive internet usage disorder and
impulsive-compulsive sexual disorder. Like substance addiction, these behaviours
may be initially driven by brain reward systems and then become habitual in nature
[22]. Where these disorders lie on the impulsive-compulsive spectrum remains
controversial. Hoarding appears to be a unique subtype of repetitive behaviour and
will be discussed later in this chapter.

Hollander has suggested that the lower-order repetitive behaviours, which function to mediate arousal, can progress into the cognitively mediated, higher-order
symptoms [23]. Young autistic children, for example, frequently demonstrate perseverative, self-stimulatory behaviours including hand flapping, rocking, finger
flicking, and opening and closing doors. When these children grow older, higher-
order repetitive behaviours such as counting, washing, checking, repetitive re-
questing and repetitive asking for reassurance may supplement and/or supplant
such lower-order repetitive behaviour. In a similar fashion young children with
OCD, or other OCSDs, may engage in comorbid, self-stimulatory TTM. Indeed,
developmental research has indicated a possible age-related trend for repetitive behaviours, with the earlier years being characterized by motor and sensory-related
repetitive behaviours (e.g. stereotypy, TTM) that yield to or are supplemented by
higher-order repetitive thoughts and behaviours (e.g. obsessions, rituals) in the
later years. This seems to correspond to the earlier average age of onset for disorders characterized by motor and sensory-related repetitive behaviours (e.g. autism,
TS and TTM) in comparison to the later onset for the disorders characterized by
the more cognitively mediated repetitive behaviours (e.g. OCD, BDD and OCPD;
Figure 6.3).

Determining placement of proposed OCSDs using cross-cutting domains

In 2006 the following disorders were examined by the the Research Planning Agenda for DSM-5: OCSD Work Group [24] for possible inclusion in

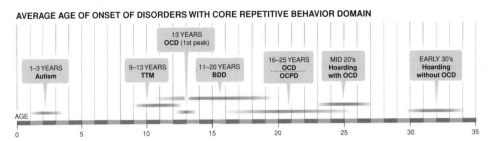

AVERAGE AGE OF ONSET OF DISORDERS WITH CORE REPETITIVE BEHAVIOR DOMAIN

Figure 6.3 Reproduced from Taylor BP, Hollander E. Autism spectrum and obsessive-compulsive disorders. In: Geschwind D, Dawson G, Amaral D (eds), *Autism Spectrum Disorders.* Oxford University Press, 2010 (2011). With kind permission from Oxford University Press.

the newly proposed OCSD category: OCD, OCPD, TS, paediatric autoimmune neuropsychiatric disorder associated with streptococcus (PANDAS), TTM, BDD, autism, eating disorders, Huntington's/Parkinson's, schizo-obsessive, ICDs and substance use disorders. The proposed DSM-5 approach to categorizing OCSDs would certainly help in the screening and diagnosis of these under-recognized and under-treated disorders. Data for each of the disorders examined by the work group were organized into endophenotyping grids, which were created for the important cross-cutting domains including phenomenology (obsessions and compulsions), comorbidity, course of illness, family history, genetic factors, brain circuitry, somatic treatments and CBT. The work group then reviewed the categorized data in order to determine the appropriate placement of each OCSD. The endophenotyping grid (Table 6.1), demonstrates the high comorbidity of OCSDs, such as BDD, TS and TTM in first-degree family members of probands with OCD [25]. Therefore, family history is contributory to establishing the relationship between various disorders and may indicate underlying genetic factors, and thus reflect underlying aetiology. The classification system in DSM-5 will attempt to integrate knowledge of the aetiologies of psychiatric disorders.

The OCSDs have been associated with abnormalities in the fronto-striatal circuitry, in particular caudate hyperactivity. Interestingly, subtle differences in the fronto-striatal-thalamic circuitry may result in different clinical presentations [26]. Further research on brain circuitry may shed light upon both how various disorders are linked and the underlying pathophysiology involved. DSM-5 will attempt to define the relationship between disorders and formulate diagnostic criteria by using measures of pathophysiology (Table 6.2).

The OCSD Work Group examined somatic treatments for each of the candidate disorders. In contrast to other mood and anxiety disorders, selective serotonin reuptake inhibitors (SSRIs) have demonstrated a selective efficacy in the treatment of OCD, whereas norepinephrine (noradrenaline) reuptake inhibitors do not help OCD [27]. Similarly, SSRIs have been shown to have some efficacy in the treatment

Table 6.1 Endophenotyping grid: comorbidity.

	OCPD (LP = 1.7–9%)	TS (LP = 7%)	TMM (LP = 3%) (%)	BDD (LP = 3%)	Eating disorders	ICDs	SUDs (alcohol LP = 12%)
OCD	–	–	13	3–37% of OCD patients had comorbid BDD	Commonly comorbid with AN and BN: 37%	KM: 7–60%; PM: 0%; PG: 1–2%; IED: 10.6%	Mixed data, approximately 14%
OCPD	–	Not associated with TS	8.3				
TS	–	–	3	LP = 3%	–		Less frequent than in OCD
BDD	–	Higher associated with OCD	–	30%	–		
ICDs	–					KM: more than OCD; PG: 22.9%; IED: commonly comorbid	Yes, more strongly than OCD
Trichotillomania	–	Higher associated with OCD	–		–	KM: more than OCD	Yes
Eating disorders	15.2–26%	No known association	9	AN: LP = 4–9%; BN: LP = 6–7%		KM: more than OCD	Yes
SUDs	29.4% alcohol and 25.7% drug	Higher in first-degree relatives of probands with tics	19%	Alcohol LP = 30–43%; other drug: LP = 22–34%	Commonly comorbid in BN, but not in AN	KM: more alcohol dependence than in OCD; PG: SUDs 40–52%, alcohol abuse 18%; IED: SUD = 48%	–

AN, anorexia nervosa; BDD, body dysmorphic disorder; BN, bulimia nervosa; ICD, impulse control disorder; IED, intermittent explosive disorder; KM, kleptomania; LP, lifetime prevalence; OCD, obsessive-compulsive disorder; OCPD, obsessive-compulsive personality disorder; PG, pathological gambling; PM, pyromania; SUD, substance use disorder; TMM, trichotillomania; TS, Tourette syndrome. TMM is separated out of the ICDs because it presents with more compulsive and fewer impulsive characteristics KM, PM and PG.

Source: reproduced from Hollander E, Braun A, Simeon D. Should OCD leave the anxiety disorders in DSM-V? The case for obsessive compulsive-related disorders. *Depress Anxiety* 2008,**25**:317–329. Courtesy of Wiley-Liss, Inc.

Table 6.2 Endophenotyping grid: brain circuitry.

OCD	OCPD	TS	TMM	BDD	Eating disorders	ICDs	SUDs
Hyperactivity in orbital frontal cortex (OFC)					AN and BN: persistent serotonin and dopamine alteration after recovery associated with anxiety and harm avoidance suggesting that these are trait-related. Some evidence implicating limbic (especially reward circuits) and caudate-associative/cognitive pathways including parietal lobe	KM: frontal lobe trauma, degeneration, parietal tumour; PG: ventro-medial PFC decreased activity, anterior cingulated gyrus, and nucleus accumbens involvement; IED: frequently reduced activity of frontal lobe and serotonergic activity; PM: no data	Yes, like OCD
Hyperactivity in caudate nucleus				Yes but leftward shift in CN asymmetry, whereas rightward shift in OCD			Yes, like OCD
Hyperactivity in thalamus				Because of impaired verbal and nonverbal memory compared to healthy controls, corticostriatal systems are implicated			Yes, like OCD

Hyperactivity in anterior
cingulated cortex
Pathological correlation of
activity in these structures
in untreated state in
treatment-responsive
patients

Same regions activated
further when symptoms
are provoked
Frontal-subcortical activity
decreased with
successful treatment
Distinct correlations with
specific symptom factors

Yes, like OCD

Additional brain regions
implicated including
amygdala, striatum
(including ventral striatum),
temporal gyri, posterior
cingulate, insula, motor
cortex, hippocampus,
cerebellum, parietal cortex,
occipital cortex, brain stem
(VTA, LC) implicated;
motivational neurocircuitry
involving cortico-striato-
thalamo-cortical circuitry
implicated

AN, anorexia nervosa; BDD, body dysmorphic disorder; BN, bulimia nervosa; CN, caudate nucleus; KM, kleptomania; LC, locus ceruleus; OCD, obsessive-compulsive disorder; OCPD, obsessive-compulsive personality disorder; PFC, prefrontal cortex; TS, Tourette syndrome; VTA, ventral tegmental area.
Source: reproduced from Hollander E, Braun A, Simeon D. Should OCD leave the anxiety disorders in DSM-V? The case for obsessive compulsive-related disorders. *Depress Anxiety* 2008,**25**:317–329. Courtesy of Wiley-Liss, Inc.

Table 6.3 Research Planning Agenda for DSM-5 Work Group suggested criteria for OCRDs.

Suggested diagnostic criteria for OCRDs
(1) Phenomenology
(a) Obsessions and/or compulsions
(b) Course
(2) Comorbidity
(3) Family history
(4) Fronto-striatal brain circuitry i.e., caudate hyperactivity
(5) Treatment response

DSM-5, Diagnostic and Statistical Manual of Mental Disorders, 5th edition (in preparation); OCRD, obsessive-compulsive-related disorder.
Source: reproduced from Hollander E, Braun A, Simeon D. Should OCD leave the anxiety disorders in DSM-V? The case for obsessive compulsive-related disorders. *Depress Anxiety* 2008,**25**:317–329. Courtesy of Wiley-Liss, Inc.

of other OCSDs such as kleptomania [28] and binge eating disorder [29]. This too may provide partial support for a grouping of OCSDs.

After much debate, the work group decided not to include behavioural addictions, such as pathological gambling, pyromania, kleptomania, compulsive buying, internet addiction, binge eating and compulsive sexual behaviour within the OCSDs. Instead, the work group created a parallel category, behavioural and substance addictions, which would encompass both substance use and ICDs/behavioural addictions. Both substance and behavioural addictions may share similarly altered brain circuitry, including deficits in frontal lobe and nucleus accumbens activity associated with reward/behavioural motivation circuitry, which may lead to impulsive choice [30,31]. This is demonstrated by opting for small, immediate reinforcement despite long-term negative consequences. After reviewing the endophenotyping grids for each of the proposed disorders, the work group decided upon five criteria for possible inclusion of a disorder into the OCSD category (Table 6.3). The strength of placement of each disorder in the overall OCSD category was determined by using these criteria (Table 6.4).

Obsessive-compulsive spectrum nosology

Once the category of OCSDs has been established, the question remains how these disorders should be considered in relation to other psychiatric disorders. There are multiple possible formulations. For example, the OCSDs can be considered as an isolated group of disorders. Alternatively, the OCSDs can be assigned to the anxiety disorders category, although there are several arguments against such a placement. While anxiety is a symptom in many OCSDs, it is also a common

Table 6.4 List of DSM-5 OCRDs, denoting each disorder's strength of placement within this category based on examination of the endophenotyping grids (Tables 6.1–6.2).

DSM-5 obsessive-compulsive-related disorders	Strength of placement
OCD	Very strong
OCPD	Moderate
Tourette syndrome	Strong
Grooming disorders	Moderate
Trichotillomania	Moderate
Excoriation (picking)	Mild
Nail biting	Mild
BDD	Strong
Eating disorders	Moderate

BDD, body dysmorphic disorder; DSM-5, Diagnostic and Statistical Manual of Mental Disorders, 5th edition (in preparation); OCD, obsessive-compulsive disorder; OCRD, obsessive-compulsive-related disorder.
Source: reproduced from Hollander E, Braun A, Simeon D. Should OCD leave the anxiety disorders in DSM-V? The case for obsessive compulsive-related disorders. *Depress Anxiety* 2008,**25**:317–329. Courtesy of Wiley-Liss, Inc.

symptom in mood and psychotic disorders making it relatively non-specific. But whereas anxiety is the core phenomenological feature of the anxiety disorders, the core phenomenological features of the OCSDs are the repetitive thoughts and behaviours. In terms of neurocircuitry, the OCSDs appear to be predominantly mediated by abnormal functioning of fronto-striatal circuits whereas abnormal functioning of the amygdala-centred 'fear-circuitry' appears to drive the anxiety disorders. These respective circuits appear to be regulated by different, but overlapping, neurotransmitter systems. While serotonin and dopamine predominate in the fronto-striatal circuits, serotonin, norepinephrine and gamma-aminobutyric acid (GABA) primarily mediate the amygdala-centred fear circuitry. Much of what we know about the neurotransmitters mediating these circuits is derived from medication studies, which also highlight important differences between the OCSDs and the anxiety disorders. As mentioned previously SSRIs have selective efficacy in the treatment of OCD. This appears to be the case in BDD as well, with both disorders being non-responsive to selective norepinephrine reuptake inhibitors [32]. This is in contrast to the anxiety disorders, which respond to both serotonergic and non-serotonergic antidepressants. The response to benzodiazepines also separates OCD proper from the remaining anxiety disorders as benzodiazepines have clear efficacy in a wide range of anxiety disorders with the noted exception of OCD. This also appears to be the case for BDD. Furthermore, both OCD and BDD commonly require higher doses and longer duration of antidepressant treatment before a response is seen compared to the anxiety disorders. These differences in

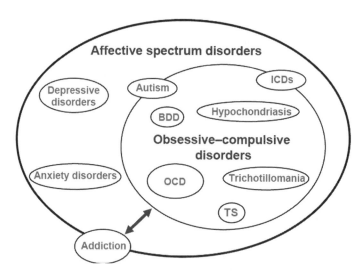

Figure 6.4 Reproduced from Hollander E, Kim S, Khanna S *et al.* Obsessive-compulsive disorder and obsessive-compulsive spectrum disorders: diagnostic and dimensional issues. *CNS Spectr* 2007;**12**(2 Suppl. 3), pp. 5–13. With kind permission from MBL Communications, Inc.

phenomenology, neurocircuitry, neurotransmitters and treatment response suggest that the OCSDs should not be placed within the anxiety disorders category.

Another option is to place the OCSDs in a larger, supraordinate group alongside the anxiety disorders, post-traumatic stress disorder (PTSD), and the dissociative disorders. This would be more consistent with the current International Classification of Diseases, Tenth Revision (ICD-10) classification in which the category neurotic, stress-related and somatoform disorders is a supraordinate group under which the separate categories consisting of anxiety disorders, OCD, somatoform disorders, dissociative disorders and adjustment disorders are subsumed. One may also view the OCSDs as part of a larger supraordinate grouping of 'affective spectrum disorders', which would include the anxiety disorders as well as the depressive disorders (Figure 6.4). One of the more interesting alternatives would be to view the OCSDs as a group of disorders bridging the affective disorders and the addiction disorders (Figure 6.5). In this model, the more cognitive, higher order OCSDs, like BDD and OCD proper, are positioned closer to the affective end and the more motoric, lower order OCSDs, like TTM and TS, are placed closer to the addictive end. The ICDs can be conceptualized as a group that bridges the OCSDs and the addictive disorders.

Obsessive-compulsive disorder, the prototypical OCSD, has several core characteristics, such as loss of voluntary control, repetitiveness, compulsiveness, reinforced behaviours, aberrant habit learning and uncertainty, which resemble addictive behaviour and suggest that similar brain mechanisms may be involved in OCD and behavioural addictions. [33]. Additionally, addiction researchers highlight the

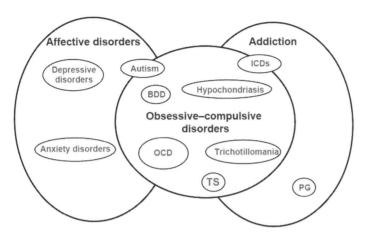

Figure 6.5 Reproduced from Hollander E, Kim S, Khanna S *et al.* Obsessive-compulsive disorder and obsessive-compulsive spectrum disorders: diagnostic and dimensional issues. *CNS Spectr* 2007;**12**(2 Suppl. 3), pp. 5–13. With kind permission from MBL Communications, Inc.

'compulsive' nature of addictions, and look to OCD as a model of addictions: 'In particular, ritualistic-compulsive actions share similarities with addictive behaviour' [33]. Although the role of serotonin has been the focus of most research and theorizing about OCD, accumulating evidence suggests abnormal dopamine activity may play a key role in compulsive/addictive elements of OCD, so OCD and addictions may share similar abnormalities in cortico-striato-thalamic circuitry modulated by ascending dopaminergic innervation.

The likely importance of dopamine has been noted over the years [34,35] and recently Denys and his colleagues [33,36] reviewed the extensive evidence that has become available and described dopaminergic models of OCD, two of which are of interest here: the behavioural addiction model and the cortico-striatal model.

The behavioural addiction model of OCD is particularly intriguing as it fits with the phenomenology and behavioural features of OCD, as well as with the cognitive behavioural model of OCD, which is based in learning theory, and with the biological findings. OCD and addictions have many similarities. On the surface the compulsive rituals of OCD are behaviourally similar to established addictions; these similarities include the loss of voluntary control, as well as the compulsiveness and repetitiveness of habits. Although the motivations may seem dissimilar (i.e., OCD rituals seek to avoid or neutralize harm and addictive behaviours seem to seek pleasure), in both cases the goal of the behaviours is reward. Additionally, it has been observed that addictions change over time, from the initial stages where the individual is seeking pleasure to later stages where there is a loss of control over the behaviour and it becomes compulsive. Thus, over time, addictions seem to become very similar to OCD. Everitt and Robbins [37] have argued, based on biological findings and explained by basic pavlovian and instrumental learning principles, that this change in the character of addiction results from a shift from prefrontal cortical to striatal control over drug-seeking and drug-taking behaviour and a progression from ventral to more dorsal striatal areas involving dopaminergic innervation. Conversely over time the compulsions in OCD may become reinforcing and a shift could possibly be seen from more dorsal to more ventral striatal areas. It is clear that midbrain dopamine is positively reinforcing and plays a role in addictions; likewise, the reinforcing nature of OCD rituals may be due to increased dopamine transmission. The hypothesis of increased midbrain dopamine neurotransmission is consistent with the corticostriatal model of OCD [33]. This widely endorsed model posits an imbalance of the direct versus the indirect pathways, resulting in a hyperactive circuit that leads to the repetitive behavioural rituals of OCD [38]. The importance of dopamine in the pathophysiology of OCD is evident from many different areas of research. These areas include: pharmacological treatment and challenges; animal models; imaging; genetics; and neuropsychology.

OCD SUBTYPES: UNDERSTANDING THE HETEROGENEITY OF OCD

Obsessive-compulsive disorder continues to fascinate the public, as well as clinicians and researchers, in large part due to the seemingly endless variation in OCD symptom presentation. Some experts see this heterogeneity as evidence that OCD is actually not a singular entity. Subtyping is an attempt to parse a heterogeneous group into more homogeneous subgroups. As explained by Robins and Guze in their seminal article on diagnostic validity in psychiatric illness, 'homogenous diagnostic grouping provides the soundest base for studies of etiology, pathogenesis, and treatment. The roles of heredity, family interactions, intelligence, education and sociological factors are most simply, directly and reliably studied when the group studied is as homogenous as possible' [39]. Multiple systems of subtyping OCD have developed throughout the years. Three candidate subtypes that are currently under consideration for inclusion in DSM-5 are tic-related OCD, early-onset OCD and PANDAS. As each of these subtypes is associated with onset in childhood, they will be described in Chapter 7.

Dimensional approach

One of the most studied systems of subtyping is commonly referred to as the 'dimensional approach'. The dimensional approach to subtyping is based on the observation that while the variety of different symptom presentations in OCD seems endless, in fact the thematic content of obsessions and compulsions appears to fall into some predictable themes or 'symptom dimensions'. Factor analysis of the the Y–BOCS Symptom Checklist was originally done by Baer in 1994 [40]. In a sample of 107 patients, he found that symptoms loaded primarily on three factors: symmetry/hoarding, contamination/cleaning and pure obsessions. Since that time, multiple other factor analyses of the Y–BOCS Symptom Checklist have been done in both adults and children, with some finding as few as three or as many as six factors. In a systematic meta-analalyis that included 5124 patients from 21 different studies, Bloch *et al.* [41] found that symptoms loaded on four dimensions: forbidden thoughts (harm, aggressive, sexual, religious and somatic obsessions and checking compulsions); symmetry/ordering; contamination/cleaning; and hoarding symptoms. This dimensional approach to OCD offers to address the apparent heterogeneity and temporal stability of symptoms and provides an innovative method to enhance research in comorbidity, response to treatment, and genetic, familial and neurological studies. Using this method, several studies have indicated assocations between certain comorbid disorders and shared symptom domains.

Due to variability in OCD aetiology, determining genetic markers of the disorder is difficult. This approach of breaking down the heterogeneous phenotypes into symptom dimensions may facilitate new methods of studying genetic susceptibility. While the research in this area is sparse, there have been some significant findings. For example, the OCD Collaborative Genetics Study Group found robust sibling-sibling intraclass correlations for both the hoarding and forbidden thoughts dimensions. Both the contamination/cleaning and symmetry/ordering dimension also showed significant familiality, albeit smaller [42] (for more details, see Chapter 11).

Neuropsychological studies of OCD symptom dimensions have shown that those with high scores in the hoarding domain had poor decision-making, and OCD patients scoring high in symmetry and ordering symptoms had impaired set-shifting [43]. While neuroimaging studies have consistently shown orbitofrontal cortex involvement in obsessive-compulsive symptoms, the contribution of other areas of brain circuitry in OCD is less clear. Applying the symptom dimensions approach may help account for differences between individuals as suggested in some studies that show correlations between obsessive-compulsive symptoms and different neural activities, which may in turn mediate the manifestation of these symptoms. One study of OCD patients with predominantly contamination/cleaning symptoms showed activation in both the visual regions of the brain and the insular cortex when shown washer-relevant pictures [44]. Both of these regions have been linked to disgust perception (for more details, see Chapter 5, Table 5.2).

The heterogeneity of OCD can also be seen when looking at differences in response to treatment. Studies incorporating the dimensional approach may help determine predictors of treatment response. For example, some studies have shown that the presence of sexual obsessions is a predictor of non-response to SSRIs [45–47], while aggressive obsessions without the presence of sexual obsessions was predictive of good response to SSRIs or clomipramine [48]. Multiple studies have shown that high scores on the symmetry/ordering dimension are correlated with a poorer response to SSRIs and clomipramine alone [48–51]. These data are not surprising in light of the fact that the tic-related subtype of OCD, which has been reported to have a high incidence of symmetry/ordering obsessions and compulsions, may have better response to augmentation with neuroleptics than non-tic OCD [52,53]. The hoarding dimension has classically been known to have a poor response to treatment with serotonin reuptake inhibitors (SRIs). While some studies have supported this assertion [54–56], others have found no difference in response to SRIs between hoarding and non-hoarding OCD patients [45,46,57, 58]. In terms of psychotherapy, hoarding has been consistently shown to have poorer response to CBT [26,59–62], which is the gold standard for treatment of OCD.

The dimensional approach has some limitations, including appropriate tools for measurement of symptoms, methods of analysis, and questions on the validity of the Y–BOCS Symptom Checklist.

Associated symptom domains

Thus far, we have examined the issues of the obsessive-compulsive spectrum and of OCD subtypes separately. Alternatively, they can both be viewed through the lens of core and associated symptom domains. The core symptom domain of both the OCD subtypes and OCSDs are repetitive thoughts and behaviours while the associated symptom domains may include features such as impulsivity, insight, tics (motor and/or sensory), reward sensitivity, attention, mood instability, anxiety and social functioning (Figure 6.6). Each of these associated domains can affect phenotypic expression of the core symptom domain as well as the course of illness, comorbidity and treatment response.

As opposed to a completely categorical approach, we may instead view each of these associated domains as a dimensional construct. For example, 'a patient might score high on tics, low on insight, and high on impulsivity; this pattern of symptoms could be used to describe many patients who are currently classified (arguably only artifactually) as having OCD comorbid with a motor tic disorder' [63], which is currently being considered for DSM-5 as an OCD subtype. A patient with autism would also score high on impulsivity and tics (motor and/or sensory) as well as on anxiety, but would score low on attention and social functioning. This approach has clear implications for clinical practice. It would remind clinicians to assess for these associated symptom domains as opposed to ending their inquiry prematurely after making a categorical diagnosis. This would, in turn, increase the likelihood of treatment for these associated domains, the lack of which may contribute to treatment resistance of core symptoms. This approach leads to a more individually tailored treatment focusing on each patient's unique clinical presentation.

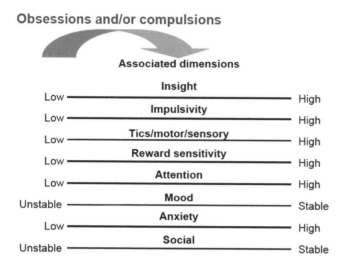

Figure 6.6 Reproduced from Hollander E, Kim S, Khanna S *et al.* Obsessive-compulsive disorder and obsessive-compulsive spectrum disorders: diagnostic and dimensional issues. *CNS Spectr* 2007;**12**(2 Suppl. 3), pp. 5–13. With kind permission from MBL Communications, Inc.

Compulsive hoarding: OCPD, OCD subtype, dimension, OCSD or something else?

The nosology of hoarding is a complex issue due to hoarding's historical association with certain disorders and its heterogeneity of phenomenology. In the *Diagnostic and Statistical Manual of Mental Disorders, Fourth Edition, Text Revision* (DSM-IV-TR), hoarding is listed as one of the eight criteria for OCPD. While commonly considered a symptom of OCD as well, hoarding is conspicuously absent from the examples of obsessive-compulsive symptoms listed in the DSM-IV-TR description of OCD. However, in the differential diagnosis section on OCPD, it states that if hoarding is extreme, a diagnosis of OCD should be considered. So is hoarding a symptom of both OCPD and OCD? An increasing amount of evidence suggests that in most cases of hoarding the answer is usually neither.

Is hoarding a symtom of OCPD? Data from a sample of 2237 patients from a Norwegian network of psychotherapeutic day hospitals that specialized in the treatment of personality disorders, was studied by Hummelen *et al.* [64]. They found only weak correlations between the hoarding criterion and the remaining OCPD criteria. They concluded that the removal of hoarding behaviour, as well as miserliness, may improve the OCPD construct. Similar conclusions were drawn from other studies [65,66]. Pertussa *et al.* [67] looked at four patient groups, which included patients who exhibited symptoms of hoarding minus OCD, OCD plus hoarding, OCD minus hoarding, and anxiety disorders. They found that once the hoarding criterion was removed from OCPD, the number of patients who fulfilled

OCPD criteria was comparable in the four patient groups. These results correspond to similar findings by Frost *et al.* [68]. Both studies lend further credence to the position that compulsive hoarding and OCPD are unrelated conditions. This conclusion is in line with the ICD-10, in which Anancastic Personality Disorder (which corresponds with the DSM-IV diagnosis of OCPD) does not include hoarding or miserliness in its criteria.

Is hoarding a symptom dimension and/or a subtype of OCD? In recent studies of OCD symptom dimensions, hoarding has consistently been found to be an independent factor within OCD. This was recently confirmed in a meta-analyis of over 5000 OCD patients by Bloch *et al.* [41]. They found hoarding to be a distinct factor in both adult and paediatric patients. However, such studies still do not indicate whether hoarding is truly a dimension/subtype of OCD, for several reasons. First, it is unclear how many of these patients would still be diagnosed with OCD if hoarding symptoms were not counted towards the diagnosis. We also know that these studies focus on patients with a diagnosis of OCD and therefore a large number of patients who hoard but do not exhibit other OCD symptoms are often not included. Lastly, we do not know in patients who have both hoarding and other OCD symptoms whether the hoarding symptoms are part of the OCD or a distinct comorbid conditon.

Multiple studies have shown that the majority of patients with hoarding display no other OCD symptoms [68–70]. The most striking of these was an epidemiological study by Samuels *et al.* of compulsive hoarding [70], which found that not one of the participants with compulsive hoarding fulfilled the diagnostic criteria for OCD. This suggests that hoarding is not a symptom of OCD. Differences in the phenomenology of compulsive hoarding and OCD also suggest that hoarding is neither a symptom nor a subtype of OCD. One such difference is the fact that hoarding is an ego-syntonic behaviour [71], which can often bring pleasure and is therefore positively reinforced. This positive reinforcement is the type of conditioning that we see in impulse control disorders. This is in contrast to the compulsions seen in OCD, which are classically ego-dystonic and negatively reinforced due to their ability to reduce anxiety. A study by Frost *et al.* provides further evidence of a link between hoarding and ICDs [72]. This study found that 61% of compulsive hoarders met criteria for a diagnosis of compulsive buying and approximately 85% reported excessive acquisition, with family informants indicating that nearly 95% exhibited excessive acquisition. Furthermore, Samuels *et al.* found OCD patients with hoarding showed greater comorbidity with trichotillomania and skin picking than those without hoarding [73].

Neuroimaging studies have also suggested that hoarding is a distinct entity from OCD [74]. In a study using [18F]-fluorodeoxyglucose positron emission tomography (FDG-PET), Saxena *et al.* found that medication-free compulsive hoarders had a different pattern of baseline cerebral glucose metabolism than both non-hoarding OCD patients and controls [75]. Compulsive hoarders did not demonstrate the hypermetabolism in the orbitofrontal cortex, caudate and thalamus that has been associated with non-hoarding OCD patients [75,76]. Instead, significantly lower metabolism in the posterior cingulate cortex (PCC) was evident among the compulsive hoarders group compared to controls. An additional finding was that lower activity in the dorsal anterior cingulate cortex (ACC) and anterior medial thalamus significantly correlated with greater hoarding severity [75].

In an effort to replicate their findings, Saxena *et al.* conducted another FDG-PET study involving 20 medication-free adults with compulsive hoarding syndrome and 18 age- and gender-matched healthy controls [77]. In comparison to controls, the study showed that compulsive hoarders had significantly lower glucose metabolism in the bilateral dorsal and ventral ACC, while no differences were found in the brain regions commonly associated with OCD. Similar to their previous study, the authors found that greater hoarding severity was significantly correlated with lower relative activity in the right dorsal ACC, as well as in the right PCC and bilateral putamen. They concluded from their findings that compulsive hoarding appears to be a neurobiologically distinct disorder with unique abnormalities in brain function that do not overlap with those seen in non-hoarding OCD. More on brain imaging can be found in Chapter 10.

It would appear that while often comorbid with OCD, compulsive hoarding is in fact a distinct disorder. However, in a minority of cases of hoarding comorbid with OCD the hoarding does appear to be a symptom of the OCD. In a study looking at hoarders with and without comorbid OCD, Pertusa *et al.* [78] found that the majority of hoarding behaviour was phenomenologically similar in both groups and in line with a distinct compulsive hoarding disorder in which things of sentimental and/or intrinsic value were hoarded. However, the authors found that the hoarding of a subgroup, comprising approximately one-quarter of the subjects in the hoarding with OCD group, was of a significantly different character. These subjects often hoarded bizarre items and their hoarding behaviour appeared to be associated with symptoms typically found in OCD, including checking rituals, magical thinking regarding feared consequences, and the need for symmetry. The hoarding in these patients was more severe and disabling. Pertusa *et al.* stated that it is unclear whether the hoarding in this subgroup of patients represents a primary symptom dimension of OCD or a behaviour that is secondary to other OCD symptom dimensions [78].

Is compulsive hoarding an OCSD? As previously noted, compulsive hoarding phenomenologically has similarities to the impulse control disorders in that hoarding behaviour is ego-syntonic, often pleasurable and positively reinforced. This is quite different from the compulsions of OCD, which are classically ego-dystonic and negatively reinforced due to their ability to reduce anxiety. In addition, the vast majority of compulsive hoarders indulge in excessive acquisition or compulsive buying, which despite the descriptor of 'compulsive', appears to be more impulsive than compulsive. Yet some symptoms seen in compulsive hoarding do appear similar to those found in OCD. Patients' fears of discarding something of importance, which leads to hoarding behaviour, can be viewed as equivalent to OCD obsessions, while the avoidance of discarding objects and the urge to save items can be viewed as compulsions [78]. A recent study by Frost *et al.* [79] demonstrated that while hoarders had a high level of comorbidity with OCD (18%), they also had high levels of comorbidity with major depression (53%), generalized anxiety disorder (24%), and social phobia (24%) [79]. These data, along with the very high comorbidity of compulsive buying with hoarding [67], make it difficult to draw any conclusions about the nosology of hoarding based on comorbidity. However, in looking at a sample of OCD patients with and without hoarding, Samuels *et al.* [73] found hoarders to have a greater prevalence of symmetry obsessions, counting compulsions and ordering compulsions. Furthermore, hoarding and tics were more frequently encountered in the first-degree relatives of hoarding probands in comparison to non-hoarding probands. This relationship with tics and symmetry obsessions may be evidence of a link between hoarding and the proposed tic-related OCD subtype in which patients commonly have symmetry obsessions. This relationship therefore may be seen as evidence that hoarding should be considered an OC spectrum condition.

This section has presented the complexities in the nosology of hoarding and its unclear relationship with OCD. While hoarding seems to involve different neurocircuitry and may respond to treatment differently than OCD, there is a clear clinical overlap between them, as described above. Nevertheless, it may be premature to assign hoarding to the OCSD group as it also has been linked to affective/anxiety disorders and ICDs. Since hoarding has been predominantly studied in patients who have OCD, research in the non-OCD population may provide further direction in the classification of hoarding.

CONCLUSION

This chapter reviews various approaches to conceptualizing OCSDs, which including describing disorder clusters, distinct repetitive behaviour subtypes, and associated symptom domains. The appropriate placement of these OCSDs in relation to other neuropsychiatric disorders is also discussed as well as different methods of subtyping OCD. Lastly, this chapter explores the complicated nosology of hoarding. Our understanding of the OCSDs, OCD subtypes and hoarding continues to grow and will likely be advanced in the future through endophenotyping research. Such research may be the key to understanding the biological underpinnings of these complex disorders, leading to new and improved treatments, and this translational approach may also impact the diagnosis and classification of such conditions in future versions of the DSM.

REFERENCES

1. Hollander E. *Obsessive-Compulsive Related Disorders.* Washington, DC: American Psychiatric Press, 1993.

2. Hollander E, Friedberg JP, Wasserman S *et al.* The case for the OCD spectrum. In: Abramowitz JS, Houts AC (eds), *Handbook of Controversial Issues in Obsessive-Compulsive Disorder.* New York: Kluwer Academic Press, 2005; pp. 95–118.

3. Jenike MA. Illnesses related to obsessive-compulsive disorder. In: Jenike ME, Baer LB, Minichiello WE (eds), *Obsessive Compulsive Disorders: Theory and Management,* 2nd edn. Chicago: Year Book Medical Publishers, 1990; pp. 39–60.

4. McElroy SL, Phillips KA, Keck PE. Obsessive compulsive spectrum disorder. *J Clin Psychiatry* 1994;**55**(Suppl.):33–51.

5. Stein DJ. Neurobiology of the obsessive-compulsive spectrum disorders. *Biol Psychiatry* 2002;**47**:296–304.

6. Hollander E, Wong CM. Obsessive-compulsive spectrum disorders. *J Clin Psychiatry* 1995;**56**(Suppl.):3–6.

7. Blaszczynski A. Pathological gambling and obsessive-compulsive spectrum disorders. *Psychol Rep* 1999;**84**:107–113.

8. Dale RC. Autoimmunity and the basal ganglia: New insights into old diseases. *Q J Med* 2003;**96**:183–191.

9. Peterson BS, Thomas P, Kane MJ *et al.* Basal ganglia volumes in patients with Gilles de la Tourette syndrome. *Arch Gen Psychiatry* 2003;**60**:415–424.

10. Sears LL, Vest C, Mohamed S *et al.* An MRI study of the basal ganglia in autism. *Prog Neuropsychopharmacol Biol Psychiatry* 1999;**23**:613–624.

11. Cath DC, Spinhoven P, Hoogduin CA *et al.* Repetitive behaviors in Tourette's syndrome and OCD with and without tics: What are the differences? *Psychiatry Res* 2001;**101**:171–185.

12. McDougle CJ, Kresch LE, Goodman WK *et al.* A case-controlled study of repetitive thoughts and behavior in adults with autistic disorder and obsessive-compulsive disorder. *Am J Psychiatry* 1995;**152**:772–777.

13. El Mansari M, Blier P. Mechanisms of action of current and potential pharmacotherapies of obsessive-compulsive disorder. *Prog Neuropsychopharmacol Biol Psychiatry* 2006;**20**:362–373.

14. Hollander E, Kwon JH, Stein DJ *et al.* Obsessive-compulsive and spectrum disorders: overview and quality of life issues. *J Clin Psychiatry* 1996;**53**:3–6.

15. Zohar J, Westenberg HGM, Stein DJ *et al.* Poster at 61st Annual Convention and Scientific Program Vulnerability and Resilience: Implications for Psychiatric Disorders, May 2006, Toronto, Canada.

16. Fineberg NA, Potenza M, Chamberlain SR *et al.* Probing compulsive and impulsive behaviors, from animal models to endophenotypes: a narrative review. *Neuropsychopharmacology* 2009;**35**:592.

17. Hollander E, Baker BR, Kahn J *et al.* Conceptualizing and assessing impulse-control disorders. In: Hollander E, Stein DJ (eds), *A Clinical Manual of Impulse Control Disorders.* Washington, DC: American Psychiatric Publishing, Inc., 2005; pp. 1–18.

18. Joel D, Stein DJ, Schreiber R. Animal models of obsessive-compulsive disorder: from bench to bedside via endophenotypes and biomarkers. In: McArthur RA, Borsini F (eds), *Animal and Translational Models for CNS Drug Discovery,* Vol. 1: Psychiatric Disorders. Amsterdam: Elsevier, 2008; pp. 133–154.

19. Stein DJ, Grant JE, Franklin ME *et al.* Trichotillomania (hair pulling disorder), skin picking disorder, and stereotypic movement disorder: towards DSM-V. *Depress Anxiety* 2010;**27**:611–626.

20. Hollander E, Kim S, Zohar J. OCSDs in the forthcoming DSM-V. *CNS Spectr* 2007;**12**:320–323.

21. Potenza MN, Koran LM, Pallanti S. The relationship between impulse-control disorders and obsessive-compulsive disorder: a current understanding and future research directions. *Psychiatry Res* 2009;**170**:22–31.

22. Grant JE, Brewer JA, Potenza MN. The neurobiology of substance and behavioral addictions. *CNS Spectr* 2006;**11**:924–930.

23. Taylor BP, Hollander E. Comorbid Obsessive-Compulsive Disorders. In: Geschwind D, Dawson G, Amaral D (eds), *Autism Spectrum Disorders*. New York: Oxford University Press, 2011; pp. 270–284.

24. Hollander E, Zohar J, Sirovatka PJ *et al.* (eds). *Obsessive-Compulsive Spectrum Disorders: Refining The Research Agenda for DSM-V*. Arlington, VA: American Psychiatric Association, 2011.

25. Bienvenu OJ, Samuels JF, Riddle MA *et al.* The relationship of obsessive-compulsive disorder to possible spectrum disorders: results from a family study. *Biol Psychiatry* 2000;**48**:287–293.

26. Mataix-Cols D, Conceicao do Rosario-Campos M, Leckman JF. A multidimensional model of obsessive-compulsive disorder. *Am J Psychiatry* 2005;**162**:228–238.

27. Goodman WK, Price LH, Delgado PL *et al.* Specificity of serotonin reuptake inhibitors in the treatment of obsessive-compulsive disorder. Comparison of fluvoxamine and desipramine. *Arch Gen Psychiatry* 1990;**47**:577–585.

28. Dannon PN, Aizer A, Lowengrub K. Kleptomania: differential diagnosis and treatment modalities. *Curr Psychiatry Rev* 2006;**2**:281–283.

29. Carter WP, Hudson JI, Lalonde JK *et al.* Pharmacologic treatment of binge eating disorder. *Int J Eat Disord* 2003;**34**:S74–S88.

30. Cardinal RN, Pennicott DR, Sugathapala CL *et al.* Impulsive choice induced in rats by lesions of the nucleus accumbens core. *Science* 2001;**292**:2499–2501.

31. Volkow ND, Fowler JS, Wange GW. The addicted human brain viewed in the light of imaging studies: brain circuits and treatment strategies. *Neuropharmacology* 2004;**47**:3–13.

32. Hollander E, Allen A, Kwon J *et al.* Clomipramine vs desipramine crossover trial in body dysmorphic disorder selective efficacy of a serotonin reuptake inhibitor in imagined ugliness. *Arch Gen Psychiatry* 1999;**56**:1033–1039.

33. Denys D, Zohar J, Westenberg HG. The role of dopamine in obsessive-compulsive disorder: preclinical and clinical evidence. *J Clin Psychiatry* 2004;**65**(Suppl. 14):11–17.

34. Goodman WK, McDougle CJ, Price LH *et al.* Beyond the serotonin hypothesis: a role for dopamine in some forms of obsessive compulsive disorder? *J Clin Psychiatry* 1990;**51**(Suppl.):36–43.

35. Goodman WK, McDougle CJ, Price LH. The role of serotonin and dopamine in the pathophysiology of obsessive compulsive disorder. *Int Clin Psychopharmacol* 1992;**7**(Suppl. 1):35–38.

36. Westenberg HG, Fineberg NA, Denys D. Neurobiology of obsessive compulsive disorder: Serotonin and beyond. *CNS Spectr* 2007;**12**(Suppl. 3):14–27.

37. Everitt BJ, Robbins TW. Neural systems of reinforcement for drug addiction: from actions to habits to compulsion. *Nat Neurosci* 2005;**8**:1481–1489.

38. Saxena S, Brody AL, Schwartz JM *et al*. Neuroimaging and frontal-subcortical circuitry in obsessive-compulsive disorder. *Br J Psychiatry* 1998;**35**(Suppl.):26–37.
39. Robins E, Guze SB. Establishment of diagnostic validity in psychiatry illness: its application to schizophrenia. *Am J Psychiatry* 1970;**126**:983–987.
40. Baer L. Factor analysis of symptom subtypes of obsessive-compulsive disorder and their relation to personality and tic disorders. *J Clin Psychiatry* 1994;**55**:18–23.
41. Bloch MH, Landeros-Weisenberger A, Rosario MC *et al*. Meta-analysis of the factor structure of obsessive-compulsive disorder. *Am J Psychiatry* 2008;**165**:1532–1542.
42. Hasler G, Pinto A, Greenberg BD *et al*. Familiality of factor analysis-derived YBOCS dimensions in OCD-affected sibling pairs from the OCD Collaborative Genetics Study. *Biol Pyschiatry* 2007;**61**:617–625.
43. Lawrence NS, Wooderson S, Mataix-Cols D *et al*. Decision making and set shifting impairments are associated with distinct symptom dimensions in obsessive-compulsive disorder. *Neuropsychology* 2006;**20**:409–419.
44. Phillips ML, Marks IM, Senior C *et al*. A differential neural response in obsessive-compulsive patients with washing compared with checking symptoms to disgust. *Psychol Med* 2000;**30**:1037–1050.
45. Alonso MP, Menchon JM, Pifarre J *et al*. Long-term follow-up and predictors of clinical outcome in obsessive-compulsive patients treated with serotonin reuptake inhibitors and behavioral therapy. *J Clin Psychiatry* 2001;**65**:535–540.
46. Shetti CN, Reddy YC, Kandavel T *et al*. Clinical predictors of drug nonresponse in obsessive-compulsive disorder. *J Clin Psychiatry* 2005;**66**:1517–1523.
47. Ferrão YA, Shavitt RG, Bedin NR *et al*. Clinical features associated to refractory obsessive-compulsive disorder. *J Affect Disord* 2006;**94**:199–209.
48. Landeros-Weisenberger A, Bloch MH, Kelmendi B *et al*. Dimensional predictors of response to SRI pharmacotherapy in obsessive-compulsive disorder. *J Affect Disord* 2010;**121**:175–179.
49. Stein DJ, Andersen EW, Overo KF. Response of symptom dimensions in obsessive-compulsive disorder to treatment with citalopram or placebo. *Revista Bras Psiquiatr* 2007;**29**:303–307.
50. Stein DJ, Carey PD, Lochner C *et al*. Escitalopram in obsessive-compulsive disorder: response of symptom dimensions to pharmacotherapy. *CNS Spectr* 2008;**13**:492–498.
51. Matsunaga H, Nagata T, Hayashida K *et al*. A long-term trial of the effectiveness and safety of atypical antipsychotic agents in augmenting SSRI-refractory obsessive-compulsive disorder. *J Clin Psychiatry* 2009;**70**:863–868.
52. Bloch MH, Landeros-Weisenberger A, Kelmendi B *et al*. A systematic review: antipsychotic augmentation with treatment refractory obsessive-compulsive disorder. *Mol Psychiatry* 2006;**11**:622–632.
53. Ipser JC, Carey P, Dhansay Y *et al*. Pharmacotherapy augmentation strategies in treatment-resistant anxiety disorders. *Cochrane Database Syst Rev* 2006;(4): CD005473.
54. Black DW, Monahan P, Gable J *et al*. Hoarding and treatment response in 38 nondepressed subjects with obsessive-compulsive disorder. *J Clin Psychiatry* 1998;**59**:420–425.
55. Winsberg ME, Cassic KS, Koran LM. Hoarding in obsessive-compulsive disorder: a report of 20 cases. *J Clin Psychiatry* 1999;**60**:591–597.

56. Mataix-Cols D, Rauch SL, Manzo PA *et al.* Use of factor-analyzed symptom dimensions to predict outcome with serotonin reuptake inhibitors and placebo in the treatment of obsessive-compulsive disorder. *Am J Psychiatry* 1999;**156**:1409–1416.
57. Erzegovesi S, Cavallini MC, Cavedini P *et al.* Clinical predictors of drug response in obsessive-compulsive disorder. *J Clin Psychopharmacol* 2001;**21**:488–492.
58. Saxena S, Brody AL, Maidment KM *et al.* Paroxetine treatment of compulsive hoarding. *J Psychiatr Res* 2007;**41**:481–487.
59. Leckman JF, Rauch SL, Mataix-Cols D. Symptom dimensions in obsessive-compulsive disorder: implications for the DSM-V. *CNS Spectr* 2007;**12**:376–387, 400.
60. Abramowitz JS, Franklin ME, Foa EB. Empirical status of cognitive-behavioral therapy for obsessive-compulsive disorder: a meta-analytic review. *Rom J Cogn Behav Psychother* 2002;**2**:89–104.
61. Mataix-Cols D, Marks IM, Greist JH *et al.* Obsessive-compulsive symptom dimensions as predictors of compliance with and response to behaviour therapy. *Psychother Psychosom* 2002;**71**:255–262.
62. Abramowitz JS, Franklin ME, Schwartz SA *et al.* Symptom presentation and outcome of cognitive-behavioral therapy for obsessive-compulsive disorder. *J Consult Clin Psychol* 2003;**71**:1049–1057.
63. Zohar J, Hollander E, Stein DJ *et al.* Consensus statement. *CNS Spectr* 2007; **12**(Suppl. 3):59–63.
64. Hummelen B, Wilberg T, Pedersen G *et al.* The quality of the DSM-IV obsessive-compulsive personality disorder construct as a prototype category. *J Nerv Ment Dis* 2008;**196**:446–455.
65. Grilo CM. Diagnostic efficiency of DSM-IV criteria for obsessive compulsive personality disorder in patients with binge eating disorder. *Behav Res Ther* 2004;**42**: 57–65.
66. Ansell EB, Pinto A, Edelen MO *et al.* Structure of Diagnostic and Statistical Manual of Mental Disorders, fourth edition criteria for obsessive-compulsive personality disorder in patients with binge eating disorder. *Can J Psychiatry* 2008;**53**:863–867.
67. Pertusa A, Fullana MA, Singh S *et al.* Compulsive hoarding: OCD symptom, distinct clinical syndrome, or both? *Am J Psychiatry* 2008;**165**:1289–1298.
68. Frost R, Steketee G, Williams L. Hoarding: a community health problem. *Health Soc Care Community* 2000;**8**:229–234.
69. Frost R, Steketee G, Tolin D *et al.* Diagnostic issues in compulsive hoarding. Paper presented at the European Association of Behavioural and Cognitive Therapies, Paris, France, 2006.
70. Samuels J, Bienvenu OJ, Grados MA *et al.* Prevalence and correlates of hoarding behavior in a community-based sample. *Behav Res Ther* 2008;**46**:836–844.
71. Steketee G, Frost R. Compulsive hoarding: current status of the research. *Clin Psychol Rev* 2003;**23**:905–927.
72. Frost RO, Tolin DF, Steketee G *et al.* Excessive acquisition in hoarding. *J Anxiety Disord* 2009;**23**:632–639.
73. Samuels JF, Bienvenu OJ, Riddle MA *et al.* Hoarding in obsessive compulsive disorder: results from a case-control study. *Behav Res Ther* 2002;**40**:517–528.
74. Saxena S. Neurobiology and treatment of compulsive hoarding. *CNS Spectr* 2008; **13**(Suppl. 14):29–36.

75. Saxena S, Brody A, Maidment KM *et al.* Cerebral glucose metabolism in obsessive-compulsive hoarding. *Am J Psychiatry* 2004;**161**:1038–1048.
76. Saxena S, Bota RG, Brody AL. Brain-behavior relationships in obsessive-compulsive disorder. *Sem Clin Neuropsychiatry* 2001;**6**:82–101.
77. Saxena S, Maidment KM, Baker SK *et al.* Anterior cingulate cortex dysfunction in compulsive hoarding. Paper presented at the Annual Meeting of the American College of Neuropsychopharmacology, Boca Raton, FL, 2007.
78. Pertusa A, Frost RO, Fullana MA *et al.* Refining the diagnostic boundaries of compulsive hoarding: a critical review. *Clin Psychol Rev* 2010;**30**:371–386.
79. Frost, RO, Steketee G, Tolin D *et al.* Diagnostic comorbidity in hoarding and OCD. Paper presented at the World Congress of Behavioral and Cognitive Therapies, Boston, MA, 2010.

CHAPTER 7

Paediatric OCD: Developmental Aspects and Treatment Considerations

Daniel A. Geller,[1,2] Alyssa L. Faro,[1] Ashley R. Brown[1] and Hannah C. Levy[3,4]

[1]The OCD and Related Disorders Program, Department of Psychiatry, Massachusetts General Hospital; [2]Harvard Medical School; [3]Department of Psychology; [4]Department of Psychology, Concordia University, Montreal, QC, Canada

INTRODUCTION

Obsessive-compulsive disorder (OCD) is one of the most prevalent psychiatric disorders and is projected by the World Health Organization to be among the 10 leading causes of global disability [1]. It affects children, adolescents and adults, suggesting continuity across the lifespan. Although OCD is frequently considered a unitary disorder with little consideration of age at onset, the bimodal incidence of the disorder, which includes a preadolescent peak of onset, and a number of specific clinical characteristics seen in children, suggest that a developmental subtype of OCD exists. Here we highlight those aetiological and clinical features unique to paediatric OCD that support this hypothesis.

EPIDEMIOLOGY

The high prevalence of OCD in youths was not generally recognized until the first epidemiological study just over 20 years ago [2]. Prevalence rates of paediatric OCD found in epidemiological studies are around 1–2% in the United States and elsewhere [2–6]. In the 2003 British Child Mental Health Survey of over

Obsessive-Compulsive Disorder: Current Science and Clinical Practice, First Edition. Edited by Joseph Zohar.
© 2012 John Wiley & Sons, Ltd. Published 2012 by John Wiley & Sons, Ltd.

10 000 5–15-year-olds, the point prevalence was 0.25% and the majority of cases identified had been undetected and untreated. In this study, lower socioeconomic and intelligence quotients were associated with OCD in youth [7]. There are two peaks of *incidence* (new-onset cases) for OCD across the lifespan, one occurring in preadolescent children with a mean age of onset of 9–10 years [8] and a later peak in early adult life [9]. It is this earlier cohort that is the focus of this chapter. If all paediatric cases of OCD persisted in adulthood, we would expect an increasing cumulative prevalence of OCD across the lifespan as more cases (new incidents) are added to the population. However, the anticipated cumulative increase in prevalence does not occur because of the variable outcome of childhood-onset OCD, with a substantial number becoming subclinical over time [10]. The finding of a bimodal incidence of OCD raises important questions regarding aetiology and underlying pathophysiology of the paediatric subtype.

AETIOLOGICAL CONSIDERATIONS

Genetic factors

Early onset increases familial risk

In the last decade our knowledge of paediatric OCD has increased with large-scale genetic and family studies. The contribution of genetic factors to the development of OCD has been explored in twin, family genetic and segregation analysis studies [11–16]. While family studies consistently demonstrate that OCD is familial [11,15, 17–20], the morbid risk of OCD in first-degree relatives appears to be much greater for index cases with a childhood onset. For example, in their multi-site family study of OCD, Nestadt *et al.* [12] found a risk for OCD of around 12% in first-degree relatives, while relatives of paediatric OCD probands have shown age-corrected morbid risks from 24% to 26% in more recent studies [21–24], with the last two studies including control samples. These findings suggest a greater genetic loading in paediatric-onset OCD. A further substantial proportion of relatives (5–15%) are affected with subthreshold OC symptoms that speak to genetic influences [11,12] but may also be relevant to family functioning.

Because early-onset OCD is a more familial form of the disorder, several researchers have used families ascertained from childhood-onset OCD cases to look for genetic causes. More specifically, investigations have focused on identifying common polymorphisms in several serotonin transmitter system genes, but have found only nominal association in two serotonin genes previously reported to have shown association in single studies. Although no single study showed replication, a pooled analysis of five replication studies found the marker *SLC6A4* HTTLPR, a functional length polymorphism found in the promoter region of *SLC6A4*, which encodes the serotonin transporter protein, to show significant association [25]. More recently, interest in glutamatergic mechanisms in the pathophysiology of OCD has led to study of the glutamate transporter gene *SLC1A1* [26–29]. Large-scale genome-wide association studies that target trios with paediatric-onset probands are underway in the United States and globally (through the International OCD Genetics Consortium) providing testimony to the expectation of a higher genetic yield in early-onset cases.

Tic- and ADHD-related OCD in youth

Many investigators have reported a higher than expected frequency of OCD among Tourette syndrome (TS) patients [30–34]. Gilles de la Tourette himself anecdotally reported OCD symptoms in one of his original patients. In addition, very high comorbidity between attention-deficit hyperactivity disorder (ADHD) and TS has been reported in almost every study of paediatric patients with TS [35–37]. There is considerable empirical support for an aetiological and genetic link between ADHD and OCD, with Tourette syndrome (TS) hypothesized as a link between these two disorders. Twin studies implicate genetic factors as important for the expression of all three disorders [38–44]. Family studies have also demonstrated that TS and OCD as well as TS and ADHD often co-occur and co-segregate within families [11,13,22,23,33,45]. Given the frequent comorbidity that has been observed between TS, OCD and ADHD in children, it is also plausible that there are common susceptibility genes for some components of these three conditions in which several overlapping neurologically mediated behaviours could occur. In a familial risk analysis examining the genetic association between OCD and ADHD in children, Geller *et al.* [46] found that: (i) relatives of children with OCD with and without ADHD had similar and significantly higher rates of OCD than did relatives of non-OCD comparison children; (ii) the risk for ADHD was elevated *only* among relatives of OCD + ADHD probands; (iii) there was evidence of co-segregation between OCD and ADHD in affected relatives; and (iv) there was no evidence of non-random mating between parents affected with OCD and ADHD. These findings are most consistent with the hypothesis that, in children, OCD that is comorbid with ADHD represents a distinct familial subtype (Figure 7.1).

Obsessive-compulsive disorder that is comorbid with tic disorders and ADHD may not only represent a distinct familial subtype that can inform genetic studies, but also, from a clinical perspective, children and their relatives affected with OCD plus comorbid tics and/or ADHD appear to have differing treatment responses and outcomes compared with their non-comorbid counterparts (see section on 'Clinical features and treatment' below). They may also manifest more OCD *spectrum* disorders that involve greater degrees of impulsivity such as pathological gambling, trichotillomania, skin picking or binge eating disorders [47] (see also Chapter 6).

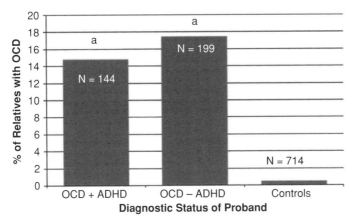

^a p < 0.001 versus Control group

(a) Kaplan–Meier estimates of obsessive-compulsive disorder (OCD) among first-degree
     relatives of OCD probands with and without ADHD and control probands with neither disorder.

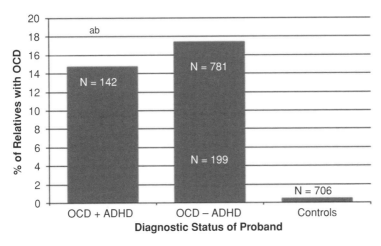

^a p < 0.001 versus Control group
^b p = 0.005 versus OCD-ADHD group

(b) Kaplan–Meier estimates of attention-deficit/hyperactivity disorder (ADHD) among first-degree
     relatives of OCD probands with and without ADHD and control probands with neither disorder.

Figure 7.1   Rate of obsessive-compulsive disorder (OCD) among relatives with and
without attention-deficit hyperactivity disorder (ADHD). Reprinted from Geller D,
Petty C, Vivas F, Johnson J, Pauls D, Biederman J. Examining the relationship between
obsessive-compulsive disorder and attention-deficit/hyperactivity disorder in children
and adolescents: A familial risk analysis. *Biol Psychiatry*. 2007;**61**:316–321, with
permission from Elsevier.

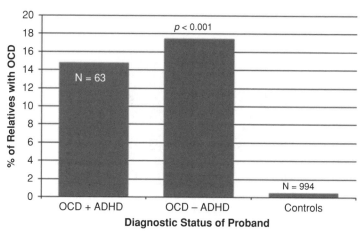

(c) Kaplan-Meier estimate of obsessive-compulsive disorder (OCD) among relatives
     with and without attention-deficit/hyperactivity disorder (ADHD).

Figure 7.1 (*Continued*)

Non-genetic factors

Adverse perinatal factors

Besides genetic factors, the above studies also point to major effects of *non-genetic* influences in the expression of OCD. In a cross-cultural sample of 4246 twin pairs, Hudziak *et al.* [48] used structural equation modelling to examine the influence of both genetic (45–58%) and unique environmental (42–55%) factors and concluded that both types of factors are about equally important. Indeed, many if not most cases of OCD arise *without* a positive family history of the disorder – so called 'sporadic' cases. It is generally assumed that sporadic cases have less genetic loading than familial cases. Information regarding environmental triggers of the disorder may be especially relevant for the sporadic form since the OCD cannot be explained by the presence of an affected relative. To date studies have focused on perinatal (intrauterine, birth and postnatal) experiences of affected children and immune-mediated neuropsychiatric models of illness. The intrauterine environment also includes exposure to potential teratogens such as alcohol and tobacco.

Lensi *et al.* [49] collected perinatal histories from 263 patients as part of a study of gender differences in OCD and found a higher rate of *perinatal trauma* (defined by dystocic delivery, use of forceps, breech presentation or prolonged hypoxia) in males with an earlier onset of OCD. In another study of 60 paediatric probands with Tourette syndrome (TS), Santangelo *et al.* [50] found that TS probands with comorbid OCD ($n = 33$) were almost eight times more likely to have been delivered by forceps than those without OCD, and five times more likely to have been regularly exposed to coffee, cigarettes and alcohol *in utero*. A similar study by Mathews *et al.*

[51] also identified drug exposure *in utero* as a significant predictor of increased tic severity and comorbid OCD status in a sample of 180 probands (ages 3 to 59) with TS. Geller *et al.* [52] reported that in a sample of 130 children and adolescents with OCD and 49 matched controls, children with OCD had mothers with significantly higher rates of illness during pregnancy requiring medical care ($\chi^2 = 8.61, p = 0.003$) and more birth difficulties (induced labour, forceps delivery, nuchal cord, or prolonged labour) ($\chi^2 = 7.51, p = 0.006$). Among the OCD-affected children they reported significant associations between adverse perinatal experiences and earlier age at onset, increased OCD severity and increased risk for comorbid ADHD, chronic tic disorder, anxiety disorder and major depressive disorder [52].

Paediatric autoimmune neuropsychiatric disorders associated with streptococcus (PANDAS)

The emergence of research on immune-based neuropsychiatric causes (PANDAS) applies uniquely to children based on the epidemiology of group A beta-haemolytic streptococcus (GABHS). Since its original description [53], perhaps no issue in paediatric OCD remains as controversial (and confusing) as the debate around PANDAS. The central hypothesis of PANDAS derives from observations of neurobehavioural disturbance accompanying Sydenham chorea, a sequel of rheumatic fever. An immune response to GABHS infections leads to cross-reactivity with, and inflammation of, basal ganglia with a distinct neurobehavioural syndrome that includes OCD and tics (and perhaps ADHD-like symptoms as well). Diagnostic criteria laid out by Swedo *et al.* [54]) (Table 7.1), have been used in a variety of antibiotic prophylaxis studies [55,56], but detractors argue that GABHS is but one of many non-specific physiological stressors that can trigger an increase in tics or OCD [57]. The weight of evidence at this time supports the belief that a subset of children with OCD and tic disorders can have both onset and clinical exacerbations

Table 7.1 Diagnostic criteria for paediatric autoimmune neuropsychiatric disorders associated with streptococcus (PANDAS).

1. Presence of obsessive-compulsive disorder and/or a tic disorder
2. Prepubertal onset between 3 and 12 years of age, or Tanner I (prepubertal) or II (first stage puberty)
3. Episodic course (abrupt onset and/or exacerbations)
4. The symptom onset or exacerbations are temporally related to *two* documented GABHS infections
5. Association with neurological abnormalities (motor hyperactivity, choreiform movements and/or tics)

Criteria for PANDAS diagnosis, as used in multiple antibiotic prophylaxis studies (Swedo *et al.*, 1997).
GABHS, group A beta-haemolytic streptococcus.

linked to GABHS [58]. In a 2-year prospective longitudinal case-control study of children with putative PANDAS-linked OCD and TS, clinical exacerbations linked to GABHS were significantly elevated in PANDAS-identified children. However, in these children, assessment of multiple immune markers did not demonstrate any differences between PANDAS and non-PANDAS cases [59]. Much is yet to be understood about the immunology of streptococcus and its role in infection-triggered neuropsychiatric symptoms.

Systematic research on PANDAS has been impeded by scepticism and confusion, but recent efforts to forge a consensus on this issue have involved disentangling the syndromatic presentation of an acute neurobehavioural disturbance [60] (OCD, tics, change in motor activity or coordination, behavioural regression, urinary frequency) from specific aetiological infective agents such as GABHS, opening the possibility that other immune triggers may be studied [61].

The role of the family in paediatric OCD

Children are embedded in families and, not surprisingly, families may become deeply enmeshed in their children's OCD. Parents are often intimately involved in their children's OC symptoms and may unwittingly reinforce compulsive behaviours by providing verbal reassurance or other 'accommodation' to children (e.g. handling objects that children avoid such as opening doors, laundering 'contaminated' clothes and linens excessively, even wiping children on the toilet who will not do it themselves). Since OCD and other anxiety disorders are highly familial, disentangling parental psychopathology from disturbed family functioning associated with the child's OCD is critical, especially in the younger patient whose parents control many contingencies of their daily behaviour and who are therefore dependent on parents for many activities of daily living. The very high intensity of affect and irritability displayed by some affected children engaged in ritualistic behaviours makes it difficult for parents to react with the supportive yet detached responses needed for effective behavioural management. Increasingly, the central role of family (both for maintenance of pathology as well as therapeutic agents) in children affected with OCD has been recognized and is reflected in both broader assessment that evaluates family function, and newer models of treatment intervention. Flessner *et al.* [62] reported that accommodation is ubiquitous among families of children with OCD and provided information regarding specific predictors in children and parents.

'Trauma' and stress in paediatric OCD

While the extant literature supports an association between psychological trauma and the development of OCD in adults [63,64], and this link is a plausible mediator for environment–gene interactions leading to phenotypic expression of OCD in genetically vulnerable individuals, little is understood regarding the role of stressful life events and onset of OCD in youth. A 2011 paper [65] explored the relationship between OCD and traumatic life events in children and adolescents, and found that the rate of PTSD and trauma exposure was higher in children with OCD than in a comparable control group of non-OCD youth matched for age, gender and socioeconomic status (SES). Children with concurrent PTSD had more intrusive fears and distress and less control over their rituals than children with OCD but without PTSD. Total symptom scale scores were higher in those with concurrent PTSD. Based on these findings, careful consideration and quantification of psychologically stressful life events are needed in clinical populations of youths with OCD.

Aetiology: summary

In summary, several aetiological considerations of youths with obsessive-compulsive disorder support a distinct paediatric subtype. While a specific gene pathway has yet to be discovered, there is considerable empirical support for a genetic link between OCD and the prototypical neurodevelopmental disorders, ADHD, and Tourette syndrome (TS). Non-genetic factors including perinatal injury may also be associated with paediatric OCD. While controversial, there is evidence to suggest that paediatric OCD may be caused by group A beta-haemolytic streptococcus (GABHS) infections (i.e. PANDAS) representing a specific post-infectious encephalopathic neuropsychiatric syndrome. Similar to adults, there is growing empirical support for an association between psychological trauma exposure and development of OCD in children.

CLINICAL FEATURES

Although classified among the anxiety disorders in the DSM-IV-TR [66], a variety of affects (e.g. disgust) may drive the symptoms of OCD in youths. Additionally, these emotions are frequently hidden or poorly articulated in young children, making paediatric OCD an under-recognized, underdiagnosed and undertreated disorder [7]. Despite apparent continuity in the phenotypic presentation of children and adults, issues such as limited insight and evolution of symptom profiles that follow developmental challenges over time differentiate children from adults with OCD [67–70]. In addition, children with OCD frequently display compulsions without well-defined obsessions, and symptoms other than typical washing or checking rituals (e.g. blinking and breathing rituals) [71]. One review of paediatric OCD [8] found that although the majority of children exhibit both obsessions and compulsions (mean number over lifetime was 4.0 and 4.8, respectively [68]), children were more likely to endorse only compulsions compared to adolescents.

Often children's obsessions centred upon fear of a catastrophic family event (e.g. death of a parent). These studies also reported that although OCD symptoms tended to wax and wane, they persisted in the majority of children but frequently changed over time so that the presenting symptom constellation was not maintained [71]. In many studies, parents are noted to be intimately involved in their child's rituals, especially in reassurance seeking, a form of 'verbal checking' [62]. Another study that examined effects of age on symptom constellation [67] found that religious and sexual obsessions were selectively over-represented in adolescents compared with children and adults. Only hoarding was seen more often in children than in adolescents and adults. These findings provide evidence for developmental influences in the phenotypic expression of the disorder and may be understood in the context of conflict and anxiety negotiating expected stages of attachment, autonomy, and sexual and moral development. As a corollary, rates of separation anxiety disorder appear inversely proportional to age and as high as 56% in childhood subjects [67].

Gender and age at onset

Unlike adult OCD, paediatric OCD is characterized by male predominance [72]. In a review of studies reporting on 419 childhood OCD patients, all but one study reported a male predominance, with an average 3:2 male to female ratio [8]. Two reports found that boys had an earlier age of onset of OCD than girls. Adult gender patterns appear in late adolescence. In a review of clinical studies, age of onset of paediatric OCD ranged from 7.5 to 12.5 years (mean 10.3 years, SD 2.5 years) and the mean age at ascertainment ranged from 12 to 15.2 years (mean 13.2 years) [8]. This means that age at assessment generally lagged 2.5 years after age at onset, a finding of considerable clinical importance and consistent with the secretive nature of the disorder.

Elaboration of phenotypic dimensions

Factor or cluster analytic methods take into account the broad phenotypic heterogeneity of OCD by identifying consistent symptom *'dimensions'* rather than a categorical (present/not present) diagnostic approach. Stewart *et al.* [73] conducted an exploratory principal components analysis of OC symptoms in children and adolescents with OCD to identify dimensional phenotypes. A four-factor solution emerged explaining 60% of symptom variance characterized by: (i) symmetry/ordering/repeating/checking; (ii) contamination/cleaning/aggressive/somatic, (iii) hoarding; and (iv) sexual/religious symptoms; this suggested fairly consistent covariation of OCD symptoms across the lifespan. The dimensional approach to phenotyping OCD provides a new research method that may yield important biological signals in genetic, translational and treatment studies where more traditional DSM-IV/ICD-10 approaches do not.

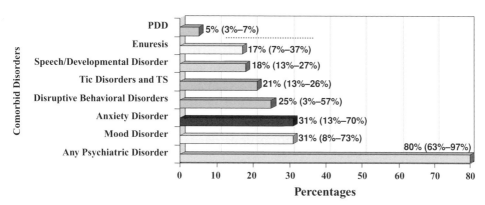

Figure 7.2 Comorbid disorders in paediatric obsessive-compulsive disorder (OCD). PDD, pervasive developmental disorder; TS, Tourette syndrome.

Comorbid conditions

Obsessive-compulsive disorder in youth is usually accompanied by other psychopathology that may complicate the assessment and treatment of affected children. Even cases derived from epidemiological studies that avoid the referral bias inherent in many clinical studies, demonstrate comorbid psychiatric diagnoses in over 50% of children with OCD [5,74]. Furthermore, while OCD symptoms in children are usually chronic, this comorbid psychopathology often shows a distinct chronology so that assessment and treatment approaches must evolve with time. A review of clinical studies consistently reported not only high rates of tic disorders, but also mood, anxiety, ADHD, disruptive behaviour, specific developmental disorders and enuresis in youths with OCD [8] (Figure 7.2).

In addition to an increased association with tics and Tourette syndrome [11, 75], many investigators have reported a higher frequency of learning disabilities (LD) [69] and frequent comorbidity with disruptive behaviour disorders [76,77]. Irrespective of age at ascertainment, an earlier age at onset predicts increased risk for ADHD and other anxiety disorders. In contrast, mood and psychotic disorders are associated with increasing chronological age and are more prevalent in adolescent subjects. Tourette syndrome is associated with both age at onset (earlier onset is more likely to be associated with comorbid TS) and chronological age (adolescents usually show remission of tics).

Whether comorbid psychiatric symptoms in youths are artifacts of, or 'secondary' to OCD or whether they reflect true comorbid states may be determined by family and genetic studies that examine the prevalence and segregation of comorbid diagnoses in relatives of children ascertained with OCD as the primary disorder [78]. How much comorbid disorders modify the expression or outcome of paediatric OCD when they occur is uncertain although there is some evidence that certain disorders may adversely moderate treatment response (see 'Treatment' below, and also Chapters 2, 5 and 6). By contrast, the OCD phenotype appears independent of the presence or absence of ADHD in its symptoms, patterns of comorbid disorders, or OCD-specific functional impairment [79]. In any case, the presence (or absence) of comorbid psychopathology is important for clinicians to identify, not only because it may require treatment in its own right, but because of its relevance to the course and outcome as well as treatment response.

Neuropsychological endophenotypes

Although not part of the core diagnostic symptoms, interest in the neuropsychological 'endophenotype' of children with OCD has grown over the last several years out of clinical and anecdotal experience that many children have academic difficulties that are not wholly explained by their primary disorder. Given the potential involvement of frontostriatal systems in OCD, several aspects of neuropsychological performance have been especially relevant to its study, especially measures of visuospatial integration, short-term memory, attention and executive functions. Few studies have examined neuropsychological processes among children with the disorder [80]. A handful of early studies of children with OCD yielded inconsistent results, with deficits in executive functioning, visuospatial performance and attention implicating basal ganglia dysfunction [81,82], and deficits in verbal IQ, working memory, processing speed and executive functioning [83], while other studies failed to find significant neuropsychological deficits among youths with OCD [5,84–86]. In a related line of research, Rosenberg and colleagues examined cognitive functions associated with the prefrontal cortex, using an oculomotor paradigm, and found that paediatric OCD subjects demonstrated higher response suppression failures than controls, which were correlated with impairments of frontostriatal functioning [87,88]. In 2007, Andres *et al.* [89] examined the neuropsychological performance of children and adolescents with OCD and found impairment in visual memory, visual organization and 'velocity' (processing speed). Although not yet well characterized, deficits in visuospatial performance and processing speed appear common and may underlie academic dysfunction in affected children.

Clinical features: summary

In summary, clinical features of paediatric OCD vary from the phenotypic expression of the disorder in adults. There is evidence to suggest that the nature of obsessions and compulsions differs in youth (e.g. poorly defined obsessions, blinking rituals), as well as gender patterns, comorbid conditions (e.g. learning disabilities) and possible neuropsychological deficits (e.g. visual memory). These specific features may adversely affect treatment response and are thus important to identify in children with OCD.

CLINICAL ASSESSMENT

The symptoms of OCD may range from mild to moderate in severity, be prominent in one setting and not another, wax and wane over time, and be hidden from others, including family members. Basic probes can be derived from the diagnostic criteria of the DSM-IV and include direct questions such as, 'Do you ever have repetitive, intrusive or unwanted thoughts, ideas, images or urges that upset you or make you anxious and that you cannot suppress?' Questions may be rephrased for younger children, 'Do you have worries that just won't go away?' A similar probe for compulsions might be: 'Do you ever have to do things over and over, even though you don't want to or you know they don't make sense, because you feel anxious or worried about something?' Phrased for younger children, the question might be, 'Do you do things over and over or have habits you can't stop?' By observing behaviours in their children, adults sometimes are left to infer obsessions that are not articulated or even acknowledged. Avoidance behaviours may imply concerns about some normal activity such as entering a room or handling an object.

A reliable instrument such as the Children's Yale–Brown Obsessive Compulsive Scale (CY–BOCS) best captures a standardized inventory of symptoms and scalar assessment of severity [90]. The CY–BOCS is a 10-item anchored ordinal scale (0–4) that rates the clinical severity of the disorder by scoring the time occupied, degree of life interference, internal resistance, subjective distress, and degree of control, for both obsessions and compulsions. Its use has been validated for paediatric subjects [90]. A symptom checklist of over 60 symptoms of obsessions and compulsions categorized by the predominant theme involved, such as hoarding, washing, contamination and checking, is included in the CY–BOCS. Though the CY–BOCS is the present standard assessment tool for paediatric OCD, there are several important limitations to this scale. For example, avoidance behaviour is not included in the quantitative score of the scale, which may therefore underestimate severity when avoidance is an impairing feature of the presenting behaviour. Additionally, the heterogeneous nature of OCD is such that the CY–BOCS symptom checklist may fail to capture atypical symptoms. Examples include behaviours motivated by sensory unease or fear of 'transformation' into other people or of acquiring an unwanted personality trait from another person (an uncommon form of contamination). The scale is not linear and is less sensitive to treatment effects in milder cases (see also Chapter 1).

Other validated OCD scales with psychometric properties deemed acceptable include the Leyton Obsessional Inventory [91], the Children's Obsessive Compulsive Inventory (CHOCI) [92], the children's Florida Obsessive Compulsive Inventory (FOCI) [93], and the Obsessive Compulsive Inventory – Child Version (OCI-CV) [94]. Interviews that more broadly assess for internalizing symptoms [95] and anxiety, including the Pediatric Anxiety Rating Scale (PARS) [96], Anxiety Disorders Interview Schedule (ADIS-C) [97], Screen for Child Anxiety Related

Emotional Disorders (SCARED) [98] and Multidimensional Anxiety Scale for Children (MASC) [99], may also be beneficial.

The presence of comorbid psychiatric symptoms should be given careful consideration in the assessment and management of OCD subjects at all ages because psychiatric comorbidity is the rule in youths with OCD, seen in both specialty and non-specialty child psychiatry settings [100]. Comorbid eating disorders are rare in preadolescent children with OCD but become more prevalent during adolescence [100,101]. Medical considerations outweigh other concerns of psychopathology (except suicidality) and must be addressed and stabilized to permit mental health interventions in these children. A 'spectrum' of compulsive/impulsive habit disorders such as compulsive nail biting, trichotillomania, skin picking and other forms of self-injury share important features with OCD but significant differences as well and are discussed in Chapter 6 in this book.

It is critical to assess the role of individual family members in maintenance and management of OC symptoms. The familial nature of anxiety disorders and OCD is a further factor in a family's reactions to a child with OCD. Thorough and specific questions about activities of daily living may be needed to understand the sequence of OC behaviours at home. Educational and school history provides an ecologically valid and essential measure of function and of illness severity.

Medical inquiry should centre on the central nervous system during systems review with consideration of neurological symptoms (e.g. choreiform movements) and trauma (e.g. concussion). Attention to infection with group A beta-haemolytic streptococcus (GABHS) as a potential precipitant for a PANDAS-associated OCD [54] has recently increased. Inquiry regarding GABHS is indicated in acute and dramatic onsets or exacerbations in preadolescent patients or when a sudden relapse occurs in a child in remission. Antistreptococcal antibodies such as anti-DNase B and anti-streptolysin O (ASO) are present in most children by early adolescence, but a 0.2 log rise in titres is considered evidence of a recent infection.

DIFFERENTIAL DIAGNOSIS

Normal development

Toddlers and preschoolers regularly engage in ritualistic behaviour as part of normal development. Examples include bedtime or mealtime routines that are insisted upon. As a rule, interruption of the rituals does not create severe distress in the child and they do not cause impairment in family functioning.

Other psychiatric disorders

The most difficult differential diagnosis perhaps occurs in the context of a pervasive developmental disorder (PDD or 'autism spectrum' disorder). Core symptoms of these disorders include stereotypic and repetitive behaviours, and a narrow and restricted range of activities and interests that may be confused with OCD, especially in young children. A minority of children with OCD (~5%) may also meet criteria for Asperger syndrome or PDD [102]. In addition to the core social and communication insufficiencies that are a diagnostic hallmark of 'spectrum' disorders, the most helpful criterion for clinicians to differentiate PDD from OCD is whether symptoms are ego-dystonic and associated with anxiety-driven obsessional fears. Children with PDD frequently engage in stereotypic behaviours with apparent gratification and will only become upset when their preferred activities are interrupted. Another helpful feature is whether symptoms are typical of OCD (such as washing, cleaning or checking) from which one can infer some obsessional concern.

Another diagnostic predicament occurs in the context of limited insight of obsessional thoughts, which merge into overvalued ideas and even delusional thinking suggesting psychosis. In fact, insight in children with OCD is not static, but fluctuates with anxiety levels and is best assessed when anxiety is lowest. While OC symptoms may rarely herald a psychotic or schizophreniform disorder in youths, especially in adolescents, other positive or negative symptoms of psychosis will typically be present or emerge to assist in differential diagnosis, and the nature of obsessional ideation in these patients is often atypical [103].

TREATMENT

In mild to moderate cases of paediatric OCD, cognitive behavioural therapy (CBT) is generally the first treatment recommended. This reflects findings of an initial large-scale randomized controlled trial of CBT [104] and later meta-analyses of CBT trials [105] suggesting a large effect size. New approaches in behaviour therapy include intensive inpatient and outpatient treatment [106], family-based CBT [105], group CBT [107] and CBT intervention for very young children with OCD [108]. Since the publication of a CBT treatment manual that operationalized and standardized the method [109], numerous studies have reliably shown its acceptability and efficacy [110]. The protocol used by March and Foa in the National Institutes of Health (NIH)-funded Paediatric OCD Treatment Study (POTS) [104] consists of 14 visits over 12 weeks spread across five phases: (i) psychoeducation, (ii) cognitive training, (iii) mapping OCD, (iv) exposure and response prevention (ERP) and (v) relapse prevention and generalization training. All visits occur on an hourly once-per-week basis, excluding weeks 1 and 2, when patients visit twice a week. One 10-minute telephone contact between each visit is scheduled during weeks 3 through 12. Each session includes a review of the previous week, a determination of goals, the introduction of new information, therapist-assisted practice, homework assignments to be completed during the week, and monitoring procedures. ERP is typically implemented gradually (sometimes called graded exposure), with exposure targets preferably under patient control or, less desirably, under therapist control.

Different types of cognitive interventions have been used to supply the child with a 'tool kit' to facilitate compliance with ERP [109]. Each must be individualized and must consider the child's cognitive abilities and developmental stage. *Modelling* may reduce anticipatory anxiety and present an opportunity for practising constructive self-talk before and during ERP. Clinically, *positive reinforcement* (rewards) does not seem to alter OCD symptoms directly, but rather helps to encourage exposure and ultimately produces a noticeable if indirect clinical benefit. In contrast, punishment is not beneficial in the treatment of OCD. Most CBT programmes use liberal positive reinforcement for ERP and disallow contingency management procedures unless aiming at disruptive behaviour that takes place beyond the area of OCD.

Useful CBT manuals and self-help books are available for both families and therapists interested in developing mastery of these methods such as *Obsessive-Compulsive Disorders: A Complete Guide to Getting Well and Staying Well* by Fred Penzell PhD, *Talking Back to OCD: The Program that Helps Kids and Teens Say "No Way" and Parents say "Way to Go"* by John March MD, *What to do when Your Child has Obsessive-Compulsive Disorder: Strategies and Solutions* by Aureen Pinto Wagner PhD, and *Freeing Your Child from Obsessive-Compulsive Disorder* by Tamar Chansky PhD. These can all be found in the resource section on the International OCD Foundation website at www.ocfoundation.org (see also Chapter 3).

Pharmacotherapy

More severe symptoms are an indication for the introduction of medication, typically in addition to CBT. Scores of 23–26 on the CY–BOCS or scores of *marked to severe impairment* based on time occupied, subjective distress and functional limitations on the Clinical Global Impression Severity Scale (CGI-S) provide a standard for consideration of drug intervention. In addition, any situation that might obstruct the successful delivery of CBT, such as a child being too ill or refusing to engage in treatment, should be cause for earlier consideration of medication treatment. Comorbid psychopathology including multiple anxiety disorders, major mood disturbance, and disruptive behavioural disorders, including ADHD, may diminish acceptance of or adherence to CBT and may require medication in its own right. Poor insight into the irrational nature of the obsession and/or compulsion can also lead to resistance to CBT. Successful implementation of CBT will become more difficult if the need for close family involvement is present in chaotic or non-intact families. Finally, there is a critical shortage of skilled paediatric CBT practitioners with the training to deliver the highest standard of CBT in many areas, leading to medication as the default treatment of choice. Informed consent is not completely 'informed' without a discussion of CBT (which should be documented in the medical record).

Clomipramine was the first agent approved for use in paediatric populations with OCD [111] in the United States (in 1989). Subsequent industry-sponsored multi-site randomized controlled trials (RCTs) have demonstrated significant efficacy of the selective serotonin reuptake inhibitors (SSRIs) compared with placebo, including sertraline [112], fluvoxamine [113], fluoxetine [114] and paroxetine [115]. Unfortunately, no comparative treatment studies have yet been carried out and currently there is little to guide clinicians regarding their choice of SSRIs.

A meta-analysis of all published randomized controlled medication trials in children and adolescents with OCD showed an effect size (ES) (expressed as a pooled standardized mean difference (SMD) for results of all studies) of 0.46 (95% confidence interval (CI) $= 0.37–0.55$) and found a statistically significant difference between drug and placebo treatment ($z = 9.87$, $p < 0.001$) [116]. The absolute response rate (defined as $\geq 25\%$ reduction in CY–BOCS scores after treatment) differed between SSRI and placebo, with a range from 16% (sertraline and fluvoxamine) to 24% (fluoxetine) yielding a *number needed to treat* (NNT) of between 4 and 6. However, clomipramine (CMI, a non-selective SRI) was shown to be significantly superior to each of the SSRIs, while SSRIs were comparably effective [116] in a multivariate regression of drug effect controlled for other variables. However, direct comparisons (which might give a more adequate answer), performed in adults rather than children, do not support superior efficacy of CMI, as no differences emerged in head-to-head comparisons between different SSRIs and CMI [117]. Moreover, CMI is generally not used as the primary drug of choice for children due to its frequent adverse event profile [111] and concerns around monitoring possible arrhythmogenic effects [118].

Although the effect size for CBT 'appears' larger than that for medication (often defined as 1.0 or larger), meta-analysis cannot determine whether CBT or medication is a more effective treatment, as major differences in design (e.g. placebo-control vs wait-list condition) and study population, rather than differences in efficacy of interventions, could account for differences in observed effect sizes. In the POTS study [104] there was no statistically significant difference between CBT alone and sertraline alone, and both were better than placebo. Fewer long-term studies have been carried out, but they suggest that there is a cumulative benefit over longer periods of drug exposure with gradually declining scalar scores and rising rates of remission for sertraline [119] up to periods of one year.

Moderating effect of comorbid conditions

The influence of psychiatric comorbidity on response and relapse rates in children and adolescents treated with paroxetine for OCD [120] showed that while the response rate to paroxetine in the overall treated sample was high (71%), the response rates in patients with comorbid ADHD, tic disorder or Oppositional

Defiant Disorder (ODD) (56%, 53% and 39%, respectively) were significantly less than in patients with OCD only (75%). Further, comorbidity was associated with a greater rate of relapse in the total patient population – 46% for ≥ 1 comorbid disorder ($p = 0.04$) and 56% for ≥ 2 comorbid disorders ($p < 0.05$) vs 32% for no comorbidity. More recent work has confirmed these findings. March *et al.* [121] conducted a post hoc analysis of data from POTS [104] comparative treatment trial to find the extent to which the presence of a comorbid tic disorder influenced symptom reduction on the CY–BOCS predicted score after 12 weeks of treatment. Those children with a comorbid tic disorder failed to respond to sertraline and did not separate statistically from placebo-treated patients. Response in youths with OCD but without tics, however, replicated previously published intent-to-treat outcomes. In children with tics, sertraline was only helpful when combined with CBT while CBT alone remained effective for youths with OCD only. The presence of disruptive behaviour disorders in particular may represent a therapeutic challenge for clinicians, especially those with a cognitive behavioural orientation. Storch *et al.* [122] examined the impact of psychiatric comorbidity on CBT response in children and adolescents with OCD treated systematically with standard weekly or intensive family-based CBT. Those children with one or more comorbid diagnoses had lower treatment response and remission rates with CBT relative to those without a comorbid diagnosis. As in the paroxetine study, the number of comorbid conditions was negatively related to outcome. Since certain comorbid disorders may adversely impact the outcome of both CBT and medication management of paediatric OCD, assessment and treatment of other psychiatric disorders prior to and concurrent with treatment of OCD may improve final outcome.

Multimodal treatment

For moderate to severe OCD, the greatest efficacy can be found in the combination of CBT with medication. As such, it should be considered the default option for treatment of moderate to severe paediatric OCD. Combined treatment in the POTS study showed the greatest rate of remission and decrease in symptom scores, with an effect size that was roughly the arithmetic sum of the component treatments (CBT $= 0.97$, sertraline $= 0.67$ and combined $= 1.4$). When receiving combined treatment, 54% of children achieved a complete remission (defined by CY–BOCS ≤ 10) and a decrease in the unadjusted mean of greater than or equal to 10 points on the CY–BOCS. Mediating better outcomes of CBT by decreasing anxiety and improving a child's ability to withstand ERP is possibly one of the greatest benefits of medication. Although the medication used in the POTS study was sertraline, it is reasonable to extrapolate the POTS study findings to different medications that have independently shown efficacy in children with OCD.

Medication augmentation strategies in treatment resistance

Treatment resistance can be defined as the failure of *adequate* trials of at minimum two SSRIs or one SSRI *and* a clomipramine trial, in addition to a failure of *adequately* delivered CBT. However, most children are partial responders, rather than having no response at all to treatment. When OCD presents on its own, hospitalization is infrequently recommended for the individual. Some children, however, may require inpatient care when comorbid conditions, including severe mood instability or suicidal ideation, are apparent. Standard inpatient psychiatric units and staff are not well equipped to manage young people with OCD, as their avoidance or rituals may be misinterpreted as oppositional behaviour, which can lead to unhelpful behavioural interventions.

Methods that are not supported by randomized controlled evidence include use of venlafaxine or duloxetine, which possess similar combined monoamine uptake inhibition properties to clomipramine but with less potential adverse cardiovascular effects. In one small open trial clonazepam has also been used in combination with SSRIs, but this should be used with caution in younger children [123]. In adults with OCD high-quality RCTs using atypical antipsychotics have been done and are summarized in a comprehensive meta-analysis by Bloch *et al.* [124], but *no controlled data exist* in children and only open trials and case reports are reported. Some children with treatment-resistant OCD may benefit from judicious neuroleptic augmentation, particularly children with tic disorders [125], pervasive developmental disorder symptoms and mood instability. To re-emphasize, no controlled data exist for the use of atypical antipsychotics in children with OCD. Regular metabolic, weight and Adverse Event (AE) monitoring should occur at a minimum, with baseline and follow-up assay of fasting lipid profile and serum glucose.

Novel augmentation trials are also described for stimulants, sumatriptan, gabapentin, inositol, pindolol, opiates, St John's wort and, more recently, *N*-acetyl cysteine and the glutamate antagonists riluzole and memantine – but *none of these meet minimal standards that permit recommendation for their routine use in children*. Putative PANDAS cases of OCD have also attracted experimental and novel treatment interventions. Antibiotic prophylaxis with penicillin failed to prevent streptococcal infections in one study but was successful in a subsequent study, with reduction in both infections and OCD symptoms in the year of prophylaxis compared to the previous baseline year [56]. Extant data are insufficient to meet minimal standards to suggest routine antibiotic prophylaxis for children with OCD, even when PANDAS is suspected as an aetiology. Instead standard treatments for both OCD and streptococcal infections are recommended. Intravenous immunoglobulin (IVIG) as a method to reduce putative circulating antineuronal antibodies has become more common but systematic published data are lacking and the procedure is not without significant risk. Therapeutic plasma exchange is performed in some centres yet remains an insufficiently studied intervention with significant risk and potential morbidity. D-cycloserine augmentation of CBT was reported as advantageous in a meta-analysis in adults [126] and in a recent paediatric preliminary trial [127].

Safety and tolerability

Generally, SSRI medications are well tolerated, and safer than their predecessor tricyclic antidepressants (TCAs), especially in the event of misuse or overdose. Titration schedules should be moderate, with modest increases every 3 weeks or so to allow for improvement to manifest before aggressively escalating doses. Following stabilization treatment is generally continued for 6–12 months and then *very gradually* withdrawn over several months. Two or three moderately severe relapses should lead to consideration of longer-term treatment (years).

Clinicians should be aware of behavioural side effects, which are more likely in younger children [128] and may be late-onset adverse effects appearing in conjunction with reduction in anxiety. The study by Martin *et al.* [128] found that peripubertal children exposed to antidepressants were at higher risk of conversion to mania compared with adolescents and young adults. For children with mild depression or anxiety disorders the 'number needed to harm' (NNH) was 13 (95% CI, 11–15). These side effects are sensitive to dose adjustment and the goal is to find a therapeutic window that provides a clinical response but 'acceptable' degrees of behavioural activation. If not attainable, then rotation to another SSRI is indicated. All antidepressant medications in the United States carry black box warnings from the Food and Drug Administration about suicide, but it should be noted that no suicides occurred in any of the RCTs of SSRIs. Bridge *et al.* [129], in the most comprehensive analysis of the extant data stratified by diagnosis, found no *statistically* significant increased risk of suicidal thinking or behaviour in the collective paediatric OCD trials. The pooled absolute risk difference between SSRI- and placebo-treated youths with OCD was 0.5%, with an NNH of 200. Risk appeared to be of potentially greater consequence in subjects participating in depression studies. An evaluation of the paediatric patient's medical condition and in particular, cardiac status, is mandated by the use of clomipramine. A baseline (pretreatment) electrocardiogram (ECG) should be requested.

Treatment: summary

In summary, clinicians should consider the severity of paediatric OCD symptoms before treatment is initiated. For mild to moderate OCD, CBT is recommended as the first-line treatment. When paediatric OCD symptoms escalate to more severe ranges (e.g. CY–BOCS scores of 23–26), the combination of pharmacotherapy and psychotherapy may be warranted. For these cases, the combination of SSRIs and CBT has shown the most favourable treatment outcome, with the majority (54%)

of child participants achieving full remission in one study. Safety and tolerability of medication must be considered before initiating pharmacological treatment for paediatric OCD, as some medications approved for adults may not be appropriate for children.

COURSE AND PROGNOSIS

The long-term prognosis for paediatric OCD is better than originally conceived [10,130,131] and better than described for adults. Many children will remit entirely or become clinically subthreshold over time. Adverse prognostic factors include very early age at onset, concurrent psychiatric diagnoses, poor initial treatment response, long duration of illness and a positive first-degree family history of OCD. In a review of outcome studies, Stewart *et al.* [10] applied meta-analysis regression to evaluate predictors and persistence of OCD. Sixteen study samples reported in 22 studies with a total of 521 children with OCD, and follow-up periods ranging from 1 to 15.6 years (mean 5.7 years), showed pooled mean persistence rates of 41% for *full* OCD and 60% for *full* or *subthreshold* OCD. Earlier age of OCD onset, increased duration of OCD, and inpatient treatment predicted greater persistence. Comorbid psychiatric illness and poor initial treatment response were poor prognostic factors. Concurrent psychopathology including multiple anxiety disorders, major mood disturbance and disruptive behavioural disorders may reduce acceptance of or compliance with treatment. Hence, the consideration of comorbid disorders in youths with OCD is not an academic matter. In contrast, gender, age at assessment, length of follow-up and year of publication were not reported as predictors of remission or persistence. Conclusions regarding the predictive importance of early treatment and family psychiatric history cannot yet be drawn from the extant literature. However, psychosocial function is frequently compromised; in five of the studies reviewed, subjects were less likely to live with a partner, and between 52% and 100% were unmarried. In one study 30% were still living with their parents as adults, and in another there was a marked pattern of hiding symptoms from family. These studies report high levels of social/peer problems (55–100%), isolation, unemployment (45%) and difficulties sustaining a job (20%).

CONCLUSIONS AND FUTURE RESEARCH

There is considerable support for the notion that although OCD affecting children is diagnosed using DSM-IV criteria identical to those used with adults, it is distinct in important ways from the disorder in adults.

1. OCD is common in children and adolescents and is frequently under-recognized, underdiagnosed and undertreated due to the secretive nature of its symptoms.

2. Phenotypically, OCD in children is characterized by developmentally specific symptom profiles that reflect the conflicts of the age group.
3. Families often become enmeshed in their children's rituals.
4. Most often, OCD in children is accompanied by a distinct pattern of comorbid psychopathology that has an important impact on morbid functioning and treatment outcome.
5. Tic disorders, Tourette syndrome and ADHD are selectively over-represented in children with OCD and may be genetically linked to paediatric OCD.
6. The risk of OCD in first-degree relatives of childhood cases is markedly elevated compared with adult-onset OCD.
7. An immune-mediated aetiology of neuropsychiatric symptoms that include OCD and tics is unique to childhood-onset OCD.
8. Outcome in childhood-onset OCD is better than previously recognized and generally better than the outcome in adults.

The increasing power of genome-wide association methods and of pooling data, such as made possible by the newly created International OCD Genetics Consortium, can be used to advantage by recruiting childhood probands to increase the yield in genetic studies (for more details, see Chapter 11). Ever more powerful magnets provide a non-invasive and child-safe method for endophenotypic, translational and pharmacogenomic studies that should increase specificity of treatments to improve effect sizes and decrease adverse events. Novel therapeutic approaches employing glutamatergic, GABA-ergic and peptide neurotransmitter manipulation are likely and will be informed by genetic studies. Real challenges remain in identifying environmental triggers (in genetically susceptible children) as only prospective long-term studies of as-yet-unaffected 'at-risk' children can hope to understand the complex gene–environment interactions that underlie most cases of paediatric OCD.

ACKNOWLEDGEMENTS

The authors wish to acknowledge expert contributors to the American Association of Child and Adolescent Psychiatry (AACAP) practice parameters 'Assessment and Treatment of OCD in Children and Adolescents' developed by Drs Geller and March and the AACAP Work Group on Quality Issues.

REFERENCES

1. World Health Organization. Mental health: facing the challenges, building solutions. Report from the WHO European Ministerial Conference, Helsinki, 12–15 January 2005. WHO Regional Office for Europe.

2. Flament M, Whitaker A, Rapoport J *et al.* Obsessive compulsive disorder in adolescence: An epidemiological study. *J Am Acad Child Adolesc Psychiatry* 1988;**27**:764–771.
3. Valleni-Basile L, Garrison CZ, Jackson KL *et al.* Frequency of obsessive-compulsive disorder in a community sample of young adolescents. *J Am Acad Child Adolesc Psychiatry* 1994;**33**:782–791.
4. Apter A, Fallon Jr. TJ, King RA *et al.* Obsessive-compulsive characteristics: From symptoms to syndrome. *J Am Acad Child Adolesc Psychiatry* 1996;**35**:907–912.
5. Douglass HM, Moffitt TE, Dar R, McGee R, Silva P. Obsessive-compulsive disorder in a birth cohort of 18-year-olds: Prevalence and predictors. *J Am Acad Child Adolesc Psychiatry* 1995;**34**:1424–1431.
6. Thomsen P. Obsessive-compulsive disorder in children and adolescents: Self-reported obsessive-compulsive behaviour in pupils in Denmark. *Acta Psychiatr Scand* 1993;**88**:212–217.
7. Heyman I, Fombonne E, Simmons H, Ford T, Meltzer H, Goodman R. Prevalence of obsessive-compulsive disorder in the British nationwide survey of child mental health. *Int Rev Psychiatry* 2003;**15**:178–184.
8. Geller D, Biederman J, Jones J *et al.* Is juvenile obsessive compulsive disorder a developmental subtype of the disorder?: A review of the pediatric literature. *J Am Acad Child Adolesc Psychiatry* 1998;**37**:420–427.
9. Rasmussen S, Eisen J. The epidemiology and clinical features of obsessive compulsive disorder. *Psychiatric Clin N Am* 1992;**15**:743–758.
10. Stewart SE, Geller DA, Jenike M *et al.* Long term outcome of pediatric obsessive compulsive disorder: a meta-analysis and qualitative review of the literature. *Acta Psychiatr Scand* 2004;**110**:4–13.
11. Pauls D, Alsobrook II J, Goodman W, Rasmussen S, Leckman J. A family study of obsessive-compulsive disorder. *Am J Psychiatry* 1995;**152**:76–84.
12. Nestadt G, Samuels J, Bienvenu JO *et al.* A family study of obsessive compulsive disorder. *Arch Gen Psychiatry* 2000;**57**:358–363.
13. Grados M, Riddle M, Samuels J *et al.* The familial phenotype of obsessive-compulsive disorder in relation to tic disorders: The Hopkins OCD family study. *Biol Psychiatry* 2001;**50**:559–565.
14. Reddy P, Reddy J, Srinath S, Khanna S, Sheshadri S, Girimaji S. A family study of juvenile obsessive-compulsive disorder. *Can J Psychiatry* 2001;**46**:346–351.
15. Pato M, Pato C, Pauls D. Recent findings in the genetics of OCD. *J Clin Psychiatry* 2002;**63**(Suppl. 6):30–33.
16. Hanna G, Himle JA, Curtis GC, Gillespie B. A family study of obsessive-compulsive disorder with pediatric probands. *Am J Med Genetics* 2005;**134**:13–19.
17. Lenane M, Swedo S, Leonard H, Pauls D, Sceery W, Rapoport J. Psychiatric disorders in first degree relatives of children and adolescents with obsessive compulsive disorder. *J Am Acad Child Adolesc Psychiatry* 1990;**29**:407–412.
18. Leonard HL, Lenane MC, Swedo SE, Rettew DC, Gershon ES, Rapoport JL. Tics and tourette's disorder: A 2- to 7-year follow-up of 54 obsessive-compulsive children. *Am J Psychiatry* 1992;**149**:1244–1251.

19. Bellodi L, Sciuto G, Diaferia G, Ronchi P, Smeraldi E. Psychiatric disorders in the families of patients with obsessive-compulsive disorder. *Psychiatry Res* 1992;**42**:111–120.

20. Black DW, Noyes R, Goldstein RB, Blum N. A family study of obsessive-compulsive disorder. *Arch Gen Psychiatry* 1992;**49**:362–368.

21. Chabane N, Delorme R, Millet B, Mouren M, Leboyer M, Pauls D. Early-onset obsessive-compulsive disorder: a subgroup with a specific clinical and familial pattern? *J Child Psychol Psychiatry* 2005;**46**:881–887.

22. Hanna GL, Fischer DJ, Chadha KR, Himle JA, Van Etten M. Familial and sporadic subtypes of early-onset obsessive-compulsive disorder. *Biol Psychiatry* 2005;**57**:895–900.

23. Do Rosario-Campos MC, Leckman JF, Curi M *et al*. A family study of early-onset obsessive-compulsive disorder. *Am J Med Genetics B* 2005;**136B**:92–97.

24. Geller DA, Biederman J, Petty C, Stewart SE, Haddad S, Pauls D (eds). Age-corrected risk of OCD in relatives of affected youth. In: *Joint Scientific Proceedings of the American Academy of Child and Adolescent Psychiatry and the Canadian Academy of Child and Adolescent Psychiatry*; 2005 October 18–23; Toronto, Canada.

25. Dickel D, Veenstra-VanderWeele J, Bivens N *et al*. Association studies of serotonin system candidate genes in early-onset obsessive-compulsive disorder. *Biol Psychiatry* 2007;**61**:322–329.

26. Dickel D, Veenstra-VanderWeele J, Cox N *et al*. Association testing of the positional and functional candidate gene SLC1A1/EAAC1 in early-onset obsessive-compulsive disorder. *Arch Gen Psychiatry* 2006;**63**:717–720.

27. Arnold P, Sicard T, Burroughs E, Richter M, Kennedy J. Glutamate transporter gene SLC1A1 associated with obsessive-compulsive disorder. *Arch Gen Psychiatry* 2006;**63**:717–720.

28. Hanna GL, Veenstra-VanderWeele J, Cox NJ *et al*. Genome-wide linkage analysis of families with obsessive-compulsive disorder ascertained through pediatric probands. *Am J Med Genetics B* 2002;**114**:541–552.

29. Welch JM, Lu J, Rodriguiz RM *et al*. Cortico-striatal synaptic defects and OCD-like behaviours in Sapap3-mutant mice. *Nature* 2007;**4488**:894–900.

30. Frankel M, Cummings JL, Robertson MM, Trimble MR, Hill MA, Benson DF. Obsessions and compulsions in Gilles de la Tourette's syndrome. *Neurology* 1986;**36**:378–382.

31. Pauls DL, Towbin KE, Leckman JF, Zahner GEP, Cohen DJ. Gilles de la Tourette's syndrome and obsessive-compulsive disorder: Evidence supporting a genetic relationship. *Arch Gen Psychiatry* 1986;**43**:1180–1182.

32. Robertson M, Trimble M, Lees A. The psychopathology of the Gilles de la Tourette syndrome: a phenomenological analysis. *Br J Psychiatry* 1988;**152**:383–390.

33. Pauls DL, Raymond CL, Stevenson JM, Leckman JF. A family study of Gilles de la Tourette Syndrome. *Am J Hum Genetics* 1991;**48**:154–163.

34. Eapen V, Robertson MM, Alsobrook JP 2nd, Pauls DL. Obsessive compulsive symptoms in Gilles de la Tourette syndrome and obsessive compulsive disorder: Differences by diagnosis and family history. *Am J Med Genetics* 1997;**74**:432–438.

35. Jagger J, Prussof B, Cohen D, Kidd K, Carbonari C, John K. The epidemiology of Tourette's syndrome. *Schizophrenia Bull* 1982;**8**:267–278.

36. Comings DE, Comings BG. A controlled study of Tourette syndrome. I. Attention-deficit disorder, learning disorders, and school problems. *Am J Hum Genetics* 1987;**41**:701–741.

37. Pauls DL, Leckman JF, Cohen DJ. Familial relationship between Gilles de la Tourette's syndrome, attention deficit disorder, learning disabilities, speech disorders, and stuttering. *J Am Acad Child Adolesc Psychiatry* 1993;**32**:1044–1050.

38. Price RA, Leckman JF, Pauls DL, Cohen DJ, Kidd KK. Gilles de la Tourette's syndrome: tics and central nervous system stimulants in twins and nontwins. *Neurology* 1986;**36**:232–237.

39. Hyde TM, Aaronson BA, Randolph C, Rickler KC, Weinberger DR. Relationship of birth weight to the phenotypic expression of Gilles de la Tourette's syndrome in monozygotic twins. *Neurology* 1992;**42**:652–658.

40. Carey G, Gottesman I. Twin and family studies of anxiety, phobic and obsessive disorders. In: Klien D, Rabkin J (eds), *Anxiety: New Research and Changing Concepts*. New York: Raven Press, 1981; pp. 117–136.

41. Torgersen S. Genetic factors in anxiety disorder. *Arch Gen Psychiatry* 1983; **40**:1085–1089.

42. Andrews G, Stewart G, Allen R, Henderson A. The genetics of six neurotic disorders: a twin study. *J Affect Dis* 1990;**19**:23–29.

43. Andrews G, Stewart G, Morris-Yates A, Holt P, Henderson AS. Evidence for a general neurotic syndrome. *Br J Psychiatry* 1990;**157**:6–12.

44. Faraone S. Report from the Fourth International Meeting of the Attention Deficit Hyperactivity Disorder Molecular Genetics Network. *Am J Med Genetics B* 2003; **121B**:55–59.

45. Faraone SV, Biedeman J, Mick E *et al.* Family study of girls with Attention Deficit Hyperactivity Disorder. *Am J Psychiatry* 2000;**157**:1077–1083.

46. Geller DA, Petty C, Vivas F, Johnson J, Pauls D, Biederman J. Examining the relationship between obsessive compulsive disorder and attention deficit hyperactivity disorder in children and adolescents: A familial risk analysis. *Biol Psychiatry* 2007;**61**:316–321.

47. Hollander E. Obsessive-compulsive spectrum disorders: An overview. *Psychiatr Ann* 1993;**23**:355–358.

48. Hudziak JJ, Van Beijsterveldt CE, Althoff RR *et al.* Genetic and environmental contributions to the Child Behavior Checklist Obsessive-Compulsive Scale: a cross-cultural twin study. *Arch Gen Psychiatry* 2004;**61**:608–616.

49. Lensi P, Casssano G, Correddu G, Ravagli S, Kunovack J, Akiskal HS. Obsessive-compulsive disorder. Familial-developmental history, symptomatology, comorbidity and course with special reference to gender-related differences. *Br J Psychiatry* 1996;**169**:101–107.

50. Santangelo SL, Pauls DL, Goldstein JM, Faraone SV, Tsuang MT, Leckman JF. Tourette's syndrome: What are the influences of gender and comorbid obsessive-compulsive disorder? *J Am Acad Child Adolesc Psychiatry* 1994;**33**:795–804.

51. Mathews CA, Bimson B, Lowe TL *et al.* Association between maternal smoking and increased symptom severity in Tourette's syndrome. *Am J Psychiatry* 2006;**163**:1066–1073.

52. Geller D, Wieland N, Carey K *et al.* Perinatal factors affecting expression of obsessive compulsive disorder in children and adolescents. *J Child Adolesc Psychopharmacol* 2008;**18**:373–379.

53. Swedo S, Leonard H, Mittleman B *et al.* Identification of children with pediatric autoimmune neuropsychiatric disorders associated with streptococcal infections by a marker associated with rheumatic fever. *Am J Psychiatry* 1997;**154**:110–112.

54. Swedo SE, Leonard HL, Garvey M *et al.* Pediatric autoimmune neuropsychiatric disorders associated with streptococcal infections: Clinical description of the first 50 cases. *Am J Psychiatry* 1998;**155**:264–271.

55. Garvey M, Perlmutter S, Allen A *et al.* A pilot study of penicillin prophylaxis for neuropsychiatric exacerbations triggered by streptococcal infections. *Biol Psychiatry* 1999;**45**:1564–1571.

56. Snider LA, Lougee L, Slattery M, Grant P, Swedo SE. Antibiotic prophylaxis with azithromycin or penicillin for childhood-onset neuropsychiatric disorders. *Biol Psychiatry* 2005;**57**:788–792.

57. Kurlan R, Kaplan EL. The pediatric autoimmune neuropsychiatric disorders associated with streptococcal infection (PANDAS) etiology for tics and obsessive-compulsive symptoms: hypothesis or entity? Practical considerations for the clinician. *Pediatrics* 2004;**113**:883–886.

58. Murphy TK, Sajid M, Soto O *et al.* Detecting pediatric autoimmune neuropsychiatric disorders associated with streptococcus in children with obsessive-compulsive disorder and tics. *Biol Psychiatry* 2004;**55**:61–8.

59. Kurlan R, Johnson D, Kaplan EL, Group TSS. Streptococcal infection and exacerbations of childhood tics and obsessive-compulsive symptoms: a prospective blinded cohort study. *Pediatrics* 2008;**121**:1188–1197.

60. Bernstein GA, Victor AM, Pipal AJ, Williams KA. Comparison of clinical characteristics of pediatric autoimmune neuropsychiatric disorders associated with streptococcal infections and childhood obsessive-compulsive disorder. *J Child Adolesc Psychopharmacol* 2010 Aug;**20**(4):333–340.

61. Murphy TK, Kurlan R, Leckman J. The immunobiology of Tourette's disorder, pediatric autoimmune neuropsychiatric disorders associated with Streptococcus, and related disorders: a way forward. *J Child Adolesc Psychopharmacol* 2010 Aug;**20**(4):317–331.

62. Flessner CA, Freeman JB, Sapyta J *et al.* Predictors of parental accommodation in pediatric obsessive-compulsive disorder: findings from the Pediatric Obsessive-Compulsive Disorder Treatment Study (POTS) trial. *J Am Acad Child Adolesc Psychiatry* 2011;**50**:716–725.

63. Huppert JD, Moser JS, Gershuny BS *et al.* The relationship between obsessive-compulsive and posttraumatic stress symptoms in clinical and non-clinical samples. *J Anxiety Dis* 2005;**19**:127–136.

64. Gershuny BS, Baer L, Parker H, Gentes EL, Infield AL, Jenike MA. Trauma and posttraumatic stress disorder in treatment-resistant obsessive-compulsive disorder. *Depress Anxiety* 2008;**25**:69–71.

65. Lafleur DL, Petty C, Mancuso E, McCarthy K, Biederman J, Faro A, Levy HC, Geller DA. Traumatic events and obsessive compulsive disorder in children and adolescents: is there a link? *J Anxiety Disord* 2011 May;**25**(4):513–519. Epub 2010 Dec 27.

66. American Psychiatric Association. *Diagnostic and Statistical Manual of Mental Disorders, Fourth Edition, Text Revision* (DSM-IV-TR). Washington, DC: American Psychiatric Association, 2000.

67. Geller D, Biederman J, Agranat A *et al.* Developmental aspects of obsessive compulsive disorder: Findings in children, adolescents and adults. *J Nerv Ment Dis* 2001;**189**:471–477.

68. Hanna GL. Demographic and clinical features of obsessive-compulsive disorder in children and adolescents. *J Am Acad Child Adolesc Psychiatry* 1995;**34**:19–27.

69. Sobin C, Blundell M, Karayiorgou M. Phenotypic differences in early- and late-onset obsessive-compulsive disorder. *Compr Psychiatry* 2000;**41**:373–379.

70. Thomsen PH, Jensen J. Obsessive-compulsive disorder: Admission patterns and diagnostic stability. A case-register study. *Acta Psychiatr Scand* 1994;**90**:19–24.

71. Rettew DC, Swedo SE, Leonard HL, Lenane MC, Rapoport JL. Obsessions and compulsions across time in 79 children and adolescents with obsessive-compulsive disorder. *J Am Acad Child Adolesc Psychiatry* 1992;**31**:1050–1056.

72. Fireman B, Koran LM, Leventhal JL, Jacobson A. The prevalence of clinically recognized obsessive-compulsive disorder in a large health maintenance organization. *Am J Psychiatry* 2001;**158**:1904–1910.

73. Stewart ES, Rosario MC, Brown TA *et al.* Principal components analysis of obsessive-compulsive disorder symptoms in children and adolescents. *Biol Psychiatry* 2007;**61**:285–291.

74. Flament M, Whitaker A, Rapoport J, Davies M, Berg C, Shaffer D. An epidemiological study of obsessive-compulsive disorder in adolescence. In: Rapoport J (ed.) *Obsessive-Compulsive Disorder in Children and Adolescents*. Washington, DC: American Psychiatric Press, 1989; pp. 253–267.

75. Eichstedt JA, Arnold SL. Childhood-onset obsessive-compulsive disorder: a tic-related subtype of OCD? *Clin Psychol Rev* 2001;**21**:137–157.

76. Geller D, Biederman J, Jones J, Shapiro S, Schwartz S, Park K. Obsessive compulsive disorder in children and adolescents: A review. *Harvard Rev Psychiatry* 1998;**5**:260–273.

77. Geller D, Biederman J, Griffin S, Jones J, Lefkowitz TR. Comorbidity of juvenile obsessive-compulsive disorder with disruptive behavior disorders. *J Am Acad Child Adolesc Psychiatry* 1996;**35**:1637–1646.

78. Geller D, Petty C, Vivas F, Johnson J, Pauls D, Biederman J. Further evidence for co-segregation between pediatric obsessive compulsive disorder and attention deficit hyperactivity disorder: a familial risk analysis. *Biol Psychiatry* 2007;**61**:1388–1394.

79. Geller DA, Coffey BJ, Faraone S *et al.* Does comorbid attention-deficit/hyperactivity disorder impact the clinical expression of pediatric obsessive compulsive disorder. *CNS Spectr* 2003;**8**:259–264.

80. Schultz RT, Evans DW, Wolff M. Neuropsychological models of childhood obsessive-compulsive disorder. *Child Adolesc Psychiatr Clin N Am* 1999;**8**:513–531.

81. Cox C, Fedio P, Rapoport J. Neuropsychological testing of obsessive-compulsive adolescents. In: Rapoport J (ed.), *Obsessive-Compulsive Disorder in Children and Adolescents*. Washington, DC: American Psychiatric Press, 1989; pp. 73–85.

82. Behar D, Rapoport J, Berg C *et al*. Computerized tomography and neuropsychological test measures in adolescents with obsessive compulsive disorder. *Am J Psychiatry* 1984;**141**:363–369.

83. DeGroot CM, Yeates KO, Baker GB, Bornstein RA. Impaired neuropsychological functioning in Toilette's Syndrome subjects with co-occurring obsessive-compulsive and attention deficit symptoms. *J Neuropsychiat Clin Neurosci* 1997;**9**:267–272.

84. Thomsen PH, Jensen J. Latent class analysis of organic aspects of obsessive-compulsive disorder in children and adolescents. *Acta Psychiatr Scand* 1991;**84**:391–395.

85. Beers S, Rosenberg DR, Dick EL *et al*. Neuropsychological study of frontal lobe function in psychotropic-naive children with obsessive-compulsive disorder. *Am J Psychiatry* 1999;**156**:777–779.

86. Beers SR, Rosenberg DR, Ryan CM. Dr. Beers and colleagues reply. *Am J Psychiatry* 2000;**157**:1183.

87. Rosenberg D, Averbach D, O'Hearn K, Seymour A, Birmaher B, Sweeney J. Oculomotor response inhibition abnormalities in pediatric obsessive-compulsive disorder. *Arch Gen Psychiatry* 1997;**54**:831–838.

88. Rosenberg D, Keshavan M, O'Hearn K *et al*. Frontostriatal measurement in treatment-naive children with obsessive compulsive disorder. *Arch Gen Psychiatry* 1997;**54**:824–830.

89. Andres S, Boget T, Lazaro L *et al*. Neuropsychological performance in children and adolescents with Obsessive-Compulsive disorder and influence of clinical variables. *Biol Psychiatry* 2007;**61**:946–951.

90. Scahill L, Riddle M, McSwiggin-Hardin M *et al*. Children's Yale–Brown Obsessive Compulsive Scale: reliability and validity. *J Am Acad Child Adolesc Psychiatry* 1997;**36**:844–852.

91. Berg CJ, Rapoport JL, Flament M. The Leyton Obsessional Inventory – Child Version. *J Am Acad Child Adolesc Psychiatry* 1986;**25**:84–91.

92. Shafran R, Frampton I, Heyman I, Reynolds M, Teachman B, Rachman S. The preliminary development of a new self-report measure for OCD in young people. *J Adolescence* 2003;**26**:137–142.

93. Storch EA, Bagner D, Merlo LJ *et al*. Florida Obsessive-Compulsive Inventory: development, reliability, validity. *J Clin Psychol* 2007;**63**:851–859.

94. Foa EB, Coles M, Huppert JD, Pasupuleti RV, Franklin ME, March J. Development and validation of a child version of the obsessive compulsive inventory. *Behav Ther* 2010;**41**(1):121–132.

95. Myers K, Winters NC. Ten-year review of rating scales. II: Scales for internalizing disorders. *J Am Acad Child Adolesc Psychiatry* 2002;**41**:634–659.

96. The Research Units on Pediatric Psychopharmacology Anxiety Study Group. The Pediatric Anxiety Rating Scale (PARS): Development and psychometric properties. *J Am Acad Child Adolesc Psychiatry* 2002;**41**:1061–1069.

97. Silverman WK, Albano AM. *The Anxiety Disorders Interview Schedule for DSM-IV: Child and Parent Versions*. San Antonio, TX: Psychological Corporation, 1996.

98. Birmaher B, Khetarpal S, Brent D *et al*. The Screen for Child Anxiety Related Emotional Disorders (SCARED): scale construction and psychometric characteristics. *J Child Adolesc Psychopharmacol* 1997;**36**:545–553.

99. March JS, Parker JD, Sullivan K, Stallings P, Conners CK. The Multidimensional Anxiety Scale for Children (MASC): factor structure, reliability, and validity. *J Child Adolesc Psychopharmacol* 1997;**36**:554–565.

100. Geller D, Biederman J, Faraone SV *et al*. Clinical correlates of obsessive-compulsive disorder in children and adolescents referred to specialized and non-specialized clinical settings. *Depress Anxiety* 2000;**11**:163–168.

101. Rubenstein CS, Pigott TA, L'Heureux F, Hill JL, Murphy DL. A preliminary investigation of the lifetime prevalence of anorexia and bulimia nervosa in patients with obsessive compulsive disorder. *J Clin Psychiatry* 1992;**53**:309–314.

102. Geller D, Biederman J, Faraone SV, Bellorde CA, Kim GS, Hagermoser LM. Disentangling chronological age from age of onset in children and adolescents with obsessive compulsive disorder. *Int J Neuropsychopharmacol* 2001;**4**:169–78.

103. Geller D, March J. Practice parameter for the assessment and treatment of children and adolescents with obsessive-compulsive disorder. *J. Am. Acad. Child Adolesc. Psychiatry*, 2012;51(1):98–113.

104. March J, Foa E, Gammon P *et al*. Cognitive-behavior therapy, sertraline, and their combination for children and adolescents with obsessive-compulsive disorder: the Pediatric OCD Treatment Study (POTS) randomized controlled trial. *JAMA* 2004; **292**:1969–1976.

105. Barrett P, Healy-Farrell L, March JS. Cognitive-behavioral family treatment of childhood obsessive-compulsive disorder: A controlled clinical trial. *J Am Acad Child Adolesc Psychiatry* 2004;**43**:46–62.

106. Franklin M, Kozak M, Cashman L, Coles M, Rheingold A, Foa E. Cognitive-behavioral treatment of pediatric obsessive-compulsive disorder: an open clinical trial. *J Am Acad Child Adolesc Psychiatry* 1998;**37**:412–419.

107. Himle JA, Rassi S, Haghighatgou H, Krone KP, Nesse RM, Abelson J. Group behavioral therapy of obsessive-compulsive disorder: seven vs. twelve-week outcomes. *Depress Anxiety* 2001;**13**:161–165.

108. Freeman JB, Choate-Summers ML, Moore PS *et al*. Cognitive behavioral treatment for young children with obsessive-compulsive disorder. *Biol Psychiatry* 2007;**61**:337–343.

109. March JS, Mulle K. *OCD in Children and Adolescents: A Cognitive-Behavioral Treatment Manual*. New York: Guilford Press, 1998.

110. Watson HJ, Rees CS. Meta-analysis of randomized, controlled treatment trials for pediatric obsessive-compulsive disorder. *J Child Psychol Psychiatry* 2008;**49**:489–498.

111. Flament MF, Rapoport JL, Berg CJ *et al*. Clomipramine treatment of childhood obsessive-compulsive disorder: A double-blind controlled study. *Arch Gen Psychiatry* 1985;**42**:977–983.

112. March JS, Biederman J, Wolkow R *et al*. Sertraline in children and adolescents with obsessive-compulsive disorder: A multicenter randomized control trial. *JAMA* 1998;**280**:1752–1756.

113. Riddle MA, Reeve EA, Yaryura-Tobias JA *et al*. Fluvoxamine for children and adolescents with obsessive-compulsive disorder: A randomized, controlled, multicenter trial. *J Am Acad Child Adolesc Psychiatry* 2001;**40**:222– 229.

114. Geller DA, Hoog SL, Heiligenstein JH *et al*. Fluoxetine treatment for obsessive-compulsive disorder in children and adolescents: A placebo-controlled clinical trial. *J Am Acad Child Adolesc Psychiatry* 2001;**40**:773–779.

115. Geller DA, Wagner KD, Emslie G *et al*. Paroxetine treatment in children and adolescents with obsessive-compulsive disorder: A randomized, multicenter, double-blind, placebo-controlled trial. *J Am Acad Child Adolesc Psychiatry* 2004;**43**:1387–1396.

116. Geller DA, Biederman J, Stewart SE *et al*. Which SSRI? A meta-analysis of pharmacotherapy trials in pediatric obsessive compulsive disorder. *Am J Psychiatry* 2003;**160**:1919–1928.

117. Zohar J, Judge R, Investigators OPS. Paroxetine versus clomipramine in the treatment of obsessive-compulsive disorders. *Br J Psychiatry* 1996;**169**:468–474.

118. Biederman J. Sudden death in children treated with a tricyclic antidepressant: A commentary. *J Am Acad Child Adolesc Psychiatry* 1991;**30**:495–497.

119. Wagner KD, Cook EH, Chung H, Messig M. Remission status after long-term sertraline treatment of pediatric obsessive-compulsive disorder. *J Child Adolesc Psychopharmacol* 2003;**13**(Suppl. 1):S53–60.

120. Geller DA, Biederman J, Stewart SE *et al*. Impact of comorbidity on treatment response to paroxetine in pediatric obsessive compulsive disorder: is the use of exclusion criteria empirically supported in randomized clinical trials? *J Child Adolesc Psychopharmacol* 2003;**13**(Suppl. 1):S19–29.

121. March J, Franklin M, Leonard H *et al*. Tics moderate treatment outcome with sertraline but not cognitive-behavior therapy in pediatric obsessive-compulsive disorder. *Biol Psychiatry* 2007;**61**:344–347.

122. Storch EA, Geffken G, Merlo L *et al*. Family-based cognitive-behavioral therapy for pediatric obsessive-compulsive disorder: Comparison of intensive and weekly approaches. *J Am Acad Child Adolesc Psychiatry* 2007;**46**:469–478.

123. Leonard HL, Topol D, Bukstein O, Hindmarsh D, Allen AJ, Swedo SE. Clonazepam as an augmenting agent in the treatment of childhood-onset obsessive-compulsive disorder. *J Am Acad Child Adolesc Psychiatry* 1994;**33**:792–794.

124. Bloch MH, Landeros-Weisenberger A, Kelmendi B, Coric V, Bracken MB, Leckman JF. A systematic review: antipsychotic augmentation with treatment refractory obsessive-compulsive disorder. *Mol Psychiatry* 2006;**11**:622–632.

125. McDougle C, Epperson C, Pelton G, Wasylink S, Price L. A double-blind placebo-controlled study of risperidone addition in serotonin-reuptake inhibitor-refractory obsessive-compulsive disorder. *Arch Gen Psychiatry* 2000;**57**:794–801.

126. Norberg MM, Krystal JH, Tolin DF. A meta-analysis of D-cycloserine and the facilitation of fear extinction and exposure therapy. *Biol Psychiatry* 2008;**63**:1118–1126.

127. Storch EA, Murphy TK, Goodman WK *et al*. A preliminary study of D-cycloserine augmentation of cognitive-behavioral therapy in pediatric obsessive-compulsive disorder. *Biol Psychiatry* 2010;**68**:1073–1076.

128. Martin A, Young C, Leckman JF, Mukonoweshuro C, Rosenheck R, Douglas L. Age effects of antidepressant-induced manic conversion. *Arch Pediatr Adolesc Med* 2004;**158**:773–780.

129. Bridge J, Iyengar S, Salary CB *et al.* Clinical response and risk for reported suicidal ideation and suicide attempts in pediatric antidepressant treatment: A meta-analysis of randomized controlled trials. *JAMA* 2007;**297**:1683–1696.

130. Masi G, Millepiedi S, Mucci M, Bertini N, Milantoni L, Arcangeli F. A naturalistic study of referred children and adolescents with obsessive-compulsive disorder. *J Am Acad Child Adolesc Psychiatry* 2005;**44**:673–681.

131. Sukhodolsky DG, Rosario-Campos MC, Scahill L *et al.* Adaptive, emotional, and family functioning of children with obsessive-compulsive disorder and comorbid attention deficit hyperactivity disorder. *Am J Psychiatry* 2005;**162**:1125–1132.

Research Spotlights

Methodological Issues for Clinical Treatment Trials in Obsessive-Compulsive Disorder

Samar Reghunandanan¹ and Naomi A. Fineberg²

¹*National OCD Treatment Service, Hertfordshire Partnership NHS Foundation Trust, Queen Elizabeth II Hospital, Welwyn Garden City, UK, AL7 4HQ;*
²*National OCD Treatment Service, Hertfordshire Partnership NHS Foundation Trust, Queen Elizabeth II Hospital, Welwyn Garden City, UK, AL7 4HQ and University of Hertfordshire, College Lane, Hatfield, UK, AL10 9AB*

INTRODUCTION

Obsessive-compulsive disorder (OCD) is a common and chronic lifespan mental disorder. It affects between 2 and 3% of the adult population and up to 1% of children, regardless of nationality or socioeconomic status [1]. Females are somewhat over-represented, though males tend to show an earlier onset of illness and a poorer treatment outcome. Individuals with OCD are secretive and the illness often goes unrecognized. Patients tend to have been ill for many years before presenting for clinical treatment [2], and the magnitude of psychosocial impairment associated with OCD is recognized to be high [3]. Compared with other mental disorders, the range of treatments that are effective in OCD is limited. Selective serotonin reuptake inhibitors (SSRIs) or cognitive behaviour therapy (CBT) are recommended in most guidelines [2], but the success rate for either treatment, even when conservatively assessed, is only around 60%. It remains to be established whether combining treatment is more effective than monotherapy. For those patients who do not respond to existing OCD therapies, there is little additional evidence-based treatment available. Furthermore, there are few data to predict who will respond better to which treatment modality. Thus, there is a great need for properly powered

Obsessive-Compulsive Disorder: Current Science and Clinical Practice, First Edition. Edited by Joseph Zohar.
© 2012 John Wiley & Sons, Ltd. Published 2012 by John Wiley & Sons, Ltd.

clinical trials to explore the effects of new and potentially efficacious compounds as well as to determine the optimal existing treatment strategies. Identification of clinical biomarkers that may correlate with treatment outcomes and which may be used to build prediction models to guide personalized treatment constitutes an additional important research goal.

To date, research into OCD has been poorly developed, compared with other mental disorders that carry a similar health burden, such as schizophrenia [4]. Recently published guidelines provide a comprehensive checklist for designing and reporting observational studies in disorders such as OCD [5]. In this chapter, we explore methodological strategies for *clinical treatment trials* in OCD that may be used to demonstrate the acute and sustained long-term efficacy and tolerability of new and existing treatments, across the age range. Well-conducted randomized controlled trials (RCTs) remain the most important method for demonstrating treatment efficacy in OCD [2]. In this chapter, we address some of the key practical questions for designing RCTs in OCD, including how best to select patients for recruitment, how long the trial should last, which control treatments to choose, which rating scales detect clinically relevant changes and how to determine if an efficacious treatment protects against relapse. In addition, we consider the theoretical challenges to researchers that this illness poses, including nosological uncertainties, the problem of comorbidity and the lack of agreement on criteria for response, remission and relapse. Our overall objective is to encourage the development of pragmatic and valid research protocols, including strategies to identify predictors of treatment response and resistance, that may advance personalized healthcare for this relatively underexplored, chronic, major mental disorder.

RANDOMIZED CONTROLLED TRIALS

The guiding principle behind the introduction of a new treatment is that the treatment should have a benefit:risk balance at least as good as that of existing treatments [6]. Trials need to be designed with this in mind. Any new treatment needs to be evaluated against a standard so that this comparison can be made. To be recommended, a treatment must have shown its efficacy in double-blind RCTs that fulfil certain methodological requirements, including standard diagnostic criteria, adequate sample size, a fairly matched control group, randomized allocation to treatment, double-blind conditions, sensitive psychometric rating scales and appropriate statistical tests. Good clinical practice (GCP) criteria [7] need to be fulfilled, and approval obtained from a properly constituted ethics committee [8].

The customary design is a parallel group comparison, but a crossover design may be acceptable, provided that the treatment is randomly ordered and carry-over effects are taken into account. The evaluation of response is usually made using an analysis of variance with the initial severity of OCD as the covariate. Categorical response analysis is sometimes undertaken as well, although there are no generally agreed criteria for defining a responder [9]. Since many of the treatments tested involve an appreciable drop-out rate, it is important to undertake an intent-to treat analysis that includes all those who entered the study, to address the bias associated with evaluating the 'completers', who naturally tend to be responders [10]. As OCD is often a chronic disorder, and there are as yet no reliable predictors of episodic disease, treatment usually needs to continue long term [11]. Therefore, studies examining longer-term efficacy and relapse prevention, as well as acute-phase studies, are important elements of validating OCD treatments.

Double-blind RCTs can be distinguished according to the choice of the control. The placebo-controlled design, which compares the investigational agent with one that lacks an active ingredient, is favoured when there is no established treatment for the illness. When an established treatment exists – e.g. in the case of OCD, an SSRI or clomipramine – the new treatment ought also to be compared with this reference agent (comparator trial). Equivalence of efficacy is a reasonable argument for the introduction of a new treatment, depending upon the relative tolerability, adverse effect profile, and such like. Usually, non-inferiority (equivalence) trials are used, that is, determining whether the new treatment is no less effective than the reference comparator. In order to establish equivalence, the trial attempts to exclude inferiority, which is predetermined by a margin of difference within which the outcome of the two treatments must fall. Such studies carry the the risk that the inferiority of the new treatment to the reference treatment may be missed due to the relatively low statistical power of such studies to detect the equivalent efficacy of active compounds. However, non-inferiority trials are usually preferred over superiority trials, which tend to require even larger sample sizes. In non-inferiority trials, the optimal sample size depends on the definition of a clinically meaningful margin of difference and in disorders such as OCD this definition may be arbitrary. Furthermore, a comparator trial lacking a placebo control may not be regarded as a sufficiently stringent test of a new compound as it lacks 'assay sensitivity', that is, evidence that either treatment is performing better than an inactive treatment. Table 8.1 lists some of the advantages and disadvantages associated with controlled trials comparing active compounds.

Establishing equivalence in an active comparator study does not prove efficacy. It just means both treatments were either equally efficacious or equally inefficacious in the population tested. However, the general assumption is that if the comparator agent already has proven efficacy, the novel agent is also efficacious. In this respect, the choice of the compound and dose that constitutes the active comparator is of crucial importance. All commonly used SSRIs have shown efficacy in OCD with no convincing evidence that any one treatment is superior to another. Higher doses of SSRI appear to be more clinically efficacious, though they are associated with a greater burden of adverse effects. SSRIs are better tolerated than clomipramine, and are no less effective [11] and are therefore the preferred choice. Placebo-controlled investigation has revealed that the lowest efficacious dose of paroxetine is 40 mg, and therefore doses below this should probably be avoided in comparator trials. A

Table 8.1   Advantages and disadvantages of active controlled trials.

Advantages
- Patients not subjected to ineffective placebo
- Directly compares tolerability with existing treatments
- Easier to recruit where patients perceive they are not exposed to placebo

Disadvantages
- Large numbers required to avoid type II error and false equivalence
- Numbers rise as estimated efficacy of treatment falls
- Numbers far exceed those required in placebo-controlled trials
- Larger numbers exposed to a novel agent than if it were tested against placebo
- Tendency to conflate response rates for both treatments
- Untoward events automatically considered to be side effects leading to higher than expected dropout rates

(All limit the 'assay sensitivity' of the study)

Table 8.2   Expert consensus recommendations for a non-inferiority trial, adapted for obsessive-compulsive disorder (OCD). Adapted from Nutt et al., 2008 [12].

- Inclusion of a placebo arm to ensure 'assay sensitivity'
- Both active treatments should be superior to placebo by an accepted and clinically meaningful difference on a specific rating scale (e.g. ≥ 2 points on the Yale–Brown Obsessive-Compulsive Scale (Y–BOCS)
- Both active treatments should be superior to placebo in terms of response rate (e.g. $\geq 10\%$ better than placebo), while response may be defined as a $\geq 25\%$ improvement on the Y–BOCS
- The non-inferiority margin, i.e. the difference between the active treatments on the main efficacy measure (e.g. Y–BOCS), should be <50% of the mean difference between the reference treatment and placebo in previous randomized controlled trials
- The response rate for the new treatment should be no more than 5% lower than for the reference treatment
- The one-sided 97.5% confidence interval of the non-inferiority margin should fall within an a priori defined interval on the Y–BOCS

consensus among experts in the field has evolved regarding the requirements for a non-inferiority trial that could be adapted for OCD (Table 8.2) [12]. Ethical issues are, however, still under debate [13].

THE RATIONALE OF PLACEBO

There has been considerable debate about the ethics of using placebo in disease areas such as OCD, where effective pharmacological and psychological treatments are already well established [11]. Importantly, placebo-controlled studies expose recipients to an ineffective treatment that may sometimes precipitate adverse consequences. Studies comparing a novel treatment with an already established approach, by contrast, do not. Ethical review bodies have therefore become reluctant to sanction the use of placebos, preferring as an alternative, trials that use a known active treatment for comparison, so it is relevant and timely to question whether there are still good methodological and ethical grounds to support the continued use of placebo-controlled studies.

It is known that the number of patients required to discriminate between two interventions increases as the effect size diminishes. In other words, the smaller the difference in benefit between two treatments, the greater the number of subjects needed to demonstrate that benefit. In active-comparator studies, the measurable benefit of one intervention over a well-established treatment is usually quite small and so these studies may require very large numbers to demonstrate superiority or even equivalence. While placebo-controlled studies are not completely immune to this problem, they generally require considerably fewer participants than active-comparator studies. For example, in the treatment of OCD there has been a striking trend towards increasing placebo response rates over three decades. Such increases inevitably reduce the power of placebo studies. Figure 8.1 shows the changes measured by the Yale–Brown Obsessive-Compulsive Scale (Y–BOCS) [14,15] on placebo and active drug treatment in RCTs that were published from 1989 to 2007. Nonetheless, the sample sizes required to test efficacy against placebo remain favourable compared to those required for comparator-controlled studies, and by using placebo, fewer subjects overall are likely to be subjected to a treatment that

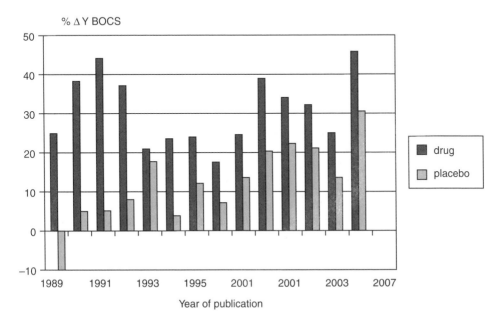

Figure 8.1 Mean reduction of baseline Yale–Brown Obsessive-Compulsive Scale (Y–BOCS) comparing serotonin reuptake inhibitor (SRI) with placebo in obsessive-compulsive disorder (OCD) trials.

might not turn out to be effective. Stein *et al.* [16] identified predictors of placebo response within clinical trials databases for escitalopram in three anxiety disorders (not OCD). Placebo responses were greater in European Union (EU) trials and less severe anxiety disorders. Predictors of placebo response rate differed for different disorders. For generalized anxiety disorder, the placebo response rate was higher in trials with several factors including EU location, GP setting, flexible dose design, and increased number of treatment arms. Given that maximizing drug–placebo differences improves trial design, researchers may consider these factors to be of relevance when planning a placebo-controlled trial in OCD.

Placebo-controlled trials are, therefore, on the whole smaller, quicker and cheaper to run. The economic burden of developing new treatments is substantial, and by reducing impediments to testing, the pharmaceutical industry is more likely to undertake development work with drugs that have novel mechanisms of action. Trial cost and feasibility are not ethical issues and it is important to keep them separate. However, taking a longer-term perspective, the importance of a commercial incentive in the development of medical treatments cannot be overlooked. One other important advantage of placebo-controlled studies is that, by referencing a new drug to placebo, we can derive clinically relevant constants for the drug such as its 'effect-size', and the 'number needed to treat'. These approaches permit absolute, rather than relative, comparisons with other established treatments.

The methodological advantages of including a placebo arm need to be offset, however, against ethical issues [17]. Primarily, patients are necessarily exposed to inefficacious treatments. Of course this does not mean they will not improve; in OCD, for example, placebo response rates regularly exceed 20% reduction in baseline severity (Figure 8.1), but they are unlikely to improve as much on placebo as on an effective treatment. Other harmful consequences of an inadequately treated disorder include prolonged psychosocial impairment (e.g. job loss, family breakdown) and even suicidal behaviour. Importantly, patients entering treatment studies are usually screened to exclude those judged to be at risk of suicidality and those with comorbidities may be excluded as well.

If we accept the methodological and pragmatic arguments for continuing to use placebos in treatment trials, we should safeguard patients to ensure they are not subjected to unacceptable risk (Table 8.3). Any placebo-controlled study should be designed to limit the numbers exposed and the duration of exposure to placebo. Moreover, attention to the study recruitment criteria becomes paramount. Patients at high risk of suicidal behaviour or who are unlikely to tolerate the rigours of being in a placebo study should not be included. This may indirectly restrict the illness severity of the sample under test. Informed written consent, explaining the method for randomization, allocation of treatment and use of placebo, and the patient's non-prejudicial right to withdraw at any time and receive conventional treatment, is a prerequisite. Patients need to be monitored carefully. This usually means more frequently than for conventional clinical practice, and research staff must be available for consultation between appointments if necessary. Explicit withdrawal criteria are needed either for non-response or adverse effects, and

Table 8.3 Recommended safeguards for placebo-controlled trials.

- Power calculations to limit numbers exposed to placebo as far as possible within limits of study validity
- Shorten participants' exposure to placebo as far as possible within limits of study validity
- Exclude cases at high suicide risk or who appear unable to tolerate the rigours of a trial
- Ensure participant gives informed, written consent
- Emphasize participant's non-prejudicial right to withdrawal
- Frequent monitoring of participant's progress
- Explicit withdrawal criteria in case of non-response or adverse events
- Protocol for follow-up after study ends

there should be a protocol for following up and treating those individuals who leave the study early, or who remain symptomatic at the end of the trial. In the absence of viable alternatives, placebo-referenced studies offer some convincing advantages over active-controlled trials in acute and long-term OCD studies. Safe use of placebos requires careful planning, and techniques for limiting exposure to ineffective treatment within the context of treatment trials should be explored. We review some of these strategies in the next paragraphs.

RECRUITMENT CRITERIA

Aside from the safety exclusions required in the case of testing against placebo (see above), a balance needs to be struck between recruitment criteria that are *strict enough* to achieve homogeneous groups of individuals with well-defined OCD without the potentially confounding effect of other coexisting illnesses, and who are therefore best placed to respond to a putative actively anti-obsessive treatment, but that are not *too narrow* to ensure that the study sample remains representative of patients seen in daily practice. In order to detect specific response predictors, there also needs to be sufficient clinical variability at baseline for associations with treatment outcome to be identified. Naturally fluctuating or unstable illness has a confounding effect on the ability to detect treatment-related changes in symptom severity, and for this reason, treatment trials usually require a 'diagnostically stable' disorder, for whom clinically relevant OCD has been continually present for at least 12 months.

DIAGNOSIS

Most treatment trials are based upon a diagnosis made according to the *Diagnostic and Statistical Manual of Mental Disorders, Fourth Edition* (DSM-IV) [18]. However, shortcomings in the existing DSM-IV criteria for OCD, such as problems with the diagnostic threshold, subtypes and stability, that may lead to biological heterogeneity, have been identified and the criteria are currently undergoing review (ref. Phillips etc.) [19]. The WHO *International Classification of Disorders, Tenth Revision* (ICD-10) diagnostic criteria [20] are broadly consistent with those of DSM-IV, but are arguably more flexible and less prescriptive. For instance, the ICD-10 does not expressly exclude 'worries about real life problems' and does not require obsessions to be time consuming, which could result in an increase in 'sub-threshold' cases. The issue of sub-threshold OCD is particularly intriguing as there are no treatment trials in this condition and no recognized diagnostic criteria.

OCD DIMENSIONS AND SUBTYPES

One approach to reducing nosological heterogeneity has been to attempt to define and select/deselect OCD subtypes or dimensions that may impact upon the treatment outcome. Data from factor analysis, genetic, functional imaging and treatment studies have highlighted the clinical relevance of a dimensional model of OCD [21]. Of the dimensions so far identified, hoarding is perhaps the best researched and may even constitute a separate syndrome [21]. Analysis of a large trials database suggests that a 'hoarding/symmetry' dimension predicts a poorer outcome to SSRI treatment compared to other factors within OCD [22]. Imaging studies additionally hint at a separate neurobiology for hoarding [23]. For this reason, treatment trials may reasonably choose to exclude cases where hoarding is the most prominent or the exclusive symptom.

The DSM-IV classifies 'poor insight' as a relatively rare 'subtype' of OCD. However, recent research suggest that poor insight is common in OCD, affecting about one-quarter of cases and positively correlates with severity, duration, age of onset, the number of obsessive-compulsive symptoms, and comorbidity (especially major depression) and negatively correlates with treatment success [24]. The presence of overvalued ideas in OCD has been theoretically linked to poorer treatment outcome with CBT [25]. However, other data suggest that the presence or absence of insight has little effect on treatment outcome with SSRIs [26]. Indeed, insight varies between different OCD subjects and within the same subject at different stages of the illness and may represent a proxy marker of illness severity [27,28]. OCD with poor insight has not so far demonstrated differentiating psychobiological features [21]. Thus, arguments for specifically excluding poor-insight OCD in psychopharmacological treatment trials are not strong. However, detailed assessment of insight using specific scales, such as item II on the Y–BOCs) [14,15] or the Brown Assessment of Beliefs Scale [29], may be helpful in defining more homogeneous patient groups and for prediction modelling.

Motor signs, such as tics, and soft neurological signs are common in OCD and may require special assessment. OCD with tics may constitute another biologically relevant subtype and is particularly common in males with early-onset illness [30].

Two studies report a poor response to anti-OCD agents in tic-related OCD [31,32], and the Expert Committee of the DSM-5 judged OCD with tics to represent a relatively treatment-resistant form of illness [33]. Thus, there are grounds for excluding from treatment trials OCD cases with tics. However, tics are very common in OCD [30], and although they tend to recede with age they are still observed, albeit in an attenuated form, in a large proportion of adult cases. Moreover, Shavitt *et al.* [34] noted a good response to clomipramine in these patients. For practical purposes, while Tourette syndrome is usually disallowed, patients with tics are often included in OCD trials. The Yale Global Tic Severity Scale (YGTSS) [35] measures the severity of tic symptoms across a range of dimensions. Using the YGTSS and the Y–BOCS, the fluctuation of tics and OCD were correlated over time, and found to demonstrate a degree of synchronicity [36]. Moreover, the YGTSS accurately identified symptom exacerbation, suggesting it represents a clinically meaningful instrument for assessing tics in individuals with OCD.

In contrast to tics, neurological soft signs are non-localizing deviant performances on motor and sensory tests, without evidence of focal neurological dysfunction. These include abnormalities in motor coordination, involuntary movement and sensory and visuo-spatial functioning. There appears to be a negative correlation between the severity of neurological soft signs in OCD and treatment outcome [37]. The Neurological Soft Sign Examination [38] is based upon a structured neurological examination and is able to differentiate patients with OCD from healthy controls, suggesting possible value in the trial scenario.

Research into the 'early-onset' OCD subtype has been hampered by the use of different age limits for its definition [21] and uncertainty around the developmental stability of OC symptoms. OCD that develops following a streptococcal infection is another putative, biologically homogeneous subtype for which evidence is accruing [39]. In addition, behavioural avoidance is a common OCD symptom that is given relatively little importance in the current diagnostic criteria [21] but that contributes substantially to psychosocial dysfunction, and is a focus for CBT that could potentially constitute a clinically meaningful dimension for classifying OCD. For factors such as these, improved assessment instruments are required to allow studies to establish their clinical relevance and effect on treatment outcome.

THE PROBLEM OF COMORBIDITY

A substantial lifetime comorbidity between OCD and other major mental disorders has been identified, including depression, which develops in approximately two-thirds of cases presenting for treatment, specific phobia (22%), social anxiety disorder (or social phobia; 18%), eating disorders (17%), alcohol dependence (14%), panic disorder (12%) and Tourette syndrome (7%) [40]. Patients with these comorbidities are usually excluded from treatment trials, because the presence of the additional disorder may confound the efficacy of the treatment under

202 OBSESSIVE-COMPULSIVE DISORDER

study. Indeed, psychiatric comorbidity is recognized to contribute towards greater treatment resistance in OCD [9]. In the case of depression, an upper limit for depressive symptoms is often set according to a cut-off score on a depression rating scale; for example, ≤24 on the Montgomery and Asberg Depression Rating Scale (MADRS) [41]. Suicidality may be excluded by reference to item 10 on the MADRS or using the suicidal item on the Mini International Neuropsychiatric Interview (MINI) [42]. The Columbia Suicide Severity Rating Scale (C-SSRS) [43] (http://www.maps.org/mdma/mt1_docs/c-ssrs1-14-09-baseline.pdf) is currently recommended by the Division of Psychiatry Products and the US Food and Drug Administration, for the prospective monitoring of suicidal ideation in treatment trials. Although these strategies theoretically improve the homogeneity of the OCD sample, and thereby the reproducibility of the results, by the same token they may diminish the 'generalizability' of the findings to the clinical scenario, where patients are mainly presenting for treatment with many of these comorbidities. The stringent exclusion of depressive symptoms may indirectly lead to the exclusion of more severe cases of OCD, who might otherwise respond well to active treatment and less well to placebo [44], and therefore this procedure could reduce the power of a comparator study to demonstrate efficacy. Moreover, there is a differential impact of obsessions, compulsions and comorbid depression on health-related quality of life (HRQoL), correlations with HRQoL being most pronounced for depression severity and the number of OCD symptoms [3]. These findings imply that OCD-related HRQoL may be most meaningfully assessed in treatment trials where depression is not too strictly excluded.

There are several other, less well-recognized and relatively uncommon disorders that, on the basis of phenomenological similarities, course of illness, family history, comorbidity and treatment response, have been termed OCD-spectrum disorders [45] and that may be misdiagnosed as OCD or show high levels of comorbidity with OCD. These include body dysmorphic disorder, hypochondriasis, Tourette syndrome, paediatric autoimmune neuropsychiatric disorders associated with streptococcal infections (PANDAS), Sydenham chorea, trichotillomania, pathological gambling and obsessive-compulsive personality disorder. In order to better understand their impact on the OCD treatment response, researchers need to actively screen for these comorbidities at baseline. Although there is no single diagnostic tool for all these disorders, versions of the Schedule for Affective Disorders and Schizophrenia (SADS) [46,47] capture many of the symptoms and syndromes associated with adult and childhood OCD, including depressive disorders, anxiety disorders, conduct disorders, oppositional defiant disorders, attention-deficit hyperactivity disorder (ADHD), autism spectrum disorders, tic disorders and post-traumatic stress disorder (PTSD). To obtain a dimensional measure of autistic disorders, the Autism Spectrum Screening Questionnaire (ASSQ) [48] can be used, while the Structured Clinician-Administered Interview for the Diagnosis of Obsessive-Compulsive Spectrum Disorders (SCID-OCSD) [49] captures pathological gambling.

RATING SCALES FOR OCD TRIALS

An ideal rating tool needs to be relatively brief yet sensitive enough to detect small but clinically relevant treatment-related changes. Over the past three decades, the Y–BOCS [14,15] has emerged as the pivotal rating scale for OCD and has been used to endorse efficacy for most of the available pharmacological treatments. The Y–BOCS is a 10-item observer-rated instrument that can be adapted as a self-rated tool and that measures the overall severity of obsessions and compulsions separately and in combination. Items include duration, interference, distress, ability to resist and control. Of these, the item measuring resistance is the least reliable, but various attempts to revise the psychometric properties of the scale have not met with general support and it remains largely in its original form. Post-randomization changes in the Y–BOCS are usually used as the primary outcome measure in treatment trials. The children's Y–BOCS includes age-appropriate modifications and has become the standard tool for OCD in children aged as young as 4 years of age [50]. Complementary scales that are also sensitive to change in OCD populations, and that may be used as secondary outcome measures, include the National Institute for Mental Health Global Obsessive-Compulsive Scale [51], the Clinical Global Impression Severity and Improvement Scales [52], the Sheehan Disability Scale (SDS) [53] and the Short-Form-36 (SF-36) [54]; these respectively measure global OCD severity, global illness severity and improvement, psychosocial impairment and health-related disability.

One of the main problems of the Y–BOCS is the subdivision into obsessions and compulsions. Many patients are not able to describe separate obsessions and compulsions. In addition, core concepts such as obsessionality, compulsivity and avoidance are disregarded. Furthermore, changes in severity of symptoms cannot be fully captured because the Y–BOCS contains classes that are too broad. For example, similar Y–BOCS ratings will be scored when a patient spends 4 hours instead of 7 hours per day on OC symptoms. New scales such as the promising Dutch Dimensional Obsessive Compulsive Scale (D-DOCS), a 10-item observer-rated scale that measures the severity of OC symptoms according to time, distribution, fixation, feeling of obligation, control, fear, distress, dysfunction, avoidance and ego-dystony, are in the process of being validated [55]. The Y–BOCS may also be criticized for failing to take account of the cognitive and executive impairments known to be associated with OCD [56]. The Cognitive Assessment Instrument of Obsessions and Compulsions (CAIOC) [57] is a novel 13-item tool. Its clinician- and self-rated versions appear to be valid and reliable measures of the severity of functional impairment associated with OCD. Further validation, including research into the relationship of the CAIOC-13 with laboratory measures of cognitive impairment and evaluation of its sensitivity to change with treatment, is indicated.

Other OCD instruments may fulfil certain roles. For example, the Obsessive Compulsive Inventory (OCI) [58] captures the richness of the complexity of OCD phenomenology, and the shortened version (OCI-R) [59] shows sensitivity to treatment-related change and may be suitable for naturalistic outcome studies; the Padua Inventory [60] seems particularly valid in distinguishing between worries and obsessions, and the Maudsley Inventory [14,15], although not sensitive in detecting treatment effects, may be useful for quantifying specific obsessions and compulsions in non-clinical samples [61].

EVALUATING ANXIETY AND DEPRESSION IN OCD

The reliable assessment of the severity of anxiety and depression is a key issue for OCD research. To date, the drugs noted to be efficacious in OCD are effective in depression and anxiety as well. The Y–BOCS has been reported to show excellent discriminant validity and low convergent validity [62] compared to the Spielberger State Trait Anxiety Inventory (STAI) [63] and the Hamilton Depression Rating Scale (HDRS) [64], suggesting that in OCD research one should include separate measures to adequately discriminate changes in depression and anxiety independently from OCD. In the absence of rating scales that are specifically validated for the OCD population, anxiety may be evaluated using the Hamilton Anxiety Rating Scale [64] and depression by the HDRS [65] or the MADRS [66], each of which have been shown to be sensitive to response in OCD treatment trials. As a tool for measuring depression within OCD, the MADRS may be more sensitive and specific than the HDRS because it contains fewer anxiety items that might confound the rating. Indeed, while all the MADRS items are sensitive to treatment response, the same is not true of the HDRS [67]. One problem with this approach is that it treats comorbid anxiety and affective symptoms, that may be secondary or integral to OCD, as though they are indistinguishable from the non-comorbid disorder. In fact, analysis of depressive symptoms in OCD patients using the MADRS revealed a different profile of symptoms compared with a group of patients with pure major depressive disorder of similar severity [68], suggesting the need for a modified depression scale to evaluate this syndrome. In the OCD depressives, anxiety, pessimistic and suicidal thoughts were more prominent while sleep and appetite disturbance were less pronounced. Surprisingly, perhaps, the anxiety syndrome that is associated with OCD is not well characterized, though worry, apprehension and avoidance are common. It is noteworthy that the Hamilton Anxiety Rating Scale focuses less on cognitive symptoms such as worry, that tend to characterize OCD, and more on somatic anxiety, which may be difficult to differentiate from adverse effects of trial medication and thereby susceptible to confound.

The STAI [63] is a self-report inventory that measures state and trait anxiety separately and thus might allow for a proper discrimination of anxiety symptoms that are secondary to OCD (state anxiety) from anxiety that is long standing and temporally more stable. The STAI may find application in studies exploring the presence of state/trait anxiety, for example in first-degree relatives, and its effect on OC beliefs/behaviour of patients [69] or in differentiating anxious and obsessive responses in acute pharmacological challenge studies [70]. However, the STAI has been shown to distinguish poorly between anxiety states and other disorders such as depression [71].

Visual analogue scales are quick and easy to administer and do not require prior training. They provide a subjective perception of the severity of the disorder and show a relatively high level of sensitivity to change; thus, in addition to pharmacological challenge studies, they may be especially useful in assessing the early response to treatment in trials at a point where small changes may not be captured by standard instruments [72].

MEASURING RESPONSE AND REMISSION

The response to treatment in OCD is slow and incremental, extending over weeks and months to reach its maximum effect. The magnitude of the treatment response may be expressed as the mean change in baseline Y–BOCS scores on active drug compared with placebo (e.g. 8.2 points in a recent meta-analysis of clomipramine [73]). Alternatively, the results can be expressed dichotomously, as the number of treatment responders in each treatment arm. It is important to remember that open-label trials are usually associated with higher rates of response because patients know that they are taking an active treatment, whereas studies based at specialist centres tend to attract resistant cases for which the response rate will naturally be lower.

There remains controversy over the optimal definition of response, remission and relapse in OCD research [9]. An adequate trial of treatment needs to be at least 12 weeks in duration, since studies so far have noted symptom remission occurring at around week 12, with further incremental improvements up to week 24 [74]. Table 8.4 represents a systematic review of the response rates for all the available SSRI trials in OCD. An adequate *clinical response* could be defined as a 35% improvement on the Y–BOCS and/or a score of 2 or less (much or very much improved) on the CGI-I, following randomization. Though a 25% improvement on the Y–BOCS is not the ultimate goal of treatment, this threshold is capable of discriminating responders from non-responders on the SDS and SF-36 and therefore represents a clinically relevant achievement. However, a 25% Y–BOCS decrease alone does not always appear to be stringent enough. For example, large-scale placebo-controlled studies such as that of Stein *et al.* [74] noted that a majority of patients in all treatment arms showed this degree of improvement, yet only about one-third were much or very much improved on the CGI. Furthermore, the clinical response rate on escitalopram reached 70% only after 24 weeks of sustained treatment, highlighting the need for acute-phase trials to be long enough to produce a representative outcome. Pallanti *et al.* [9] suggested that a 35% improvement is necessary to denote a full treatment response and that a 25–35% Y–BOCS reduction represents only a *partial response*. The response criterion of

Table 8.4 Rate of clinical response in placebo-controlled studies of selective serotonin reuptake inhibitors (SSRIs) for patients with obsessive-compulsive disorder (OCD).

Drug (duration, weeks)	Definition of clinical response				Study
	Much or very much improved on CGI-I (Criterion A)	>25% improved on baseline Y-BOCS (Criterion B)	>35% improved on baseline Y-BOCS	Criteria A&B	
Citalopram 20 mg (12)	57.4%				Montgomery et al. (2001) [118]
Citalopram 40 mg (12)	52%				
Citalopram 60 mg (12)	65%				
Clomipramine (12)	55.3%				Zohar and Judge (1996) [119]
Escitalopram 10 mg (24)	40%	75%			Stein et al. (2007) [74]
Escitalopram 20 mg (24)	38%	78%			
Fluvoxamine (8)	9/21				Goodman et al. (1989) [120]
Fluvoxamine (10)	33.3%				Goodman et al. (1996) [121]
Fluvoxamine CR (12)	34% from graph	63%	45%		Hollander et al. (2003) [75]
Fluvoxamine (10)		42% (C-YBOCS)			Riddle et al. (2001) [122]
Fluoxetine 20 mg (8)				36%	Montgomery et al. (1993) [123]
Fluoxetine 40 mg (8)				48%	
Fluoxetine 60 mg (8)				47%	
Fluoxetine 20 mg (13)			32%		Tollefson et al. (1994) [124]
Fluoxetine 40 mg (13)			34%		
Fluoxetine 60 mg (13)			35%		
Fluoxetine (13)	55%				Geller et al. (2001) [125]
Fluoxetine (16)	57%				Liebowitz et al. (2002) [126]
Paroxetine (12)	55.1%				Zohar and Judge (1996) [119]
Paroxetine 40 mg (24)	31%	69%			Stein et al. (2007) [74]
Sertraline (12)	41%				Kronig et al. (1999) [127]
Sertraline (12)	38.9%				Greist et al. (1995) [128]
Sertraline (12)	42%				March et al. (1998) [129]

CGI-I, Clinical Global Impression – Improvement (Scale); CY–BOCS, Children's Yale–Brown Obsessive-Compulsive Scale; Y–BOCS, Yale–Brown

35% is clearly more conservative than the 50% reduction required on the Ham-D in depression trials. Indeed, using the 35% criterion, Hollander *et al.* [75] reported a relative over-representation of fluvoxamine-Controlled-release (CR) responders (46%) compared with the CGI evaluation (34%) in the same trial cohort, implying that a higher Y–BOCS response criterion would be more credible. Despite such a modest criterion, response rates in acute-phase OCD trials rarely exceed 60%, emphasizing the partial efficacy of conventional treatments for this disorder. The CGI-I captures the larger clinical picture, though it lacks specificity – and perhaps to some extent sensitivity. For example, in a study of escitalopram, both 10 mg and 20 mg dosed groups separated from placebo using the Y–BOCS criterion whereas using the CGI-I criterion only escitalopram 20 mg separated from placebo. Combining the Y–BOCS with the CGI-I may produce a reasonable compromise for optimizing discriminatory power [76].

Remission is a higher hurdle than response, representing the absence of syndromal disorder [76], and there is even more debate about its definition. Unlike other disorders, such as depression, a return to a state of no illness may be a rare event in OCD. Five percent of cases may follow a naturally episodic course [77] where the term 'recovery' may fit better, whereas remission may be a more appropriate goal in non-episodic OCD. Studies have adopted categorical remission criteria using Y–BOCS scores ranging from <16 to <7 [78–82]. A total score of 16 is generally considered too high to represent meaningful remission, whereas a score of 7 is too low to be achieved by all but a very few cases. Thus while Simpson *et al.* [76] were unable to discriminate active from placebo treatments using a categorical Y–BOCS threshold of 7, the multicentre studies by Stein *et al.* [74] and Fineberg *et al.* [83] achieved the same with a Y–BOCS score of ≤10.

RELAPSE PREVENTION

Studies investigating the short-term effects of discontinuing clomipramine or SSRIs under double-blind placebo-controlled conditions showed a rapid and incremental worsening of symptoms [84], implying that treatment needs to be continued to remain effective. Evaluating whether SRIs protect against relapse requires a lengthy and complicated design involving the selection of treatment responders, usually following unblinded treatment, and randomizing them either to remain on active treatment or to switch to placebo, using graduated dose reduction to minimize discontinuation effects that might unblind the study, and under survival analysis conditions. The definition of the relapse criterion is crucial in this regard [85]. Criteria for determining relapse in reported trials have varied from the 'return to pre-treatment severity' to a predefined measure of worsened outcome. Such measures include a five-point worsening of baseline Y–BOCS scores [83], a Y–BOCS score >19, and CGI-I scores of 'worse/much worse'. If relapse criteria are too stringent [86,87] or need to be repeated over many visits [86], the number of endorsable relapses becomes artificially reduced and studies may fail through lack of statistical power. In the study by Fineberg *et al.* [83], a five-point worsening of Y–BOCS occurring at a single visit, or lack of efficacy as judged by the investigator, was used as the relapse criterion and clearly differentiated continuation of active treatment from placebo over the 16-week randomization phase. Patients relapsing using this criterion were also seen to show significant loss of health-related quality of life as measured on the SF-36, providing further justification for the clinical relevance of this criterion [88].

TREATMENT-RESISTANT OCD

Previous failure to respond to a recognized treatment is a strong predictor of future resistance. Recruitment to a RCT of a new OCD treatment needs to exclude, as far as possible, SSRI-resistant cases that are less likely to respond. In contrast, other treatment trials focus specifically on developing treatment for SSRI-resistant illness. A common strategy for SSRI-resistant OCD is to add a second treatment on to the first. The inclusion of patients responding partially but slowly to first-line treatments is likely to confound both active and placebo arms, and some trials may have been hampered by failing to apply stringent enough entry criteria for resistance [89]. However, the application of overly stringent criteria may result in the selection of patients who are too refractory to respond to any treatment whatsoever [90].

Research into treatment-resistant OCD has been hampered by the lack of consensus on its definition. Arguably, this depends on the goal of treatment – that is, whether the failure is in achieving response, or remission or recovery. An ideal definition of resistance should take into account the number of SSRI trials, role of clomipramine, duration of each trial, psychological therapy and measures of non-response as reflected by ratings on both the Y–BOCS and CGI. Such definitions should also include measures of well-being, HRQoL and level of functioning, for example using the SDS and SF-36. In the absence of a clear operational definition, terms such as non-response/refractory/resistance are used synonymously [9], and published studies have continued to use a variety of different criteria; some studies included only extremely refractory cases who had failed to respond to successive sustained treatments with more than one SRI, whereas others included those who had made a partial response to treatment with a single SRI drug. Unfortunately, there are no RCTs that allow estimation of the chance of response following a single failed trial of an SSRI. According to the most comprehensive definition to date [9], failure to respond by at least 25% from baseline on the Y–BOCS, after treatment with at least one course of SSRI given at maximally tolerated dose levels for at least 12 weeks, may constitute clinically meaningful SSRI resistance. Some studies additionally require the patient to fail a second course of SSRI [91], or to exceed a severity threshold on the Y–BOCS. For example, Simpson *et al.* [92] and

McDougle *et al.* [93] set a Y–BOCS score of ≥ 16 as the criterion for refractoriness in trials that managed to differentiate active drug from placebo.

Definitions such as these assume equivalence for all SSRIs in OCD. However, recent experience in depression, where a hierarchy of antidepressant efficacy is recognized [94,95] cautions that in the absence of properly constituted trials, we cannot assume that all SSRIs are the same in OCD [96,97]. Future definitions may equate resistance to certain SRIs in preference to others. Better understanding of the diagnostic boundaries and the relevance of subthreshold symptoms could also potentially improve the way we define treatment response and resistance in OCD. Other research has focused attention on symptom dimensions as a valid construct for assessment of resistance [98–102]. For example, the hoarding/symmetry dimension may specifically predict SSRI resistance [103] and, therefore, studies may need to screen carefully for this factor when selecting patients to enter treatment trials. Importantly, the role of psychological therapy in defining resistance has not been adequately explored, and treatment trials investigating CBT-resistant OCD are lacking. The UK National Service for Resistant OCD defines psychotherapy-resistant cases, for clinical purposes, as those who have failed to respond to two full courses of therapist-aided CBT that includes *in vivo* exposure and response prevention with home-based elements, delivered by certified CBT therapists.

PSYCHOLOGICAL TREATMENT TRIALS

The introduction of CBT for OCD was a key advance in the treatment of the disorder. The efficacy of CBT involving exposure and response prevention (ERP) has been demonstrated in Western and Eastern settings [104,105], in both individual and group formats, with improvements approximating to those seen on medication in acute-phase trials [2]. However, RCTs comparing ERP with psychological placebo, using an intent-to-treat analysis, seem to be rare and there are no adequately controlled long-term or relapse prevention trials. Hence, there remains a degree of uncertainty as to the magnitude of the clinical response that can be attributed to the specific effect of psychological therapy (akin to the effect size in pharmacological trials), and the degree of CBT resistance, non-adherence and premature discontinuation require further exploration [21].

Psychological therapies are vulnerable to a range of non-specific therapeutic effects including therapist and patient factors. It is especially relevant, therefore, that psychological therapy trials are conducted with properly matched and well-defined psychological controls. Wait list, or non-specific 'treatment as usual' that do not match these variables can no longer be considered acceptable. Stress management training, which involves either relaxation or problem-solving, could be considered to be a suitable control for attention, time, homework effort and other non-specific therapeutic effects. While it may be difficult to guarantee true study 'blindness' among the study participants, it is possible to ensure that the degree of therapist commitment to the control treatment is equivalent to that of the active therapy. Raters should be independent from the therapists and blind to the treatment allocation. Manualized protocols, ideally with video monitoring to ensure adherence within the session, offer a practical and transparent strategy to achieve this. Additional measures of patient adherence to treatment between sessions (e.g. via homework diaries) are informative. This degree of complexity requires careful training and supervision to minimize discrepancies between different therapists, and multicentre psychological treatment trials may be particularly vulnerable to site effects, which need to be monitored for.

Using randomized controlled strategies, it appears that psychological placebo response rates may be higher than in pharmacological treatment trials and may approximate to the effect of the active treatment under investigation. For example, a study comparing the effects of group CBT versus relaxation noted that patients on group CBT and group relaxation improved to roughly the same extent, suggesting that benefits accrued from non-specific group interaction rather than CBT itself, though the percentage of dropouts in the relaxation condition (35%) exceeded the number in the CBT condition (4%), implying superior acceptability for CBT [106]. Thus, properly constituted psychological treatment trials may need careful powering and substantial recruitment to avoid type II error. As we have already discussed for pharmacological trials, while there are valid grounds to use 'placebo-controlled' trials to test the efficacy of alternative forms of psychological treatment in OCD, the addition of an active comparator arm, such as ERP, may provide a valuable extra benchmark.

INTEGRATED PHARMACOLOGICAL AND PSYCHOLOGICAL TREATMENTS IN OCD

We know that SRIs and behavioural therapy are individually effective in OCD, and it would therefore seem likely that the combination of both treatments would produce even better efficacy. To date, few studies have compared pharmacotherapy, psychotherapy and combined therapy systematically [2,104] and the evidence remains incomplete. Meta-analyses [107] have not succeeded in addressing the question of relative efficacy of interventions, partly because this approach cannot adequately correct for the changes that have occurred between individual trials over the years, such as rising placebo response rates (Figure 8.1). Head-to-head comparisons of the effect of combination treatment with drug or behavioural monotherapy are preferable, and it is regrettable that so few properly controlled studies have been performed [108]. For example, a relatively large trial that randomized children and adolescents with OCD to pill placebo, sertraline, CBT, and combined sertraline with CBT (but omitted psychological placebo), was able to demonstrate that all three active treatments were superior to pill placebo, but was unable to differentiate any one active treatment from another [109]. Moreover, optimistic claims from uncontrolled case series that CBT may prevent relapse following discontinuation of SSRI [110], although intuitively persuasive, need to be explored further under properly controlled conditions. A recent, well-crafted trial that randomized SSRI partial- or non-responders to add-on treatment with intensive CBT with ERP or anxiety management, suggests adjunctive CBT may be effective in patients refractory to pharmacotherapy [92]. This finding raises the interesting question of whether the sequence in which treatments are applied affects the outcome. Future research may look towards sophisticated, randomized designs to address such complex issues.

HEALTH-RELATED QUALITY OF LIFE

Another unresolved issue is the accurate translation of Y–BOCS changes into clinically meaningful improvements in *functioning and quality of life*. Indeed, constructs such as HRQoL, disability, impairment and subjective well-being may need to be incorporated into future definitions of treatment response and remission, since they may not be adequately captured by the Y–BOCS. The SF-36 is the most frequently used measure to assess HRQoL in OCD studies. An advantage of this instrument is that it is sensitive to change, with its added ability to discriminate active from inactive OCD treatments [111]. The relationship between functional disability, HRQoL and symptom severity is not clear cut [112–116]. This could reflect a delay between the treatment-related improvement in symptoms and the improvement in psychosocial functioning [88]. Indeed, studies show that longer periods of assessment, for instance beyond 24 weeks, may be required to detect meaningful improvements in function compared to the duration required for symptomatic improvements [88]. Studies have also reported that disability, as measured by the SDS, and HRQoL, measured by the SF-36, are sensitive to baseline symptom severity, symptom improvement and symptom deterioration, and that a Y–BOCS threshold score of 26–27 correlates with a significantly greater level of overall impairment [88,117]. Thus, a total Y–BOCS score exceeding 26 may represent a clinically relevant degree of disability.

SUMMARY

Obsessive-compulsive disorder is a chronic illness with modest treatment outcomes, and RCTs of new treatments are required. Short-term and long-term efficacy studies, including those addressing treatment-resistant cases, are needed. Trial design needs to take account of the key factors contributing to heterogeneity in OCD samples that may impact on treatment outcomes, such as syndromal stability, dimensional factors, subtypes and comorbidity. Inclusion of HRQoL and disability measures may enable the development of comprehensive and clinically relevant definitions for treatment response, relapse and remission.

REFERENCES

1. Heyman I, Mataix-Cols D, Fineberg NA. Obsessive-compulsive disorder. *Br Med J* 2006;**333**:424–429.
2. National Institute For Health And Clinical Excellence. *Obsessive-Compulsive Disorder: Core Interventions in the Treatment of Obsessive-Compulsive Disorder and Body Dysmorphic Disorder.* NICE, 2006.
3. World Health Organization. The "newly defined" burden of mental problems. Fact sheet no. 217. Geneva: WHO, 1999.
4. Bobes J, González MP, Bascarán MT, Arango C, Sáiz PA, Bousoño M. Quality of life and disability in patients with obsessive-compulsive disorder. *Eur Psychiatry* 2001;**16**:239–245
5. von Elm E, Altman D, Egger M, Pocock S, Gøtzsche P, Vandenbroucke J. The Strengthening the Reporting of Observational Studies in Epidemiology (STROBE) statement: guidelines for reporting observational studies. *Lancet* 2007;**370**:1453–1457.
6. European Agency for the Evaluation of Medicinal Products (EMEA). EMEA/CPMP position statement on the use of placebo in clinical trials with regard to the revised Declaration of Helsinki. EMEA, 2001. Available at: http://www.emea.europa.eu/docs/en_GB/document_library/Position_statement/2009/12/WC500017646.pdf.
7. European Agency for the Evaluation of Medicinal Products (EMEA). Note for guidance on good clinical practice. EMEA, 2002. Available at: http://www.ema.europa.eu/docs/en_GB/document_library/Scientific_guideline/2009/09/WC500002874.pdf.
8. Bandelow B, Zohar J, Hollander E, Kasper S, Möller HJ. World Federation of Societies of Biological Psychiatry (WFSBP) guidelines for the pharmacological treatment of anxiety, obsessive-compulsive and post-traumatic stress disorders – first revision. *World J Biol Psychiatry* 2008: **9**:248–312.
9. Pallanti S, Hollander E, Bienstock C *et al.* Treatment non-response in OCD: methodological issues and operational definitions. *Int J Neuropsychopharmacol* 2002;**5**:181–191.
10. Montgomery SA, Fineberg N, Montgomery DB. The efficacy of serotonergic drugs in OCD: power calculations compared with placebo. In: Montgomery SA, Goodman WK, Goeting N (eds), *Current Approaches in Obsessive Compulsive Disorder.* Southampton, UK: Ashford Colour Press for Duphar Medical Relations, 1990; pp. 54–63.
11. Fineberg NA, Gale TM. Evidence-based pharmacotherapy of obsessive-compulsive disorder. *Int J Neuropsychopharmacol* 2005;**8**:107–129.
12. Nutt D, Allgulander C, Lecrubier Y *et al.* Establishing non-inferiority in treatment trials in psychiatry – guidelines from an Expert Consensus Meeting. *J Psychopharmacol* 2008;**22**:409–416.
13. Garattini S, Bertele V. Non-inferiority trials are unethical because they disregard patients' interests. *Lancet* 2007;**370**:1875–1877.

14. Goodman WK, Price LH, Rasmussen SA *et al*. The Yale–Brown Obsessive-Compulsive Scale. 1: Reliability. *Arch Gen Psychiatry*1989;**46**:1012–1016.

15. Goodman WK, Price LH, Rasmussen SA *et al*. The Yale–Brown Obsessive-Compulsive Scale. 2: Validity. *Arch Gen Psychiatry* 1989;**46**:1006–1011.

16. Stein DJ, Baldwin DS, Dolberg OT, Despiegel N, Bandelow B. Which factors predict placebo response in anxiety disorders and major depression? An analysis of placebo-controlled studies of escitalopram. *J Clin Psychiatry* 2006;**67**:1741–1746.

17. Fineberg NA. Editorial 89. *Rev Bras Psiquiatira* 2006;**28**:89–90.

18. American Psychiatric Association (APA). *Diagnostic and Statistical Manual of Mental Disorders*, 4th edn. Washington, DC: APA, 1994.

19. Leckman JF, Denys D, Simpson HB *et al*. Obsessive-compulsive disorder: a review of the diagnostic criteria and possible subtypes and dimensional specifiers for DSM-V. *Depress Anxiety* 2010;**27**(6):507–527.

20. World Health Organization (WHO). *The ICD-10 Classification of Mental and Behavioural Disorders. Clinical Description and Diagnostic Guidelines*. Geneva: WHO, 1992

21. Stein DJ, Denys D, Gloster TA *et al*. Obsessive compulsive disorder: Diagnostic and treatment issues. *Psychiatr Clin N Am* 2009;**32**:665–685.

22. Stein DJ, Carey PD, Lochner C *et al*. Escitalopram in obsessive-compulsive disorder: response of symptom dimensions to pharmacotherapy. *CNS Spectr* 2008;**13**:492–498.

23. Phillips ML, Mataix-Cols D. Patterns of neural response to emotive stimuli distinguish the different symptom dimensions of obsessive-compulsive disorder. *CNS Spectr* 2004;**9**:275–283.

24. Ravikishore V, Samar R, Janardhan Reddy YC. Clinical characteristics and treatment response in poor and good insight obsessive compulsive disorder. *Eur Psychiatry* 2004;**19**:202–208.

25. Kozak MJ, Foa EB. Obsessions, overvalued ideas and delusions in obsessive-compulsive disorder. *Behav Res Ther* 1994;**32**:343–353.

26. Eisen JL, Rasmussen SA, Phillips KS *et al*. Insight and treatment outcome in obsessive-compulsive disorder. *Compr Psychiatry* 2001;**42**:494–497.

27. Catapano F, Perris F, Fabrazo M *et al*. Obsessive compulsive disorder with poor insight: A 3 year prospective study. *Progr Neuropsychopharmacol Biol Psychiatry* 2010;**34**:323–330.

28. Alonso P, Menchio JM, Segaias C *et al*. Clinical implications of insight assessment in obsessive compulsive disorder. *Compr Psychiatry* 2008;**49**:305–312.

29. Eisen JL, Phillips KA, Baer L *et al*. The Brown Assessment of Beliefs Scale – reliability and validity. *Am J Psychiatry* 1998;**155**:102–108.

30. Jaisoorya TS, Janardhan Reddy YC, Srinath S *et al*. Obsessive-compulsive disorder with and without tic disorder: A comparative study from India. *CNS Spectr* 2008;**13**:705–711.

31. March JS, Franklin ME, Leonard CH *et al*. Tics moderate treatment outcome with sertraline but not cognitive-behaviour therapy in pediatric obsessive-compulsive disorder. *Biol Psychiatry* 2007;**61**:344–347.

32. McDougle CJ, Goodman WK, Leckman JF. Haloperidol addition in fluvoxamine refractory obsessive-compulsive disorder: A double blind placebo controlled study in patients with and without tics. *Arch Gen Psychiatry* 1994;**51**:302–308.

33. American Psychiatric Association. DSM-5 Development. Available at: www.dsm5
    .org.
34. Shavitt RG, Belotto C, Curi M *et al*. Clinical features associated with treatment
    response in obsessive-compulsive disorder. *Compr Psychiatry* 2006;**47**:276–281.
35. Storch EA, Murphy TK, Geffken SR *et al*. Reliability and validity of the Yale Global
    Tic Severity Scale. *Psychol Assess* 2005;**17**:486–491.
36. Roessner V, Becker A, Banaschewski T *et al*. Tic disorders and obsessive compulsive
    disorder: where is the link? *J Neural Transm Suppl*. 2005;(69):69–99.
37. Hollander E, Kaplan A, Schmeidler J *et al*. Neurological soft signs as predictors of
    treatment response to selective serotonin reuptake inhibitors in obsessive-compulsive
    disorder. *J Neuropsych Clin Neurosci* 2005;**17**:472–477.
38. Hollander E, Schiffman E, Cohen B *et al*. Signs of central nervous system dysfunction
    in obsessive-compulsive disorder. *Arch Gen Psychiatry* 1990;**47**:27–32.
39. Snider LA, Swedo SE. PANDAS: Current status and directions for research. *Mol
    Psychiatry* 2004;**9**:900–907.
40. Pigott TA, L'Heureux F, Dubbert B *et al*. Obsessive compulsive disorder: comorbid
    conditions. *J Clin Psychiatry* 1994;**55**(Suppl.):15–27.
41. Montgomery SA, Asberg M. A new depression scale designed to be sensitive to
    change. *Br J Psychiatry* 1979;**134**:382–389.
42. Sheehan DV, Lecrubier Y, Sheehan KH *et al*. The Mini-International Neuropsychi-
    atric Interview (M.I.N.I.): The development and validation of a structured diagnostic
    psychiatric interview for DSM-IV and ICD-10. *J Clin Psychiatry* 1998;**59**(Suppl. 20):
    22–33.
43. Posner, K. C-CASA and C-SSRS in CNS clinical trials: Development and implemen-
    tation. Presentation at the IOM Workshop on CNS Clinical Trials: Suicidality and
    Data Collection, Washington, DC, 2009 June 16.
44. Zimmerman M, Chelminski I, Posternak MA. Generalizability of antidepressant ef-
    ficacy trials: differences between depressed psychiatric outpatients who would or
    would not qualify for an efficacy trial. *Am J Psychiatry* 2005;**162**:1370–1372.
45. Hollander E, Kim S, Braun A *et al*. Cross-cutting issues and future directions for the
    OCD spectrum. *Psychiatry Res* 2009;**170**:3–6.
46. Kaufman J, Birmaher B, Brent D *et al*. Schedule for Affective Disorders and
    Schizophrenia for School-Age Children – Present and Lifetime Version (KSADS-
    PL): Initial reliability and validity data. *J Am Acad Child Adolesc Psychiatry* 1997;**36**:
    980–988.
47. Endicott J, Spitzer RL. A diagnostic interview: the schedule for affective disorders
    and schizophrenia. *Arch Gen Psychiatry* 1978;**35**:837–844.
48. Ehler S, Gillberg C, Wing L. A screening questionnaire for Asperger syndrome and
    other high-functioning autism spectrum disorders in school age children. *J Autism
    Dev Dis* 1999;**29**:129–141.
49. Du Toit PL, Van Kradenburg J, Niehaus D, Stein DJ. Comparison of obsessive-
    compulsive disorder patients with and without comorbid putative obsessive-
    compulsive spectrum disorders using a structured clinical interview. *Compr Psy-
    chiatry* 2001;**42**:291–300.
50. Storch EA, Murphy TK, Geffken GR *et al*. Psychometric evaluation of the Children's
    Yale–Brown Obsessive-Compulsive Scale. *Psychiatry Res* 2004;**129**:91–98.

51. Insel TR, Murphy DL, Cohen RM *et al*. National Institute of Mental Health Obsessive-Compulsive Scale (NIMH-OC). *Arch Gen Psychiatry* 1983;**46**:5–12.

52. Guy W. *ECDEU: Assessment Manual for Psychopharmacology, Revised*. US Dept Health, Education and Welfare Publication (ADM). Rockville, MD: National Institute of Mental Health, 1976; pp. 76–338.

53. Sheehan DV, Harnett-Sheehan K, Raj BA. The measurement of disability. *Int Clin Psychopharmacol* 1996;**11**(suppl 3):89–95.

54. Ware JE, Sherbourne CD. The MOS 36-item short-form health survey(SF-36). I. Conceptual framework and item selection. *Med Care* 1992;**30**:473–483.

55. Denys *et al*. Dutch Dimensional Obsessive Compulsive scale (in preparation).

56. Chamberlain SR, Blackwell AD, Fineberg NA *et al*. The neuropsychology of obsessive compulsive disorder: the importance of failures in cognitive and behavioral inhibition as candidate and endophenotypic markers. *Neurosci Biobehav Rev* 2005;**29**:399–419.

57. Dittrich WH, Johansen T, Fineberg NA *et al*. The cognitive assessment instrument of obsessions and compulsions (CAIOC). *Psychiatry Res* 2011;**187**:283–290.

58. Mataix-Cols D, Rosario-Campos MC, Leckman JF. A multi-dimensional model of obsessive-compulsive disorder. *Am J Psychiatry* 2005;**162**:228–238.

59. Abramowitz JS, Tolin DF, Diefenbach GJ. Measuring change in OCD: sensitivity of the Obsessive-Compulsive Inventory – Revised. *J Psychopathol Behav Assess* 2005;**27**:317–324.

60. Burns GL, Keortge SG, Formea GM *et al*. Revision of the Padua Inventory of obsessive compulsive disorder symptoms: Distinctions between worry, obsessions and compulsions. *Behav Res Ther* 1996;**34**:163–173.

61. Sternberger LG, Burns GL. Maudsley obsessive compulsive inventory: Obsessive-compulsive symptoms in a non-clinical sample. *Behav Res Ther* 1990;**28**:337–340.

62. Mataix-Cols D, Fullana MA, Alonso P *et al*. Convergent and discriminant validity of the obsessive compulsive scale symptom checklist. *Psychother Psychosom* 2004;**73**:190–196.

63. Spielberger CD. Theory and research on anxiety. In: Spielberger CD (ed.), *Anxiety and Behaviour*. New York: Academic Press, 1966; pp. 3–20.

64. Hamilton M. The assessments of anxiety states by rating. *Br J Med Psychol* 1959;**32**:50–55.

65. Hamilton M. A rating scale for depression. *J Neurol Neurosurg Psychiatry* 1960;**23**:56–62.

66. Montgomery SA, Asberg M. A new depression scale designed to be sensitive to change. *Br J Psychiatry* 1979;**134**:382–389.

67. Santen G, Gomeni R, Danhof M *et al*. Sensitivity of the individual items of the Hamilton Depression Rating Scale to response and its consequences for the assessment of efficacy. *J Psychiatric Res* 2008;**42**:1000–1009.

68. Fineberg NA, Fourie H, Gale TM *et al*. Comorbid depression in obsessive compulsive disorder: Symptomatic differences to major depressive disorder. *J Affect Disord* 2005;**87**:327–330.

69. Polman A, Bouman TK, De Jong PJ *et al*. Obsessive compulsive beliefs and behaviour: a family affair? PhD thesis, University of Groningen; 2010; dissertations.ub.rug.nl/FILES/faculties/medicine/. . .polman/06_c6.pdf.

70. Dittrich WH, Johansen T, Padhi AK *et al.* Clinical and neurocognitive changes with modafinil in obsessive-compulsive disorder: a case report. *Psychopharmacology* 2010;**212**:449–451.

71. Keedwell P, Snaith RP. What do anxiety scales measure? *Acta Psychiatr Scand* 2007;**93**:177–180.

72. Williams VSL, Morlock RJ, Feltner D. Psychometric evaluation of a Visual Analogue Scale for assessment of anxiety. *Health Qual Life Out* 2010;**8**:57.

73. Ackerman DL, Greenland S. Multivariate meta-analysis of controlled drug studies for obsessive-compulsive disorder. *J Clin Psychopharmacol* 2002;**22**:309–317.

74. Stein DJ, Andersen EW, Tonnoir B *et al.* Escitalopram in obsessive-compulsive disorder: A randomised, placebo-controlled, paroxetine referenced, fixed-dose, 24-week study. *Curr Med Res Opin* 2007;**23**:701–711.

75. Hollander E, Koran LM, Goodman WK *et al.* A double-blind, placebo-controlled study of the efficacy and safety of controlled-release fluvoxamine in patients with obsessive-compulsive disorder. *J Clin Psychiatry* 2003;**64**:640–647.

76. Simpson HB, Huppert JD, Petkova E *et al.* Response versus remission in obsessive-compulsive disorder. *J Clin Psychiatry* 2006;**67**:269–276.

77. Rasmussen SA, Eisen JL. Treatment strategies for chronic and refractory obsessive-compulsive disorder. *J Clin Psychiatry* 1997;**58**:9–13.

78. Hollander E, Allen A, Steiner M *et al.* Acute and long term treatment and prevention of relapse of obsessive compulsive disorder with paroxetine. *J Clin Psychiatry* 2003;**64**:1113–1121.

79. Eddy KT, Dutra L, Bradley R *et al.* A multidimensional meta-analysis of psychotherapy and pharmacotherapy for obsessive compulsive disorder. *Clin Psychol Rev* 2004;**24**:1011–1030.

80. Van Open P, De Haan E, Van Balkom AJ *et al.* Cognitive therapy and exposure in vivo in the treatment of obsessive-compulsive disorder. *Behav Res Ther* 1995;**33**:379–390.

81. Mclean PD, Whittal ML, Thordarson DS *et al.* Cognitive versus behaviour therapy in the group treatment of obsessive-compulsive disorder. *J Consulting Clin Psychol* 2001;**69**:205–214.

82. Cottraux J, Note I, Vao SN *et al.* A randomized controlled trial of cognitive therapy versus intensive behaviour therapy in obsessive compulsive disorder. *Psychother Psychosom* 2001;**70**:288–297.

83. Fineberg NA, Tonnoir B, Lemming O *et al.* Escitalopram prevents relapse of obsessive compulsive disorder. *Eur Neuropsychopharmacol* 2007;**17**:430–439.

84. Fineberg NA, Craig KJ. Pharmacological treatment of obsessive-compulsive disorder. *Psychiatry* 2007;**6**:234–239.

85. Simpson HB, Rosen W, Huppert JD *et al.* Are there reliable neuropsychological deficits in obsessive-compulsive disorder? *J Psychiatric Res* 2006;**40**:247–257.

86. Koran LM, Hackett E, Rubin A *et al.* Efficacy of sertraline in the long term treatment of obsessive-compulsive disorder. *Am J Psychiatry* 2002;**159**:88–95.

87. Romano S, Goodman W, Tamura R *et al.* Long term treatment of obsessive-compulsive disorder after an acute response: a comparison of fluoxetine versus placebo. *J Clin Psychopharmacol* 2001;**21**:46–52.

88. Hollander E, Stein DJ, Fineberg NA *et al.* Functional and health related quality of life outcomes in obsessive-compulsive disorder – relationship to treatment response and symptom relapse. *J Clin Psychiatry* 2010 Jun;**71**(6):784–92. Epub 2010 May 4.

89. Carey PD, Vythilingum B, Seedat S *et al.* Quetiapine augmentation of SRIs in the treatment refractory obsessive-compulsive disorder: a double blind randomized placebo controlled study. *BMC Psychiatry* 2005;**5**:5.

90. Denys D, Fineberg NA, Carey PD *et al.* Quetiapine addition in obsessive-compulsive disorder: is treatment outcome affected by type and dose of serotonin reuptake inhibitors? *Biol Psychiatry* 2007;**61**:412–414.

91. Denys D, De Geus F, Van Megen HG. A double-blind, randomized, placebo-controlled trial of quetiapine addition in patients with obsessive-compulsive disorder refractory to serotonin reuptake inhibitors. *J Clin Psychiatry* 2004;**65**:1040–1048.

92. Simpson HB, Foa EB, Liebowitz MR *et al.* A randomized controlled trial of cognitive-behaviour therapy for augmenting pharmacotherapy in obsessive-compulsive disorder. *Am J Psychiatry* 2008;**165**:621–630.

93. McDougle CJ, Epperson CN, Pelton GH *et al.* A double-blind, placebo-controlled study of risperidone addition in serotonin reuptake inhibitor-refractory obsessive-compulsive disorder. *Arch Gen Psychiatry* 2000;**57**:794–801.

94. Montgomery SA, Baldwin S, Blier P *et al.* Which antidepressants have demonstrated superior efficacy? A review of the evidence. *Int Clin Psychopharmacol* 2007; **22**:323–329.

95. Cipriani A, Furukawa TA, Salanti G *et al.* Comparative efficacy and acceptability of 12 new-generation antidepressants: a multiple-treatments meta-analysis. *Lancet* 2009;**373**:748–758.

96. Sacchetti E, Conte G, Guarneri L. Are SSRI antidepressants a clinically homogenous class of compounds? *Lancet* 1994;**344**:126–127.

97. Salzman C. Heterogeneity of SSRI response. *Harvard Rev Psychiatry* 1996;**4**: 215–217.

98. Ruscio AM, Stein DJ, Chiu WT. The epidemiology of obsessive-compulsive disorder in the national comorbidity survey replication. *Mol Psychiatry* 2010;**15**:53–63.

99. Fullana MA, Mataix-Cols D, Caspi A *et al.* Obsessions and compulsions in the community: prevalence, interference, help-seeking, developmental stability and co-occurring psychiatric conditions. *Am J Psychiatry* 2009;**166**:329–336.

100. Mataix-Cols D, Rauch SL, Manzo PA *et al.* Use of factor-analysed symptom dimensions to predict outcome with serotonin reuptake inhibitors and placebo in the treatment of obsessive-compulsive disorder. *Am J Psychiatry* 1999;**156**:1409–1416.

101. Leckman JF, Grice DE, Boardman J *et al.* Symptoms of obsessive-compulsive disorder. *Am J Psychiatry* 1997;**154**:911–917.

102. Hasler G, Pinto A, Greenberg BD *et al.* Familiality of factor analysis-derived Y-BOCS dimensions in OCD-affected sibling pairs from the OCD Collaborative Genetics Study. *Biol Psychiatry* 2007;**61**:617–625.

103. Stein DJ, Carey PD, Lochner C *et al.* Escitalopram in obsessive-compulsive disorder: response of symptom dimensions to pharmacotherapy. *CNS Spectr* 2008;**13**:492–498.

104. Foa EB, Liebowtz MR, Kozak MJ *et al.* Randomised placebo-controlled trial of exposure and ritual prevention, clomipramine and their combination in the treatment of obsessive-compulsive disorder. *Am J Psychiatry* 2005;**162**:151–161.

105. Nakatani E, Nakagawa A, Nakao T *et al.* A randomised controlled trial of Japanese patients with obsessive-compulsive disorder: Effectiveness of behaviour therapy and fluvoxamine. *Psychother Psychosom* 2005;**74**:269–276.

106. Fineberg NA, Hughes A, Gale T. Group cognitive behavioural therapy in obsessive-compulsive disorder: a trial controlling for group effects. *World Psychiatry* 2004; **3**:281.

107. Picinelli M, Pin S, Bellantuono C *et al*. Efficacy of drug treatment in obsessive-compulsive disorder: a metaanalytic review. *Br J Psychiatry* 1995;**166**:424–443.

108. Stein DS, Fineberg NA. Psychotherapy: An integrated approach. In: Stein DJ, Hollander E (eds.), Obsessive-Compulsive Disorder. Oxford Psychiatry Library, Oxford University Press, 2007; pp. 63–74.

109. March JS. Cognitive-behaviour therapy, sertraline and their combination for children and adolescents with obsessive compulsive disorder: the Pediatric OCD Treatment Study (POTS) randomized controlled trials. *JAMA* 2004;**292**:1969–1976.

110. March JS, Mulle K, Herbel B. Behavioural psychotherapy for children and adolescents with obsessive compulsive disorder: an open trial of a new protocol-driven treatment package. *J Am Acad Child Adolesc Psychiatry* 1994;**33**:333–341.

111. Padhi A, Fineberg NA. How should we measure health-related quality of life in obsessive compulsive disorder? Poster presentation, British Association of Psychopharmacology, Summer Meeting, July 2009.

112. Moritz S, Rufer M, Fricke S *et al*. Quality of life in obsessive compulsive disorder before and after treatment. *Compr Psychiatry* 2005;**46**:453–459.

113. Tukel R, Bozkurt O, Polat A *et al*. Clinical predictors of response to pharmacotherapy in obsessive-compulsive disorder. *Psychiatry Clin Neurosci* 2006;**60**:404–409.

114. Bystritsky A, Saxena S, Maidment K *et al*. Quality-of-life changes amongst patients with obsessive-compulsive disorder in a partial hospitalization program. *Psychiatric Services* 1999;**50**:412–414.

115. Norberg MM, Calamari JE, Cohen RJ *et al*. Quality of life in obsessive-compulsive disorder: an evaluation of impairment and a preliminary analysis of the ameliorating effects of treatment. *Depress Anxiety* 2008;**25**:248–259.

116. Tenney NH, Denys DA, Van Megen HJ *et al*. Effect of a pharmacological intervention on quality of life in patients with obsessive-compulsive disorder. *Int Clin Psychopharmacol* 2003;**18**:29–33.

117. Mancebo MC, Greenberg B, Grant JE *et al*. Correlates of occupational disability in a clinical sample of obsessive-compulsive disorder. *Compr Psychiatry* 2008;**49**:43–50.

118. Montgomery SA, Kasper S, Stein DJ *et al*. Citalopram 20 mg, 40 mg and 60 mg are all effective and well tolerated compared with placebo in obsessive-compulsive disorder. *Int Clin Psychopharmacol* 2001;**16**:75–86.

119. Zohar J, Judge R. Paroxetine versus clomipramine in the treatment of obsessive-compulsive disorder. OCD Paroxetine Study Investigators. *Br J Psychiatry* 1996; **169**:468–474.

120. Goodman WK, Price LH, Rasmussen SA *et al*. Efficacy of fluvoxamine in obsessive-compulsive disorder. A double-blind comparison with placebo. *Arch Gen Psychiatry* 1989;**46**:36–44.

121. Goodman WK, Kozak MJ, Liebowitz M *et al*. Treatment of obsessive-compulsive disorder with fluvoxamine: a multicentre, double-blind, placebo-controlled trial. *Int Clin Psychopharmacol* 1996;**11**:21–29.

122. Riddle MA, Reeve EA, Yaryura-Tobias JA *et al*. Fluvoxamine for children and adolescents with obsessive-compulsive disorder: a randomized, controlled, multicenter trial. *J Am Acad Child Adolesc Psychiatry* 2001;**40**:222–229.

123. Montgomery SA, McIntyre A, Osterheider M *et al.* A double-blind, placebo-controlled study of fluoxetine in patients with DSM-III-R obsessive-compulsive disorder. The Lilly European OCD Study Group. *Eur Neuropsychopharmacol* 1993; **3**:143–152.

124. Tollefson GD, Rampey AH Jr, Potvin JH *et al.* A multicenter investigation of fixed-dose fluoxetine in the treatment of obsessive-compulsive disorder. *Arch Gen Psychiatry* 1994;**51**:559–567.

125. Geller DA, Hoog SL, Heiligenstein JH *et al.* Fluoxetine treatment for obsessive-compulsive disorder in children and adolescents: a placebo-controlled clinical trial. *J Am Acad Child Adolesc Psychiatry* 2001;**40**:773–779.

126. Liebowitz MR, Turner SM, Piacentini J *et al.* Fluoxetine in children and adolescents with OCD: a placebo-controlled trial. *J Am Acad Child Adolesc Psychiatry* 2002;**41**:1431–1438.

127. Kronig MH, Apter J, Asnis G *et al.* Placebo-controlled, multicenter study of sertraline treatment for obsessive-compulsive disorder. *J Clin Psychopharmacol* 1999; **19**:172–176.

128. Greist JH, Jefferson JW, Kobak KA *et al.* A 1 year double-blind placebo-controlled fixed dose study of sertraline in the treatment of obsessive-compulsive disorder. *Int Clin Psychopharmacol* 1995;**10**:57–65.

129. March JS, Biederman J, Wolkow R *et al.* Sertraline in children and adolescents with obsessive-compulsive disorder: a multicenter randomized controlled trial. *JAMA* 1998;**280**:1752–1756.

CHAPTER 9

Serotonin and Beyond: A Neurotransmitter Perspective of OCD

Anat Abudy, Alzbeta Juven-Wetzler, Rachel Sonnino and Joseph Zohar

Division of Psychiatry, Chaim Sheba Medical Center, Tel Hashomer, Israel

Ever since the discovery of neurotransmitters in the early twentieth century by the pharmacologist Otto Loewi (a discovery for which he was later honoured with a Nobel prize), researchers have been trying to understand how function and malfunction of neurotransmitters contribute to the development of diseases. In this chapter, we will draw the connection between various neurotransmitters and the pathophysiology of obsessive-compulsive disorder (OCD), although there is significant 'cross-talk' among the different neurotransmitters. We will discuss every neurotransmitter individually for the sake of simplicity, even though this division between neurotransmitters is, of course, artificial.

When attempting to explore the connection between neurotransmitters and the pathogenesis of a disease, for example OCD, a specific activation of the relevant system or receptor(s) could be utilized. This is actually a challenge, and if we use a compound or ligand, the procedure is coined a pharmacological challenge. A pharmacological challenge is designed to induce a set of specific and relevant chain reactions, which will (ideally) be relevant to the examined pathology (e.g. exacerbation of obsessions and compulsions in the case of OCD).

Another approach is animal models. However, animal models of OCD are inevitably based solely on alteration in motor behaviour mimicking compulsive rituals, since aberrant 'thoughts', if present at all, are not verifiable. Most of these animal models of OCD are based on pharmacological, behavioural or genetic manipulations.

Obsessive-Compulsive Disorder: Current Science and Clinical Practice, First Edition. Edited by Joseph Zohar.
© 2012 John Wiley & Sons, Ltd. Published 2012 by John Wiley & Sons, Ltd.

Yet another possibility is to employ neurochemical studies: that is, to measure concentrations of certain neurotransmitters or metabolites in probands and in healthy controls, mainly via concentrations of the metabolites in the CSF, but also via metabolite concentrations in blood and urine.

The development of radioligands for neuroimaging techniques has facilitated studies of the central neurotransmitter systems. *In vivo* neuroimaging of the central nervous system is a unique tool for testing brain function (see Chapter 10).

Last are genetic studies, aiming at understanding the pathophysiology at a molecular level. Since genetics and neuroimaging are discussed elsewhere in this book (Chapters 10 and 11), due to their growing importance in research, we will only mention them briefly in this chapter.

SEROTONIN

Serotonin (5-hydroxytryptamine, or 5-HT) is synthesized from the amino acid tryptophan. The action of 5-HT is terminated when it is destroyed by monoamine oxidase (MAO) and catechol-*O*-methyltransferase (COMT), and converted into an inactive metabolite, such as 5-hydroxyindoleacetic acid (5-HIAA). Most of the serotonin is degraded by MAO A outside the neuron (MAO B, having low affinity for serotonin, may also degrade serotonin, but to a lesser extent). Serotonin has different receptor subtypes. Several are presynaptic (5-HT_{1A}, $5\text{-HT}_{1B/D}$) and several are postsynaptic (5-HT_{1A}, $5\text{-HT}_{1B/D}$, 5-HT_{2A}, 5-HT_{2C}, 5-HT_{3}, 5-HT_{4}, 5-HT_{5}, 5-HT_{6}, 5-HT_{7}). Presynaptic 5-HT receptors are autoreceptors that downregulate 5-HT release, while the postsynaptic serotonin receptors upregulate various neural circuits [1]. Hence, serotonin links both to excitatory and inhibitory processes.

The influence of serotonin on OCD has been examined in various ways, both in patients and in animal models. Serotonin levels have been examined in the cerebrospinal fluid (CSF) of patients with OCD. The investigation of CSF levels of metabolites raised the question of the connection between what is found in the CSF and what is actually taking place in the brain, a question relevant not only for serotonin, but also for all metabolites measured in the CSF. It has become clearer that increased CSF amines, such as serotonin, dopamine and glutamate, are not exactly the same as increased neurotransmitter activity in the cortical and subcortical pathways. Different processes, such as neuronal release and transport, glial uptake, diffusion barriers, sequestration in distinct metabolic pools and degradation, may also contribute to modifications of neurotransmitter levels in CSF. Nevertheless, various studies have proposed a blood–CSF barrier to amino acids [2,3] and suggested that CSF neurotransmitter concentrations could reflect on their function within the central nervous system after all. Taking that information into account, we will now discuss findings relating to serotonin and its metabolites in the CSF.

Serotonin and metabolite concentrations in OCD – 30 years later

A serotonergic mechanism in OCD was supported by early studies showing a positive correlation between symptom improvement and the drug-induced decrease in 5-HIAA levels, the major metabolite of 5-HT, in CSF. Thorén *et al.* [4] were the first (1980) to measure concentrations of 5-HIAA in CSF before and after 3 weeks of treatment of severe OCD with clomipramine hydrochloride. They reported that patients who responded to clomipramine treatment had significantly higher CSF levels of 5-HIAA before treatment. The amelioration of obsessive-compulsive symptoms was positively correlated with the reduction of CSF concentrations of 5-HIAA during clomipramine treatment but negatively correlated with plasma concentrations of clomipramine. CSF concentrations of 5-HIAA were assumed to reflect drug action on central serotonin neurons. However, baseline 5-HIAA levels in the CSF of OCD patients have not been found to be different from control. Insel *et al.* [5] found that platelet 3H-imipramine binding and serotonin uptake were not significantly different between OCD patients and a control group. In contrast, the level of 5-HIAA in CSF was significantly higher in a small cohort of OCD patients compared with healthy volunteers [5]. In a direct test of the role of serotonin uptake in clomipramine's anti-obsessional effects, the serotonin uptake inhibitor zimelidine was compared with the noradrenergic uptake inhibitor desipramine in a double-blind controlled study. Zimelidine reduced CSF 5-HIAA, but was clinically ineffective in this group [6]. Moreover, non-responders to zimelidine or desipramine improved significantly during a subsequent double-blind trial of clomipramine [6].

Two other studies examined *urinary* 5-HIAA levels in patients with Tourette syndrome (TS) with and without OCD: Bornstein *et al.* [7] compared TS patients with high levels of OC symptoms with patients suffering from TS but without OC symptoms, focusing on urinary measures of serotonin and its inactive metabolite 5-HIAA. Both groups were compared with normal controls. Both groups of TS patients had lower levels of 5-HIAA than controls, but there was no difference between levels of serotonin and 5-HIAA in the two TS groups, supporting the hypothesis of low concentration of serotonin in those pathologies. Obsessive symptoms were related to higher levels of 5-HIAA and to a higher turnover of serotonin. De Groot *et al.* [8] examined amines and their metabolites in urine, among patients with TS and OC symptoms, and found relationships between symptom clusters and levels of catecholamine and metabolites. Taken together, 5-HIAA appeared to be the most highly correlated with the individual obsessive-compulsive symptoms, hence suggesting a role for 5-HT in the biopathology of OCD.

Peripheral blood markers of 5-HT in OCD have also been tested. Cath *et al.* [9] evaluated subjects suffering from TS without OCD, with tic + OCD, with OCD, and controls (all without serotonergic medication). Whole blood serotonin (5-HT) and platelet MAO activity were measured. Interaction between platelet MAO, 5-HT and OCD severity was found. Platelet MAO activity was elevated in tic-free OCD subjects when compared to the other groups. Whole blood 5-HT was lowered in tic + OCD patients in comparison to OCD subjects. Whole blood 5-HT and obsessive-compulsive severity were negatively correlated amongst OCD patients. Delorme *et al.* [10] assessed whole blood serotonin concentration, platelet 5-HT transporter (5-HTT) and 5-HT$_{2A}$ receptor-binding characteristics, and platelet inositol trisphosphate (IP$_3$) (a secondary messenger molecule used in signal transduction) content in a sample of OCD probands and their unaffected parents, and compared them with controls. Lower whole blood 5-HT concentration, fewer platelet 5-HTT binding sites, and higher platelet IP$_3$ content were found in OCD probands and their unaffected parents compared to controls. The only parameter that appeared to discriminate between affected and unaffected subjects was 5-HT$_{2A}$ receptor-binding characteristics, with increased receptor number and affinity in parents and no change in OCD probands. Delorme *et al.* [11] also compared 19 OCD patients before and after 8 weeks of selective serotonin reuptake inhibitor (SSRI) treatment with 19 matched controls, assessing clinical improvement and whole blood serotonin concentration, platelet 5-HTT and 5-HT$_{2A}$ receptor-binding characteristics and platelet IP$_3$ content. Before treatment, OCD patients had higher platelet IP$_3$ content and fewer 5-HTT binding sites than the controls. Treatment with SSRIs further lowered the number of 5-HTT binding sites, normalized platelet IP$_3$ contents, and lowered the number of platelet 5-HT$_{2A}$ binding sites and whole-blood 5-HT concentrations below control values. The patients who improved most following SSRI treatment had higher whole-blood 5-HT concentrations before treatment than those who improved less, implying a role of serotonin in the pathology of the disease. Hanna *et al.* [12] assessed whole blood 5-HT concentration in children and adolescents with severe OCD and in adolescent controls. They found no difference in blood 5-HT content between the OCD patients and the normal controls. Flament *et al.* [13] examined peripheral measures of serotonergic and noradrenergic function in OCD adolescents before and after 5 weeks of treatment with clomipramine. Compared with placebo, treatment with clomipramine was clinically effective and produced a marked decrease in platelet serotonin concentration, a trend towards a reduction in platelet MAO activity, and a rise in standing plasma norepinephrine (noradrenaline). Sallee *et al.* [14] found that platelet serotonin transporter protein (5-HTPR) capacity (B_{max}) is reduced in children and adolescents with OCD. Weizman *et al.* [15] assessed imipramine binding to blood platelets in untreated TS with and without OCD. The density of imipramine binding sites in TS + OCD patients was significantly lower compared with GTS – OCD patients (28%) as well as when compared with controls (31%). Marazziti *et al.* [16] found that patients with OCD had a lower number of paroxetine sites, which is inversely correlated with the Yale–Brown Obsessive-Compulsive Scale total score, than a similar group of controls. In another trial Marazziti *et al.* [17] measured platelet imipramine (IMI) binding, serotonin uptake and platelet sulfotransferase activity (enzyme that catalyzes the sulfate conjugation of many hormones and neurotransmitters) in drug-free OCD patients and an equal number of healthy controls. Their results showed a lower number of IMI binding sites and a higher level of sulfotransferase activity in OCD patients compared with controls.

In summary, the neurochemical studies tend to suggest a role for serotonin in OCD. However, in some of the studies, issues such as OCD subtypes (with or without tics, early vs late onset, etc.) or the exact condition under which the examinations were done hampered the interpretation of the results.

Pharmacological challenge tests

Zohar *et al.* [18] were the first (1987) to show a transient exacerbation of obsessive-compulsive symptoms in OCD patients by using metachlorophenylpiperazine (mCPP), a serotonergic agonist (agonist to 5-HT_{1A}, 5-HT_{2A}, 5-HT_{1B}, 5-HT_{2B}, 5-HT_{2C}, 5-HT_3, and 5-HT_7 receptors). Following mCPP, but not following placebo, patients with OCD experienced a transient but marked exacerbation of obsessive-compulsive symptoms. This effect could be prevented by pretreatment with clomipramine [19]. This effect of mCPP on OC symptoms has been replicated in some, but not all studies [20–24]. The lack of specific symptom changes following administration of lactate [25], carbon dioxide [26], yohimbine [27] and cholecystokinin receptor agonists [28] suggests that OCD patients are not sensitive to all anxiogenic challenges and that the serotonergic component of the mCPP challenge may play a critical role in the pathology of OCD (for further discussion, see Zohar *et al.* [29]). Because mCPP affects several 5-HT receptors, challenge tests with more selective agents have been conducted to dissect the possible mechanism underlying the purported induction of OC symptoms in OCD patients.

Ipsapirone, a selective 5-HT_{1A} receptor agonist, was examined among patients with OCD, but found ineffective [30]. Sumatriptan, a selective 5-HT_{1B} receptor agonist, induced an exacerbation of OC symptoms in OCD patients in some [23], but not all [31,32] studies. Zolmitriptan [33], a $5\text{-HT}_{1B/1D}$ receptor agonist with central action (has a better penetration of the blood–brain barrier than sumatriptan) did not cause an increase in OC symptoms. Neuroendocrine responses to mCPP challenge are also inconsistent. Some studies reported a blunted prolactin and/or cortisol response following mCPP administration [20], suggesting hyporesponsive 5-HT receptor in the brain regions controlling the neuroendocrine response, while other studies have shown the opposite effect [34]. Fenfluramine interacts with both the 5-HTT and dopamine transporter (DAT) [35]. Some studies have reported a blunted prolactin or cortisol response, while others have not found behavioural or neuroendocrine effects [20,35–37]. Differences in design, heterogeneity of the patient population, and small number of subjects in most studies may account for these discrepant findings. The non-selectivity of the probes used in the studies further hampers interpretation of the data (for further discussion about mCPP and influence on serotonin receptor subtypes in animal models, see 'Animal models and the role of serotonin' below).

In summary, the studies using pharmacological challenge to examine the role of serotonin in OCD patients are in line with abnormal serotonin function in OCD. Although it is difficult to conclude which serotonin receptor is involved, there are some hints for 5-HT$_{1B}$.

Pharmacotherapy

It is more than 40 years since publication of the first case report indicating that clomipramine, a tricyclic antidepressant with a potent serotonergic compound, might have some benefit in patients with OCD [38,39], and the first double-blind crossover study to compare serotonergic medication (clomipramine) with noradrenergic medication (desipramine) was published 20 years later [40]. The selectivity of clomipramine for serotonin led to the hypothesis that serotonin is implicated in the biology of OCD [9]. This 5-HT hypothesis of OCD gained further support later through the study of SSRIs in OCD. A comparison of the clinical efficacy of fluvoxamine and sertraline with that of desipramine, which replicated an earlier study [40], supports the notion that inhibition of the 5-HTT is required for antidepressants to be efficacious in OCD [40–43]. Denys and colleagues, in a small double-blind study [44], have shown that venlafaxine and paroxetine are equally efficacious in OCD. Although this study might not be powered enough to detect differences, it does suggest that inhibition of norepinephrine uptake does not contribute to the effect of antidepressants on OCD.

El Mansari and Blier [45] have argued on the basis of their electrophysiological work that the difference in onset of action between depression and OCD can be accounted for by a greater delay in the effect of SSRIs on 5-HT release in the orbital frontal cortex (OFC), a brain region supposedly implicated in OCD, as compared to other brain regions. According to these investigators, this delay in effect in the OFC might be explained by a slower desensitization of the 5-HT$_{1B}$ autoreceptors in the OFC. They also used this finding as an argument to explain why in OCD larger doses of SSRIs are needed. In line with this finding, Dannon et al. [46] have reported that pindolol hastens the effect of SSRIs in OCD patients. They also suggest that the effect of SSRIs in OCD might be explained by the delayed stimulation of the postsynaptic 5-HT$_{2A}$ receptors in the OFC. If this were to be true, one would expect mirtazapine, which among others is a 5-HT$_{2A}$ receptor antagonist, and atypical antipsychotics that also have antagonistic effects at this receptor, to attenuate the effect of SSRIs. Clinical studies with these drugs, however, have shown the opposite. Mirtazapine, although not effective by itself [47], has been shown to hasten the effect of paroxetine [48], and several studies have shown that atypical antipsychotics augment the effects of SSRIs in refractory OCD patients [49]. Moreover, mCPP, a non-selective 5-HT$_{2A}$ receptor agonist, is either not effective or causes a worsening of OC symptoms after acute administration [20–24]. This differentiation between acute and chronic is vital, since some receptors (like 5-HT_{1B}) have a slower desensitization, which might explain why in OCD a therapeutic trial with SSRIs is considered adequate only if the patients are on appropriate dose for at least 4–6 weeks.

In summary, the evidence from pharmacotherapy studies on the role of serotonin in OCD patients has, by and large, supported the hypothesis of abnormal serotonin function in OCD.

Animal models and the role of serotonin

Chou-Green et al. [50] tested the 5-HT_{2C} receptor knockout (KO) mouse, which was first described as a model for obesity. They reported that this KO mouse increased chewing on non-nutritive clay with a distinct 'neat' pattern and a reduced habituation of head dipping activity as compared to the wild type. They concluded that the 5-HT_{2C} receptor-null mutant mouse provides a model for compulsive behaviour. The data point towards a role of the 5-HT_{2C} receptor in the pathophysiology of this behaviour, but the predictive validity of this model for OCD has not been assessed properly. Tsaltas et al. [51] have described a model based on persistence in the context of rewarded spatial alteration. Using this behavioural model, they have shown that 5-HT_{2C} receptors are implicated in the mechanism underlying the 'compulsive' behaviour in this animal model for OCD. Acute administration of mCPP, a non-selective 5-HT receptor agonist, increased 'compulsive' behaviour. The effect could be prevented by chronic pretreatment with fluoxetine, but not with diazepam or desipramine. The selective 5-HT_{1B} receptor antagonist naratriptan was not effective in this animal model, supporting the role of 5-HT_{2C} receptors underlying the effect of mCPP (see discussion about the influence on humans in the previous section).

Flaisher-Grinberg et al. [52] tested the effects of 5-HT_{2A} and 5-HT_{2C} activation and blockade in the signal attenuation rat model of OCD. In this model, 'compulsive' behaviour is induced by attenuating a signal indicating that a lever-press response was effective in producing food. Systemic administration of the 5-HT_{2C} antagonist RS 102221 decreases compulsive lever-pressing, whereas systemic administration of the 5-HT_{2A} antagonist MDL11,939 or of the $5\text{-HT}_{2A/2C}$ agonist DOI did not have a selective effect on this behaviour.

Joel and Avisar [53] developed a rat model of OCD based on the hypothesis that a deficient response feedback mechanism underlies obsessions and compulsions. Rats undergoing extinction of lever-pressing for food after the attenuation of an external feedback for this behaviour exhibit excessive lever-pressing unaccompanied by an attempt to collect a reward, which may be analogous to the excessive and unreasonable behaviour seen in OCD. Using this model, Joel et al. [54] found that lesions to the rat orbital frontal cortex led to 'compulsive' lever pressing, which was paralleled by an increase in striatal 5-HT transporter density, suggesting that compulsive behaviour in this model is mediated or accompanied by alterations in the striatal serotonergic system. The predictive validity of this model is to be further explored, since it responds to acute treatment with SSRI.

In summary, along with some of the pharmacological challenges and some of the 5-HT findings, many animal models of OCD are in line with a specific role for 5-HT in OCD, a role that needs to be further elucidated.

DOPAMINE

Dopamine is synthesized from the amino acid tyrosine. There are at least five subtypes of dopamine receptors, D1 to D5. The D1 and D5 receptors are members of the D1-like family of dopamine receptors, whereas the D2, D3 and D4 receptors are members of the D2-like family. The major degradation metabolite of dopamine is homovanillic acid (HVA) (Figure 9.1).

Dopamine and metabolite concentrations in humans

Baseline measures of dopamine and its metabolite homovanillic acid (HVA) in psychotropic-naive patients may provide direct evidence for a possible role of

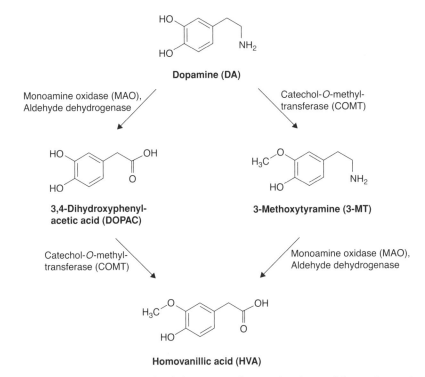

Figure 9.1 Pathways by which homovanillic acid is formed from dopamine.

dopamine in OCD. Thorén and colleagues [4] assessed levels of HVA in CSF before and after 3 weeks of treatment with clomipramine but found no change. Benkelfat and colleagues [55] found no difference between the mean plasma HVA level of 13 medication-free patients with OCD and 29 normal controls. Swedo *et al.* [56], examining CSF levels of HVA in 43 children with primary OCD, reported that CSF HVA levels were not significantly related to OCD symptoms and did not correlate with improvement following 5 weeks of treatment with clomipramine. Hollander *et al.* [57], however, observed a significant decrease in plasma HVA in 12 OCD patients relative to 10 controls following fenfluramine (serotonergic agonist) treatment, and Zahan *et al.* [58] showed that CSF metabolites of serotonin and dopamine, but not of norepinephrine, were positively correlated with electrodermal responsivity in a reaction time task in 43 adolescents and children with OCD. Marazziti *et al.* [17] measured platelet sulfotransferase activity in 17 drug-free OCD patients and an equal number of healthy controls. Sulfotransferase is an enzyme involved in the catabolism of catecholamines such as dopamine and has similar kinetic characteristics in brain and platelets. Their results showed a higher level of sulfotransferase activity in OCD patients compared with control subjects, suggesting an increased dopaminergic neurotransmission in OCD. Leckman *et al.* [6] examined the role of amines (norepinephrine, dopamine, serotonin) in the pathobiology of OCD and Tourette syndrome (TS). Concentrations of tyrosine (TYR), norepinephrine (NE), 3-methoxy-4-hydroxyphenylethylene glycol (MHPG, a metabolite of norepinephrine degradation), homovanillic acid (HVA), tryptophan (TRP) and 5-HIAA were measured in the CSF of 39 medication-free OCD patients and 44 healthy volunteers. CSF TYR concentrations were reduced ($p < 0.05$) in the OCD patients compared to the healthy subjects. After allowing for height as a covariant, CSF HVA levels were reduced ($p < 0.05$) in the OCD group compared to TS patients but not compared to the normal volunteers. No mean differences in CSF MHPG, TRP and 5-HIAA were observed in this study across the three groups. This finding provides support for the role of dopamine in the pathophysiology of OCD, since its precursor is tyrosine, and its major metabolite is HVA.

In summary, studies of the role of dopamine metabolites in OCD patients have yielded conflicting results, and hence no conclusive evidence for abnormal dopamine function in OCD can be reached at this point.

Pharmacological challenge tests

Cocaine, a dopamine transporter blocker, elevates synaptic dopamine levels and increases the dopamine transporter density [59]. It has been reported that chronic use of cocaine may be associated with stereotyped examining, searching and sorting behaviours, and an exacerbation of obsessive-compulsive symptoms [60–64]. Moreover, cocaine-abusing patients are at increased risk for the later development of OCD [65]. Methylphenidate and amphetamine have been reported to affect OCD symptoms both ways, either to exacerbate [64,66–68] or to improve [69] OCD symptoms. However, the use of cocaine, methylphenidate and amphetamine as dopaminergic probes is hampered as they also release serotonin and norepinephrine. Pitchot *et al.* [70] assessed the growth hormone (GH) response to 0.5 mg apomorphine (a dopaminergic agonist) in eight drug-free OCD patients and eight healthy male volunteers. In this study no difference in mean GH peak response was found. In contrast, Brambilla and colleagues [71,72], studying 15 patients with OCD and 15 controls, found a blunted GH response to apomorphine in OCD patients, hinting at a postsynaptic dopamine receptor subsensitivity. In the same sample, however, cortisol responses to stimulation with apomorphine were not different between the two groups. Longhurst *et al.* [73] examined the effects of catecholamine depletion in six drug-free patients with the tyrosine hydroxylase inhibitor alpha-methyl-para-tyrosine (AMPT) and found no significant changes in OC symptom severity as compared with placebo. Although bromocriptine, a selective dopamine receptor agonist, has been shown to induce stereotypies in animals, one report describes an improvement of OC symptoms in OCD patients [74].

Results from pharmacological challenge studies with dopamine receptor agonists in OCD are as yet inconsistent, yet there are indications that OC symptoms may be related to dopamine neurotransmission, at least in subsets of OCD patients.

Pharmacotherapy

Dopamine antagonists

Three years after its introduction, chlorpromazine was tested in 75 outpatients with obsessional neurosis and allied disorders in a placebo-controlled trial [75]. A significant response to chlorpromazine as compared with placebo was observed in 27 patients (36%), but it was judged to be disappointing in relieving compulsive symptoms. Since then, no placebo-controlled trial with a typical antipsychotic drug has been conducted in OCD. Except for some case reports [76–80], typical antipsychotics are considered ineffective as monotherapy in OCD, mainly on the grounds of individual clinical experience. McDougle *et al.* [81] assessed the efficacy of clozapine monotherapy in 12 adults with refractory OCD in a 10-week, open-label trial with clozapine and found no significant change. It is of note that *de novo* emergence or exacerbation of OCD symptoms during treatment with antipsychotics has been described extensively in patients with psychotic disorders [82,83]. Even though the antipsychotic medications differ in their receptor profile, emergence of OCD has not been selective to a specific antipsychotic medication but seems to emerge in most of them (risperidone [84–93], clozapine [94–97], olanzapine

[98–100], quetiapine [101–105]). However, it is most common among patients treated with clozapine [82,83].

Dopamine antagonists in addition to SSRIs

McDougle *et al.*, in a double-blind placebo-controlled study [106], demonstrated therapeutic efficacy of a small dose of D2 clear antagonist augmentation (haloperidol 1–4 g) in combination with the SSRI fluvoxamine in a group of OCD patients with tics; this was one of the first studies focusing on dopamine D2 receptor antagonists (in this study haloperidol) for augmentation of SSRIs in treatment-resistant OCD with tics [106]. With the introduction of a new generation of antipsychotic agents, these too have received attention in OCD, since they modulate both the dopamine and 5-HT function and may be associated with a lower incidence of extrapyramidal side effects. Risperidone augmentation of SSRIs in patients who failed to respond to monotherapy was shown to be effective, again particularly in the presence of tic disorder [107], in an open trial, followed by two double-blind placebo-controlled studies [108,109]. Data relating to the use of olanzapine, another atypical antipsychotic, in augmentation of treatment-resistant OCD patients are still controversial. In two open-label trials, olanzapine was shown to be effective when administered as augmentation of paroxetine and fluvoxamine, whereas testing it more thoroughly, in a double-blind placebo-controlled study, failed to indicate an advantage of adding olanzapine in fluoxetine-resistant OCD patients [108].

Modest efficacy of quetiapine as an augmentation has been suggested [110–112]. A meta-analysis [112] of existing double-blind placebo-controlled studies looking at quetiapine addition to SSRIs showed evidence of efficacy for adjunctive quetiapine. In a single-blind placebo-controlled study, this drug showed a significant improvement [113]. Supporting data also emerged from some open-label studies and a retrospective evaluation. However, another open-label trial assessing the effectiveness of quetiapine in addition to ongoing SSRI treatment suggested that a low dose of this drug may not be effective in resistant OCD patients [111].

Preliminary data are also available for aripiprazole, which is a quinolinone derivative with a high affinity for dopamine D2 and D3 receptors, as well as serotonin 5-HT$_{2A}$ and 5-HT $_{2B}$ receptors. In an open-label flexible-dose trial of aripiprazole augmentation [114], three patients out of eight (33%) met response criteria.

Amisulpride augmentation was examined in one small open-label study [115], with good results, but further investigation through randomized controlled trials is needed.

Modest usefulness of atypical antipsychotics to augment the response to SSRIs has been shown by three meta-analyses [110–112].

In summary, pharmacotherapy studies on the role of dopamine in OCD patients have, by and large, yielded evidence for a potential involvement of the dopaminergic system in OCD.

Animal models and the role of dopamine

Joel and Doljansky [116] showed that administration of the D1 antagonist SCH 23390 reduced the number of compulsive lever-presses, without affecting the number of lever-presses followed by an attempt to collect a reward. On the basis of electrophysiological data, they suggested that compulsive lever-pressing depends on a phasic decrease in stimulation of D1 receptors. Campbell and colleagues [117] have investigated the behavioural consequences of transgenic stimulation of a regional subpopulation of the dopamine neurons that express the D1 receptor in the cortex and amygdala, by generating mice that express an intracellular form of cholera toxin (CT). The study suggests that chronic stimulation of these D1-expressing neurons induces complex compulsive behaviour that resembles symptoms of OCD in humans [118]. Although these mice were resistant to behavioural inhibition by a D1 receptor antagonist and supersensitive to the D2 receptor antagonist sulpiride [119], Campbell and colleagues [120,121] suggested that chronic stimulation of cortical and limbic D1-expressing neurons may cause obsessive-compulsive behaviours. In another animal model for OCD, in which rats are chronically treated with the selective D2/3 receptor agonist quinpirole (QNP), a ritual-like set of behavioural acts resembling OCD checking behaviour has been observed [122–125]. This 'compulsive' behaviour is dependent on QNP administration, because it rapidly returns to normal behaviour when QNP administration is discontinued [126]. Postmortem analyses in these animals revealed increased tissue dopamine levels in the nucleus accumbens and right prefrontal cortex [126]. Another study [127] tried to quantify the dimensions of ritualistic 'compulsive-like' behaviour in quinpirole-induced behaviour in rats – whether the behavioural effects elicited by quinpirole sensitization remained after 2 weeks of cessation of treatment, and whether there is any effect of quinpirole treatment on the extracellular dopamine levels in the nucleus accumbens. It was found that once established, 'compulsive-like' behaviour is dependent upon quinpirole administration, as this behaviour rapidly normalized after cessation of quinpirole. Quinpirole-induced behaviour consists, unlike OCD rituals, of a smaller behavioural repertoire. As seen in patients with OCD, quinpirole-treated animals performed these behaviours with a high rate of repetition. These findings suggest that quinpirole-induced behaviour mimics only part of the compulsive behaviour as shown in OCD patients. Zor *et al.* [128] observed that ritual behaviour, such as the abundance of irrelevant or unnecessary acts in OCD rituals, was related to an increased dopamine function in the nucleus accumbens and right prefrontal cortex.

Korff *et al.* [129] conducted a study with deer mice, observing that the attenuation of stereotyped movement could be observed not only with serotonin agonist (mCPP) but also with D2 agonist. However, the putative models for OCD could be interpreted as models for other conditions, such as tic disorders, grooming and trichotillomania.

In summary, the data from the animal models of OCD examined suggest a role for dopamine, in particular of the D1 and D2 receptors, in the mechanism underlying compulsive-like behaviour.

GLUTAMATE

Glutamate is the most abundant excitatory neurotransmitter in the vertebrate nervous system (some estimate that over 90% of all the synapses in the human brain contain glutamate). In the postsynaptic cell, glutamate binds to glutamate receptors, such as the NMDA (*N*-methyl-D-aspartate) receptor. It is present in abundance in the neuroanatomical substrate implicated in OCD.

The glutamatergic influence

Recent evidence has also linked glutaminergic abnormalities with OCD. In one of the first reports (1998) implicating the glutaminergic system to OCD, Moore *et al.* [130] described striking changes in the caudate nucleus resonance on proton magnetic resonance spectroscopy in a 9-year-old boy with OCD after 12 weeks of paroxetine treatment. Rosenberg *et al.* [131] examined glutaminergic concentrations in the caudate nucleus using single-voxel proton magnetic resonance spectroscopy. They found that the glutamate concentrations were significantly greater in treatment-naive OCD patients than in controls but declined significantly after paroxetine treatment, to levels comparable with those of controls. The decrease in caudate glutamate was associated with a decrease in OCD symptom severity. In another trial, the same group [132] showed that the glutaminergic concentrations in the anterior cingulate were reduced, both in OCD and major depressive disorder patients.

Glutamate and metabolite concentrations in humans

Chakrabarty *et al.* [133] were the first (2005) to examine CSF glutamate levels in adults suffering from OCD. They found that CSF glutamate levels were significantly higher in OCD patients ($n = 21$) compared with normal controls. This preliminary study has not yet been replicated.

Animal models and the role of glutamate

McGrath *et al.* [134] showed that MK-801, a non-competitive NMDA receptor antagonist that indirectly stimulates cortico-limbic glutamate output, aggravated a transgenic-dependent abnormal behaviour (repetitive climbing and leaping) in a transgenic mouse model of comorbid TS and OCD.

In summary, it is difficult to draw conclusiions about the role of glutamate in the pathogenesis of OCD, although the studies so far suggest that the glutamate line should be further explored.

It is important to mention that there is evidence, emerging mainly from twin and family studies, that genetic risk factors are important for at least some forms of OCD. Most of the genes that have been explored are involved in the function or malfunction of the neurotransmitters mentioned above. For a thorough description about genetics and OCD the reader is referred to Chapter 11.

SEROTONIN: IS IT THE ONE TO BLAME?

The data we have summarized here raise the question of the role of serotonin in OCD. However, the findings do not necessarily point to an abnormal serotonergic system in OCD. On the contrary, several observations support the idea that inhibition of the 5-HTT, although required for antidepressants to work in OCD, is not causally related to the genesis of the disorder, for a number of reasons. First, in some patients, 5-HTT inhibition is insufficient to alleviate OC symptoms. Whether phenotypic heterogeneity may be partly related to this phenomenon is not clear. Observations such as superiority of certain SSRIs for patients with contamination fears need to be replicated in comparisons with patients with symmetry/perfectionism/hoarding [135]. Second, the doses of antidepressants necessary for OCD are substantially higher than those for depression or anxiety disorders and also substantially higher than needed to completely block the 5-HTT [136]. Actually, this unique characteristic (the length and dose of the treatment) might point to a specific serotonin subtype, since some receptors, like 5-HT$_{1B}$, appear to be somewhat 'sticky' receptors that require a longer time and higher dose for desensitization. Third, the synthesis of 5-HT depends on the availability of tryptophan in the brain. Depletion studies in depression have shown deterioration in patients on antidepressants in remission [137], but no worsening of symptoms was seen in patients with OCD who underwent a tryptophan depletion paradigm [138]. Fourth, the therapeutic effects in OCD are usually not seen within 8 weeks of starting treatment, which is much later than in patients with depression (but, as mentioned previously, it might be connected to the receptor subtype 5HT$_{1B}$). In any case, the effects of SSRIs in OCD can also be explained by taking into account the serotonin–dopamine interaction and the effects of SSRIs on dopamine release.

THE PUZZLE OF ANTIPSYCHOTICS AND OCD:
IS DOPAMINE THE ANSWER?

It is intriguing that antipsychotics in monotherapy lack efficacy in OCD, while some of the 'typicals' are associated with exacerbation of existing symptoms or induction of *de novo* OCD symptoms in schizo-obsessive patients. Moreover, some of them (e.g. risperidone or haloperidol) were shown to be efficacious in combination with SSRIs in some patients with OCD. It has been proposed that serotonin-2A (5-HT$_{2A}$) receptor antagonism exacerbates obsessive-compulsive symptoms by increasing the firing rate of the dopamine neurons, whereas D2 receptor antagonism reduces obsessive-compulsive symptoms through inhibition of the dopamine neurons [139]. Zhang *et al.* [140,141] have shown in rats that the combination of olanzapine and fluoxetine may work synergistically to increase extracellular dopamine and norepinephrine levels in the prefrontal cortex. Denys *et al.* [142] found that the combination of quetiapine and fluvoxamine may cause a synergistic dopamine increase in the prefrontal cortex and thalamus. Since the combination of antipsychotics and SSRIs does not result in augmented serotonin levels, it is unlikely that an altered serotonergic neurotransmission underlies the clinical efficacy of this combination. Additional research is warranted to determine whether changes in the extracellular dopamine levels may account for the augmentation strategy with atypical antipsychotics in OCD.

SO, IS IT A QUESTION OF LOCATION?
(OR . . . LOCATION, LOCATION, LOCATION?)

In patients with OCD the dopamine hypothesis is based on patients with dysfunction in both the prefrontal region and the basal ganglia (striatum, thalamus and amygdala). The dysfunction of the regions observed using neuroimaging techniques could be described as dopaminergic hyperfunction in the prefrontal cortex and serotonergic hypofunction or dysfunction in the basal ganglia. Some researchers propose that the ascending serotonergic projections starting from the raphe nuclei modulate the loop. Hence, serotonergic hypofunction leads to the dopaminergic loops being overactive.

Thus, dopamine and serotonin systems play key roles in the pathophysiology of OCD. A schematic role of dopaminergic hyperactivity induced by serotonergic hypoactivity in the fronto striato-thalamic circuit might be an option for the pathogenesis of neurotransmitters in OCD. The relationship between the two dominant neurotransmitters in OCD might explain the effect of SSRIs in the treatment of OCD.

The idea of multiple factors versus single factors has been gaining more attention in psychiatry. Just as the notion that in depression, multiple factors including genetic predisposition, early life adversity and stress all play important and varying, but not solo, roles, it might very well be the case for OCD as well. We propose to look not for one system, but rather at the entire picture (including non-pharmacological factors like the family role). The task ahead is not to find the cause, but to try to untie the complex knot that leads to the behavioural symptoms called OCD. A dimensional approach to individual patients, and tailoring the treatment based on each case's unique history and current presentation (whilst taking into account non-pharmacological parameters, like hidden familial support of OCD) would probably be the best avenue to pursue.

REFERENCES

1. McGrath MJ, Campbell KM, Parks CR, Burton FH. Glutamatergic drugs exacerbate symptomatic behavior in a transgenic model of comorbid Tourette's syndrome and obsessive-compulsive disorder. *Brain Res* 2000;**877**:23–30.
2. McGale EH, Pye IF, Stonier C, Hutchinson EC, Aber GM. Studies of the inter-relationship between cerebrospinal fluid and plasma amino acid concentrations in normal individuals. *Neurochemistry* 1977;**29**:291–297.
3. Rothstein JD, Martin LJ, Kuncl RW. Decreased glutamate transport by the brain and spinal cord in amyotrophic lateral sclerosis. *N Engl J Med* 1992;**326**:1464–1468.
4. Thorén P, Asberg M, Bertilsson L, Mellström B, Sjöqvist F, Träskman L. Clomipramine treatment of obsessive-compulsive disorder. II. Biochemical aspects. *Arch Gen Psychiatry* 1980;**37**:1289–1294
5. Insel TR, Mueller EA, Alterman I, Linnoila M, Murphy DL. Obsessive-compulsive disorder and serotonin: is there a connection? *Biol Psychiatry* 1985;**20**:1174–1188.
6. Leckman JF, Goodman WK, Anderson GM *et al*. Cerebrospinal fluid biogenic amines in obsessive compulsive disorder, Tourette's syndrome, and healthy controls. *Neuropsychopharmacology* 1995;**12**:73–86.
7. Bornstein RA, Baker GB. Urinary indoleamines in Tourette syndrome patients with obsessive-compulsive characteristics. *Psychiatry Res* 1992;**41**:267–274.
8. de Groot CM, Bornstein RA, Baker GB. Obsessive-compulsive symptom clusters and urinary amine correlates in Tourette syndrome. *J Nerv Ment Dis* 1995;**183**:224–230.
9. Cath DC, Spinhoven P, Landman AD, van Kempen GM. Psychopathology and personality characteristics in relation to blood serotonin in Tourette's syndrome and obsessive-compulsive disorder. *J Psychopharmacol* 2001;**15**:111–119.
10. Delorme R, Betancur C, Callebert J *et al*. Platelet serotonergic markers as endophenotypes for obsessive-compulsive disorder. *Neuropsychopharmacology* 2005; **30**:1539–1547.
11. Delorme R, Chabane N, Callebert J *et al*. Platelet serotonergic predictors of clinical improvement in obsessive compulsive disorder. *J Clin Psychopharmacol* 2004;**24**:18–23.
12. Hanna GL, Yuwiler A, Cantwell DP. Whole blood serotonin in juvenile obsessive-compulsive disorder. *Biol Psychiatry* 1991;**29**:738–744.
13. Flament MF, Rapoport JL, Murphy DL, Berg CJ, Lake CR. Biochemical changes during clomipramine treatment of childhood obsessive-compulsive disorder. *Arch Gen Psychiatry* 1987;**44**:219–225.

14. Sallee FR, Richman H, Beach K, Sethuraman G, Nesbitt L. Platelet serotonin transporter in children and adolescents with obsessive-compulsive disorder or Tourette's syndrome. *J Am Acad Child Adolesc Psychiatry* 1996;**35**:1647–1656.

15. Weizman A, Mandel A, Barber Y *et al*. Decreased platelet imipramine binding in Tourette syndrome children with obsessive-compulsive disorder. *Biol Psychiatry* 1992;**31**:705–711.

16. Marazziti D, Rossi A, Gemignani A *et al*. Decreased platelet 3H-paroxetine binding in obsessive-compulsive patients. *Neuropsychobiology* 1996;**34**:184–187.

17. Marazziti D, Hollander E, Lensi P, Ravagli S, Cassano GB. Peripheral markers of serotonin and dopamine function in obsessive-compulsive disorder. *Psychiatry Res* 1992;**42**:41–51.

18. Zohar J, Mueller EA, Insel TR *et al*. Serotonergic responsivity in obsessive-compulsive disorder. Comparison of patients and healthy controls. *Arch Gen Psychiatry* 1987;**44**:946–951.

19. Zohar J, Insel TR, Zohar-Kadouch RC *et al*. Serotonergic responsivity in obsessive-compulsive disorder. Effects of chronic clomipramine treatment. *Arch Gen Psychiatry* 1988;**45**:167–172.

20. Hollander E, DeCaria CM, Nitescu A *et al*. Serotonergic function in obsessive-compulsive disorder. Behavioral and neuroendocrine responses to oral m-chlorophenylpiperazine and fenfluramine in patients and healthy volunteers. *Arch Gen Psychiatry* 1992;**49**:21–28.

21. Charney DS, Goodman WK, Price LH *et al*. Serotonin function in obsessive-compulsive disorder. A comparison of the effects of tryptophan and m-chlorophenylpiperazine in patients and healthy subjects. *Arch Gen Psychiatry* 1988;**45**:177–185.

22. Goodman WK, McDougle CJ, Price LH *et al*. m-Chlorophenylpiperazine in patients with obsessive-compulsive disorder: absence of symptom exacerbation. *Biol Psychiatry* 1995;**38**:138–149.

23. Gross-Isseroff R, Cohen R, Sasson Y *et al*. Serotonergic dissection of obsessive compulsive symptoms: a challenge study with m-chlorophenylpiperazine and sumatriptan. *Neuropsychobiology* 2004;**50**:200–205.

24. Ho Pian KL, Westenberg HG, den Boer JA *et al*. Effects of meta-chlorophenylpiperazine on cerebral blood flow in obsessive-compulsive disorder and controls. *Biol Psychiatry* 1998;**44**:367–370.

25. Gorman JM, Liebowitz MR, Fyer AJ *et al*. Lactate infusions in obsessive-compulsive disorder. *Am J Psychiatry* 1985;**142**:864–866.

26. Perna G, Bertani A, Arancio C, Ronchi P, Bellodi L. Laboratory response of patients with panic and obsessive-compulsive disorders to 35% CO_2 challenges. *Am J Psychiatry* 1995;**152**:85–89.

27. Rasmussen SA, Goodman WK, Woods SW, Heninger GR, Charney DS. Effects of yohimbine in obsessive compulsive disorder. *Psychopharmacology (Berl)* 1987;**93**:308–313.

28. de Leeuw AS, Den Boer JA, Slaap BR, Westenberg HG. Pentagastrin has panic-inducing properties in obsessive compulsive disorder. *Psychopharmacology (Berl)* 1996;**126**:339–344.

29. Zohar J, Kennedy JL, Hollander E, Koran LM. Serotonin-1D hypothesis of obsessive-compulsive disorder: an update. *J Clin Psychiatry* 2004;**65**(Suppl. 14):18–21.

30. Lesch KP, Hoh A, Schulte HM *et al.* Long-term fluoxetine treatment decreases 5-HT$_{1A}$ receptor responsivity in obsessive-compulsive disorder. *Psychopharmacology (Berl)* 1991;**105**:415–420.

31. Ho Pian KL, Westenberg HG, van Megen HJ *et al.* Sumatriptan (5-HT1D receptor agonist) does not exacerbate symptoms in obsessive compulsive disorder. *Psychopharmacology (Berl)* 1998;**140**:365–370.

32. Stein DJ, Van Heerden B, Wessels CJ *et al.* Single photon emission computed tomography of the brain with Tc-99m HMPAO during sumatriptan challenge in obsessive-compulsive disorder: investigating the functional role of the serotonin auto-receptor. *Prog Neuropsychopharmacol Biol Psychiatry* 1999;**23**:1079–1099.

33. Boshuisen ML, den Boer JA. Zolmitriptan (a 5-HT1B/1D receptor agonist with central action) does not increase symptoms in obsessive compulsive disorder. *Psychopharmacology (Berl)* 2000;**152**:74–79.

34. de Leeuw AS, Westenberg HG. Hypersensitivity of 5-HT2 receptors in OCD patients. An increased prolactin response after a challenge with meta-chlorophenylpiperazine and pre-treatment with ritanserin and placebo. *J Psychiatr Res* 2008;**42**:894–901.

35. McBride PA, DeMeo MD, Sweeney JA *et al.* Neuroendocrine and behavioral responses to challenge with the indirect serotonin agonist dl-fenfluramine in adults with obsessive-compulsive disorder. *Biol Psychiatry* 1992;**31**:19–34.

36. Hewlett WA, Vinogradov S, Martin K *et al.* Fenfluramine stimulation of prolactin in obsessive-compulsive disorder. *Psychiatry Res* 1992;**42**:81–92.

37. Lucey JV, O'Keane V, Butcher G *et al.* Cortisol and prolactin responses to D-fenfluramine in non-depressed patients with obsessive-compulsive disorder: a comparison with depressed and healthy controls. *Br J Psychiatry* 1992;**161**:517–521.

38. Fernandez CE, Lopez-Ibor JJ. Monochlorimipramine in the treatment of psychiatric patients resistant to other therapies. *Actas luso Esp Neurol Psiq Ciec Afines* 1967;**26**:119–147.

39. Denys D, Zohar J, Westenberg HG. The role of dopamine in obsessive-compulsive disorder: preclinical and clinical evidence. *J Clin Psychiatry* 2004;**65**(Suppl. 14): 11–17.

40. Goodman WK, Price LH, Delgado PL *et al.* Specificity of serotonin reuptake inhibitors in the treatment of obsessive-compulsive disorder. Comparison of fluvoxamine and desipramine. *Arch Gen Psychiatry* 1990;**47**:577–585.

41. Zohar J, Insel TR. Obsessive-compulsive disorder: psychobiological approaches to diagnosis, treatment, and pathophysiology. *Biol Psychiatry* 1987;**22**:667–687.

42. Leonard HL, Swedo SE, Rapoport JL *et al.* Treatment of obsessive-compulsive disorder with clomipramine and desipramine in children and adolescents. A double-blind crossover comparison. *Arch Gen Psychiatry* 1989;**46**:1088–1092.

43. Hoehn-Saric R, Ninan P, Black DW *et al.* Multicenter double-blind comparison of sertraline and desipramine for concurrent obsessive-compulsive and major depressive disorders. *Arch Gen Psychiatry* 2000;**57**:76–82.

44. Denys D, van der Wee N, van Megen HJ *et al.* A double blind comparison of venlafaxine and paroxetine in obsessive-compulsive disorder. *J Clin Psychopharmacol* 2003;**23**:568–575.

45. El Mansari M, Blier P. Mechanisms of action of current and potential pharmacotherapies of obsessive-compulsive disorder. *Prog Neuropsychopharmacol Biol Psychiatry* 2006;**30**:362–373.

46. Dannon PN, Sasson Y, Hirschmann S *et al.* Pindolol augmentation in treatment-resistant obsessive compulsive disorder: a double-blind placebo controlled trial. *Eur Neuropsychopharmacol* 2000;**10**:165–169.

47. Koran LM, Quirk T, Lorberbaum JP, Elliott M. Mirtazapine treatment of obsessive-compulsive disorder. *J Clin Psychopharmacol* 2001;**21**:537–539.

48. Pallanti S, Quercioli L, Bruscoli M. Response acceleration with mirtazapine augmentation of citalopram in obsessive-compulsive disorder patients without comorbid depression: a pilot study. *J Clin Psychiatry* 2004;**65**:1394–1399.

49. Bloch MH, Landeros-Weisenberger A, Kelmendi B *et al.* A systematic review: antipsychotic augmentation with treatment refractory obsessive-compulsive disorder. *Mol Psychiatry* 2006;**11**:622–632.

50. Chou-Green JM, Holscher TD, Dallman MF, Akana SF. Compulsive behavior in the 5-HT2C receptor knockout mouse. *Physiol Behav* 2003;**78**:641–649.

51. Tsaltas E, Kontis D, Chrysikakou S *et al.* Reinforced spatial alternation as an animal model of obsessive-compulsive disorder (OCD): investigation of 5-HT2C and 5-HT1D receptor involvement in OCD pathophysiology. *Biol Psychiatry* 2005; **57**:1176–1185.

52. Flaisher-Grinberg S, Klavir O, Joel D. The role of 5-HT2A and 5-HT2C receptors in the signal attenuation rat model of obsessive-compulsive disorder. *Int J Neuropsychopharmacol* 2008;**11**:811–825.

53. Joel D, Avisar A. Excessive lever pressing following post-training signal attenuation in rats: a possible animal model of obsessive compulsive disorder? *Behav Brain Res* 2001;**123**:77–87.

54. Joel D, Doljansky J, Schiller D. 'Compulsive' lever pressing in rats is enhanced following lesions to the orbital cortex, but not to the basolateral nucleus of the amygdala or to the dorsal medial prefrontal cortex. *Eur J Neurosci* 2005;**21**:2252–2262.

55. Benkelfat C, Mefford IN, Masters CF *et al.* Plasma catecholamines and their metabolites in obsessive-compulsive disorder. *Psychiatry Res* 1991;**37**:321–331.

56. Swedo SE, Leonard HL, Kruesi MJ *et al.* Cerebrospinal fluid neurochemistry in children and adolescents with obsessive-compulsive disorder. *Arch Gen Psychiatry* 1992;**49**:29–36.

57. Hollander E, Stein DJ, Saoud JB *et al.* Effects of fenfluramine on plasma HVA in OCD (letter). *Psychiatry Res* 1992;**42**:185–188.

58. Zahn TP, Kruesi MJ, Swedo SE, Leonard HL, Rapoport JL. Autonomic activity in relation to cerebrospinal fluid neurochemistry in obsessive and disruptive children and adolescents. *Psychophysiology* 1996;**33**:731–739.

59. Little KY, Zhang L, Desmond T *et al.* Striatal dopaminergic abnormalities in human cocaine users. *Am J Psychiatry* 1999;**156**:238–245.

60. McDougle CJ, Goodman WK, Delgado PL *et al.* Pathophysiology of obsessive-compulsive disorder. *Am J Psychiatry* 1989;**146**:350–351.

61. Rosse RB, Fay-McCarthy M, Collins JP Jr *et al.* The relationship between cocaine-induced paranoia and compulsive foraging: a preliminary report. *Addiction* 1994; **89**:1097–1104.

62. Rosse RB, Fay-McCarthy M, Collins JP Jr *et al.* Transient compulsive foraging behavior associated with crack cocaine use. *Am J Psychiatry* 1993;**150**:155–156.

63. Koizumi HM. Obsessive-compulsive symptoms following stimulants. *Biol Psychiatry* 1985;**20**:1332–1333.

64. Satel SL, McDougle CJ. Obsessions and compulsions associated with cocaine abuse. *Am J Psychiatry* 1991;**148**:947.

65. Rosse RB, McCarthy MF, Alim TN *et al.* Saccadic distractibility in cocaine dependent patients: a preliminary laboratory exploration of the cocaine-OCD hypothesis. *Drug Alcohol Depend* 1994;**35**:25–30.

66. Kotsopoulos S, Spivak M. Obsessive-compulsive symptoms secondary to methylphenidate treatment. *Can J Psychiatry* 2001;**46**:89.

67. Frye PE, Arnold LE. Persistent amphetamine-induced compulsive rituals: response to pyridoxine(B6). *Biol Psychiatry* 1981;**16**:583–587.

68. Yo M, Sekine Y, Matsunaga T *et al.* Methamphetamine-associated obsessional symptoms and effective risperidone treatment: a case report. *J Clin Psychiatry* 1999; **60**:337–338.

69. Joffe RT, Swinson RP. Methylphenidate in primary obsessive-compulsive disorder. *J Clin Psychopharmacol* 1987;**7**:420–422.

70. Pitchot W, Hansenne M, Moreno AG *et al.* Growth hormone response to apomorphine in obsessive-compulsive disorder. *J Psychiatry Neurosci* 1996;**21**:343–345.

71. Brambilla F, Perna G, Bussi R *et al.* Dopamine function in obsessive compulsive disorder: cortisol response to acute apomorphine stimulation. *Psychoneuroendocrinology* 2000;**25**:301–310.

72. Brambilla F, Bellodi L, Perna G *et al.* Dopamine function in obsessive-compulsive disorder: growth hormone response to apomorphine stimulation. *Biol Psychiatry* 1997;**42**:889–897.

73. Longhurst JG, Carpenter LL, Epperson CN *et al.* Effects of catecholamine depletion with AMPT (alpha-methyl-para-tyrosine) in obsessive-compulsive disorder. *Biol Psychiatry* 1999;**46**:573–576.

74. Ceccherini-Nelli A, Guazzelli M. Treatment of refractory OCD with the dopamine agonist bromocriptine. *J Clin Psychiatry* 1994;**55**:415–416.

75. Trethowan WH, Scott PA. Chlorpromazine in obsessive-compulsive and allied disorders. *Lancet* 1955;**268**:781–785.

76. Hussain MZ, Ahad A. Treatment of obsessive-compulsive neurosis [letter]. *Can Med Assoc J* 1970;**103**:648.

77. O'Regan JB. Treatment of obsessive-compulsive neurosis. *Can Med Assoc J* 1970;**103**:650–651.

78. O'Regan JB. Treatment of obsessive-compulsive neurosis with haloperidol. *Can Med Assoc J* 1970;**103**:167–168.

79. Altschuler M. Massive doses of trifluoperazine in the treatment of compulsive rituals [letter]. *Am J Psychiatry* 1962;**119**:367–368.

80. Rivers-Bulkeley N, Hollender MH. Successful treatment of obsessive-compulsive disorder with loxapine. *Am J Psychiatry* 1982;**139**:1345–1346.

81. McDougle CJ, Barr LC, Goodman WK *et al.* Lack of efficacy of clozapine monotherapy in refractory obsessive-compulsive disorder. *Am J Psychiatry* 1995; **152**:1812–1814.

82. Mahendran R, Liew E, Subramaniam M. De novo emergence of obsessive–compulsive symptoms with atypical antipsychotics in Asian patients with schizophrenia or schizoaffective disorder: a retrospective, cross-sectional study. *J Clin Psychiatry* 2007;**68**:542–545.

83. Lykouras L, Alevizos B, Michalopoulou P, Rabavilas A. Obsessive-compulsive symptoms induced by atypical antipsychotics. A review of the reported cases. *Prog Neuropsychopharmacol Biol Psychiatry* 2003;**27**:333–346.

84. Mahendran R. Obsessional symptoms associated with risperidone treatment. *Aust N Z J Psychiatry* 1998;**32**:299–301.

85. Dryden-Edwards RC, Reiss AL. Differential response of psychotic and obsessive symptoms to risperidone in an adolescent. *J Child Adolesc Psychopharmacol* 1996;**6**:139–145.

86. Alzaid K, Jones BD. A case report of risperidone-induced obsessive-compulsive symptoms. *J Clin Psychopharmacol* 1997;**17**:58–59.

87. Chong SA, Tan CH, Lee HS. Hoarding and clozapine-risperidone combination. *Can J Psychiatry* 1996;**41**:315–316.

88. Alevizos B, Lykouras L, Zervas IM *et al.* Risperidone-induced obsessive-compulsive symptoms: a series of six cases. *J Clin Psychopharmacol* 2002;**22**:461–467.

89. Dodt JE, Byerly MJ, Cuadros C *et al.* Treatment of risperidone-induced obsessive-compulsive symptoms with sertraline. *Am J Psychiatry* 1997;**154**:582.

90. Kopala L, Honer WG. Risperidone, serotonergic mechanisms, and obsessive-compulsive symptoms in schizophrenia. *Am J Psychiatry* 1994;**151**:1714–1715.

91. Lykouras L, Zervas IM, Gournellis R *et al.* Olanzapine and obsessive-compulsive symptoms. *Eur Neuropsychopharmacol* 2000;**10**:385–387.

92. Morrison D, Clark D, Goldfarb E *et al.* Worsening of obsessive-compulsive symptoms following treatment with olanzapine. *Am J Psychiatry* 1998;**155**:855.

93. Mahendran R. Obsessive-compulsive symptoms with risperidone. *J Clin Psychiatry* 1999;**60**:261–263.

94. Steingard S, Chengappa KN, Baker RW *et al.* Clozapine, obsessive symptoms, and serotonergic mechanisms. *Am J Psychiatry* 1993;**150**:1435.

95. Levkovitch Y, Kronnenberg Y, Gaoni B. Can clozapine trigger OCD? *J Am Acad Child Adolesc Psychiatry* 1995;**34**:263.

96. Ghaemi SN, Zarate CA Jr, Popli AP *et al.* Is there a relationship between clozapine and obsessive-compulsive disorder? A retrospective chart review. *Compr Psychiatry* 1995;**36**:267–270.

97. de Haan L, Beuk N, Hoogenboom B *et al.* Obsessive-compulsive symptoms during treatment with olanzapine and risperidone: a prospective study of 113 patients with recent-onset schizophrenia or related disorders. *J Clin Psychiatry* 2002;**63**:104–107.

98. Lykouras L, Zervas IM, Gournellis R *et al.* Olanzapine and obsessive-compulsive symptoms. *Eur Neuropsychopharmacol* 2000;**10**:385–387.

99. Morrison D, Clark D, Goldfarb E *et al.* Worsening of obsessive-compulsive symptoms following treatment with olanzapine. *Am J Psychiatry* 1998;**155**:855.

100. Mottard JP, De la Sablonniere JF. Olanzapine-induced obsessive-compulsive disorder. *Am J Psychiatry* 1999;**156**:799–800.

101. Khullar A, Chue P, Tibbo P. Quetiapine and obsessive-compulsive symptoms (OCS): case report and review of atypical antipsychotic-induced OCS. *J Psychiatry Neurosci* 2001;**26**:55–59.

102. Chen CH, Chiu CC, Huang MC. Dose-related exacerbation of obsessive-compulsive symptoms with quetiapine treatment. *Prog Neuropsychopharmacol Biol Psychiatry* 2008;**32**:304–305.

103. Stamouli S, Lykouras L. Quetiapine-induced obsessive-compulsive symptoms: a series of five cases. *J Clin Psychopharmacol* 2006;**26**:396–400.
104. Ozer S, Arsava M, Ertuğrul A, Demir B. Obsessive compulsive symptoms associated with quetiapine treatment in a schizophrenic patient: a case report. *Prog Neuropsychopharmacol Biol Psychiatry* 2006;**30**:724–727.
105. Tranulis C, Potvin S, Gourgue M, Leblanc G, Mancini-Marïe A, Stip E. The paradox of quetiapine in obsessive-compulsive disorder. *CNS Spectr* 2005;**10**:356–361.
106. McDougle CJ, Goodman WK, Leckman JF, Lee NC, Heninger GR, Price LH. Haloperidol addition in fluvoxamine-refractory obsessive-compulsive disorder. A double-blind, placebo-controlled study in patients with and without tics. *Arch Gen Psychiatry* 1994;**51**:302–308.
107. Saxena S, Wang D, Bystritsky A, Baxter LR Jr. Risperidone augmentation of SRI treatment for refractory obsessive-compulsive disorder. *J Clin Psychiatry* 1996; **57**:303–306.
108. McDougle CJ, Epperson CN, Pelton GH, Wasylink S, Price LH. A double-blind, placebo-controlled study of risperidone addition in serotonin reuptake inhibitor-refractory obsessive-compulsive disorder. *Arch Gen Psychiatry* 2000;**57**:794–801.
109. Hollander E, Baldini Rossi N, Sood E, Pallanti S. Risperidone augmentation in treatment-resistant obsessive-compulsive disorder: a double-blind, placebo-controlled study. *Int J Neuropsychopharmacol* 2003;**6**:397–401.
110. Bloch MH, Landeros-Weisenberger A, Kelmendi B, Coric V, Bracken MB, Leckman JF. A systematic review: antipsychotic augmentation with treatment refractory obsessive-compulsive disorder. *Mol Psychiatry* 2006;**11**:622–632.
111. Denys D, Fineberg N, Carey PD, Stein DJ. Quetiapine addition in obsessive-compulsive disorder: is treatment outcome affected by type and dose of serotonin reuptake inhibitors? *Biol Psychiatry* 2007;**61**:412–414.
112. Fineberg NA, Stein DJ, Premkumar P *et al.* Adjunctive quetiapine for serotonin reuptake inhibitor-resistant obsessive-compulsive disorder: a meta-analysis of randomized controlled treatment trials. *Int Clin Psychopharmacol* 2006;**21**:337–343.
113. Atmaca M, Kuloglu M, Tezcan E, Gecici O. Quetiapine augmentation in patients with treatment resistant obsessive-compulsive disorder: a single-blind, placebo-controlled study. *Int Clin Psychopharmacol* 2002;**17**:115–119.
114. Pessina E, Albert U, Bogetto F, Maina G. Aripiprazole augmentation of serotonin reuptake inhibitors in treatment-resistant obsessive-compulsive disorder: a 12-week open-label preliminary study. *Int Clin Psychopharmacol* 2009;**24**:265–269.
115. Metin O, Yazici K, Tot S, Yazici AE. Amisulpride augmentation in treatment resistant obsessive-compulsive disorder: an open trial. *Hum Psychopharmacol* 2003; **18**:463–467.
116. Joel D, Doljansky J. Selective alleviation of compulsive lever-pressing in rats by D1, but not D2, blockade: possible implications for the involvement of D1 receptors in obsessive-compulsive disorder. *Neuropsychopharmacology* 2003;**28**:77–85.
117. Campbell KM, de Lecea L, Severynse DM *et al.* OCD-like behaviors caused by a neuropotentiating transgene targeted to cortical and limbic D1+ neurons. *J Neurosci* 1999;**19**:5044–5053.
118. Campbell KM, McGrath MJ, Burton FH. Behavioral effects of cocaine on a transgenic mouse model of cortical-limbic compulsion. *Brain Res* 1999;**833**:216–224.

119. Campbell KM, McGrath MJ, Burton FH. Differential response of cortical-limbic neuropotentiated compulsive mice to dopamine D1 and D2 receptor antagonists. *Eur J Pharmacol* 1999;**371**:103–111.

120. McGrath MJ, Campbell KM, Parks CR, Burton FH. Glutamatergic drugs exacerbate symptomatic behavior in a transgenic model of comorbid Tourette's syndrome and obsessive-compulsive disorder. *Brain Res* 2000;**877**:23–30.

121. Campbell KM, Veldman MB, McGrath MJ, Burton FH. TS+OCD-like neuropotentiated mice are supersensitive to seizure induction. *Neuroreport* 2000;**11**:2335–2338.

122. Einat H, Szechtman H. Perseveration without hyperlocomotion in a spontaneous alternation task in rats sensitized to the dopamine agonist quinpirole. *Physiol Behav* 1995;**57**:55–59.

123. Szechtman H, Sulis W, Eilam D. Quinpirole induces compulsive checking behavior in rats: A potential animal model of obsessive-compulsive disorder (OCD). *Behav Neurosci* 1998;**112**:1475–1485.

124. Ben-Pazi A, Szechtman H, Eilam D. The morphogenesis of motor rituals in rats treated chronically with the dopamine agonist quinpirole. *Behav Neurosci* 2001; **115**:1301–1317.

125. Szechtman H, Eckert MJ, Tse WS *et al.* Compulsive checking behavior of quinpirole-sensitized rats as an animal model of Obsessive-Compulsive Disorder(OCD): form and control. *BMC Neurosci* 2001;**2**:4.

126. Sullivan RM, Talangbayan H, Einat H, Szechtman H. Effects of quinpirole on central dopamine systems in sensitized and non-sensitized rats. *Neuroscience* 1998; **83**:781–789.

127. de Haas R, Nijdam A, Westra TA, Kas MJ, Westenberg HG. Behavioral pattern analysis and dopamine release in quinpirole-induced repetitive behavior in rats. *J Psychopharmacol* 2011;**25**:1712–1719.

128. Zor R, Keren H, Hermesh H, Szechtman H, Mort J, Eilam D. Obsessive-compulsive disorder: a disorder of pessimal (non-functional) motor behavior. *Acta Psychiatr Scand* 2009;**120**:288–298.

129. Korff S, Stein DJ, Harvey BH. Stereotypic behaviour in the deer mouse: pharmacological validation and relevance for obsessive compulsive disorder. *Prog Neuropsychopharmacol Biol Psychiatry* 2008;**32**:348–355.

130. Moore GJ, MacMaster FP, Stewart C, Rosenberg DR. Case study: caudate glutamatergic changes with paroxetine therapy for pediatric obsessive-compulsive disorder. *J Am Acad Child Adolesc Psychiatry* 1998;**37**:663–667.

131. Rosenberg DR, MacMaster FP, Keshavan MS, Fitzgerald KD, Stewart CM, Moore GJ. Decrease in caudate glutamatergic concentrations in pediatric obsessive-compulsive disorder patients taking paroxetine. *J Am Acad Child Adolesc Psychiatry* 2000;**39**:1096–1103.

132. Rosenberg DR, Mirza Y, Russell A *et al.* Reduced anterior cingulate glutamatergic concentrations in childhood OCD and major depression versus healthy controls. *J Am Acad Child Adolesc Psychiatry* 2004;**43**:1146–1153.

133. Chakrabarty K, Bhattacharyya S, Christopher R, Khanna S. Glutamatergic dysfunction in OCD. *Neuropsychopharmacology* 2005;**30**:1735–1740.

134. McGrath MJ, Campbell KM, Parks CR, Burton FH. Glutamatergic drugs exacerbate symptomatic behavior in a transgenic model of comorbid Tourette's syndrome and obsessive-compulsive disorder. *Brain Res* 2000;**877**:23–30.

135. Denys D, de Geus F, van Megen HJ *et al.* Use of factor analysis to detect potential phenotypes in obsessive-compulsive disorder. *Psychiatry Res* 2004;**128**:273–280.

136. Kent JM, Coplan JD, Lombardo I *et al.* Occupancy of brain serotonin transporters during treatment with paroxetine in patients with social phobia: a positron emission tomography study with 11C McN 5652. *Psychopharmacology (Berl)* 2002; **164**:341–348.

137. Neumeister A. Tryptophan depletion, serotonin, and depression: where do we stand? *Psychopharmacol Bull* 2003;**37**:99–115.

138. Berney A, Sookman D, Leyton M *et al.* Lack of effects on core obsessive-compulsive symptoms of tryptophan depletion during symptom provocation in remitted obsessive-compulsive disorder patients. *Biol Psychiatry* 2006;**59**:853–857.

139. Ramasubbu R. Antiobsessional effect of risperidone add-on treatment in serotonin reuptake inhibitor-refractory obsessive-compulsive disorder may be dose-dependent [letter]. *Arch Gen Psychiatry* 2002;**59**:472.

140. Zhang W, Bymaster FP. The in vivo effects of olanzapine and other antipsychotic agents on receptor occupancy and antagonism of dopamine D1, D2, D3, 5HT2A and muscarinic receptors. *Psychopharmacology (Berl)* 1999;**141**:267–278.

141. Zhang W, Perry KW, Wong DT *et al.* Synergistic effects of olanzapine and other antipsychotic agents in combination with fluoxetine on norepinephrine and dopamine release in rat prefrontal cortex. *Neuropsychopharmacology* 2000;**23**:250–262

142. Denys D, Klompmakers AA, Westenberg HG. Synergistic dopamine increase in the rat prefrontal cortex with the combination of quetiapine and fluvoxamine. *Psychopharmacology (Berl)* 2004;**176**:195–203.

CHAPTER 10

Brain Imaging

**David R. Rosenberg, Phillip C. Easter
and Georgia Michalopoulou**
*Department of Psychiatry and Behavioral Neurosciences, Wayne State University,
and the Children's Hospital of Michigan*

Obsessive-compulsive disorder (OCD) affects 1–3% of the population worldwide and is characterized by repetitive, ritualistic thoughts, interests, activities and behaviours over which the patient has very little control [1–5]. As many as 50% of all cases have their onset in childhood and adolescence, although delayed diagnosis in adulthood is not uncommon [6,7]. Advances in neuroimaging technology allow for a non-invasive structural, chemical and functional 'biopsy' of the brain and have begun to elucidate the neurobiological underpinnings of OCD, which may result in enhanced neurodiagnostic assessment and treatment. Recent investigation exploiting the emerging field of combined imaging and genetic study in the same patients with OCD offers further insight into potential mechanisms of illness and treatment response, or lack thereof, in OCD [8–10].

One of the more consistent findings in neuropsychiatry has been the identification of alterations in cortico-striatal-thalamic circuitry in adult and pediatric OCD (Figure 10.1). It should be noted, however, that recent investigation suggests that other brain regions may also be involved in the pathogenesis of OCD. In this chapter, we discuss (i) neuroimaging techniques used to examine OCD, and (ii) relevant neuroimaging and recent combined brain imaging and genetic studies conducted in OCD patients.

NEUROIMAGING MODALITIES

Structural assessment

Quantitative computerized tomography (CT) and magnetic resonance imaging (MRI) allow for measurement of brain anatomy. MRI permits enhanced

Obsessive-Compulsive Disorder: Current Science and Clinical Practice, First Edition. Edited by Joseph Zohar.
© 2012 John Wiley & Sons, Ltd. Published 2012 by John Wiley & Sons, Ltd.

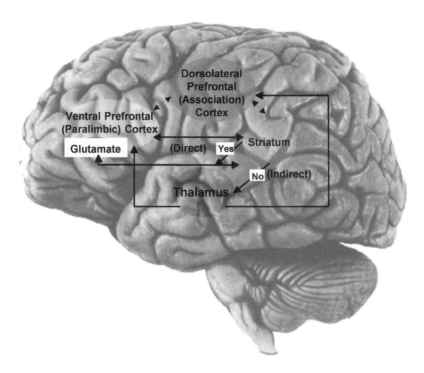

Figure 10.1 Illustration of cortico-striato-thalamo-cortico network in obsessive-compulsive disorder. Adapted from Rosenberg DR, Keshavan MS. Toward a neurodevelopmental model of obsessive-compulsive disorder. *Biol Psychiatry* 1998;**43**: 623–640; and Rosenberg DR, MacMillan S. Imaging and neurocircuitry of OCD. In: Davis KL, Nemeroff CB, Coyle J, Charney D (eds), *Neuropsychopharmacology. The 5th Generation of Progress*. Baltimore: Lippincott Williams & Wilkins, 2002; pp. 1621–1646, with permission.

three-dimensional (3D) acquisition and tissue differentiation without ionizing radiation risks. Most structural MRI studies have focused on measurement of brain volume since volumetric measures may reflect a region's function [11,12]. More recently, MRI studies have utilized (i) automated voxel-based morphometry (VBM) studies to assess for regional grey matter alterations; (ii) diffusion tensor imaging (DTI) to measure white matter tractography; and (iii) regional cortical thickness assessment.

Functional neurochemical assessment

Functional neurochemical techniques may be more sensitive than structural neuroimaging in identifying subtle brain alterations in specific psychiatric disorders [13]. Both positron emission tomography (PET) and single-photon emission computerized tomography (SPECT) measure cerebral blood flow, metabolism, and receptor and neurochemical function. PET and SPECT use ionizing radiation, which makes them less feasible in paediatric populations and for repeated study of neurodevelopmental and neurodegenerative effects. Radiation exposure is less with SPECT than with PET, although PET typically permits better resolution, which limits the usefulness of SPECT. 3D PET reduces radiation exposure significantly and may become more feasible for repeated study in neurodevelopmental and neurodegenerative disorders.

Magnetic resonance spectroscopy (MRS) allows for the direct and *in vivo* measurement of brain chemistry and important metabolites without ionizing radiation risks. In contrast to PET, however, MRS cannot currently measure serotonin or dopamine neurotransmitter and receptor systems. Functional MRI (fMRI) allows for superior temporal and spatial resolution compared to PET without any putative ionizing radiation risks [14]. Second-second temporal resolution can be achieved with event-related fMRI [15].

Magnetoelectroencephalography (MEG) combines electroencephalography (EEG) with fMRI studies [16]. This remains a modality typically used in research centres, but with advances in technology it is being increasingly used for study. This is expected to pioneer functional assessment in neuropsychiatric disorders such as OCD.

STRUCTURAL ASSESSMENT OF OCD

Total brain volume/ventricles

Total brain volume and intracranial brain volume do not differ significantly between paediatric and adult patients with OCD and controls [17–24]. Increased grey matter–white matter ratios have been observed in adult OCD patients [19,20]. Increased ventricular brain ratios (VBR), suggestive of reduced basal ganglia volume, were reported by Behar *et al.* [25] in adolescent OCD patients compared to controls. In contrast, no significant differences in VBR were observed between adult OCD patients and controls [26]. Significantly increased third ventricular but not lateral ventricular volumes were observed in 19 psychotropic-naive paediatric OCD patients compared with 19 age- and sex-matched controls [23].

Basal ganglia

Contradictory findings have been reported for basal ganglia measurement in adult OCD patients. For example, while Scarone *et al.* [27] and Robinson *et al.* [21] reported volumetric alterations in the basal ganglia of adult OCD patients compared with healthy controls, several studies reported no significant differences in basal ganglia measurement between OCD patients and controls [13,18,20,28–31]. Menzies *et al.* [32] found a significant association between impaired motor inhibition and altered caudate volume in both OCD patients and adult relatives of OCD patients. Several potential confounds may contribute to this discrepancy, such as illness duration, treatment intervention, differences in imaging methodology, region of interest and the heterogeneity of OCD.

As in adults, structural neuroimaging studies of the basal ganglia in paediatric OCD patients have always proved inconsistent. Using quantitative CT, Luxenberg *et al.* [30] found reduced caudate volume in adolescent males with OCD compared with controls. Using volumetric MRI, Rosenberg *et al.* [23] found reduced striatal (caudate + putamen) volume inversely correlated with increased OCD symptom severity, but not illness duration, in psychotropic-naive paediatric OCD patients compared with controls. Globus pallidus volume was not measured in this report. Reduced striatal volume was correlated with increased oculomotor response suppression failures in the same paediatric OCD patients [24]. In contrast, Szeszko *et al.* [33] reported reduced globus pallidus volume that correlated with increased OCD symptom severity in psychotropic-naive paediatric OCD patients in comparison with healthy paediatric controls. No significant differences in caudate or putamen volumes were observed between paediatric OCD patients and controls. Although tic disorders and Tourette syndrome were exclusionary for both the Rosenberg *et al.* [23] and Szeszko *et al.* [33] studies, the Rosenberg *et al.* [23] sample had significantly more males than females, while the Szeszko *et al.* [33] sample had significantly more females than males. Given the age range of 6 to 17 years of age in the two studies, it is possible that some of the patients, particularly males, had not yet passed through the age of risk for tic disorder and may have had premorbid and/or emerging tic/Tourette syndrome. In this regard, it is interesting to note that in the Rosenberg *et al.* [23] sample, the reduction in striatal volume in paediatric OCD patients was primarily accounted for by reduction in putamen rather than the entire striatal volume. Reduced putamen volume has been observed in patients with Tourette syndrome [34]. Case reports have also found lesions of the putamen to be associated with OCD [35,36]. Antibodies directed at the putamen are also found at significantly greater rates in paediatric OCD patients as compared to healthy paediatric controls [37].

There may also be distinct structural neuroimaging findings in the basal ganglia of paediatric patients with an autoimmune subtype of OCD, for example paediatric autoimmune neuropsychiatric disorders associated with group A beta-haemolytic streptococcal (GABHS) infections in paediatric patients (PANDAS) [38,39]. Giedd *et al.* [40,41] observed increased basal ganglia volumes (caudate, putamen and globus pallidus) in PANDAS patients compared with healthy paediatric controls. A striking association between basal ganglia volume, OCD symptom severity and response to immunotherapy was reported in an adolescent with PANDAS (Figure 10.2). Peterson *et al.* [42] found that increased antistreptolysin O antibody titres (ASO) were positively correlated with increased basal ganglia volume in

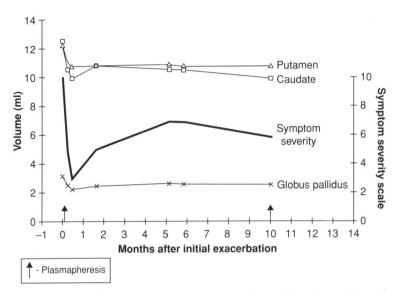

Figure 10.2 Sequential magnetic resonance imaging of basal ganglia volumes in a male adolescent undergoing plasma exchange for infection-related obsessive-compulsive disorder. Reprinted from Giedd JN, Rapoport JL, Leonard HL *et al.* Case study: acute basal ganglia enlargement and obsessive-compulsive symptoms in an adolescent boy. *J Am Acad Child Adolesc Psychiatry* 1996;**35**(7):913–915; and Rosenberg DR, MacMillan S. Imaging and neurocircuitry of OCD. In: Davis KL, Nemeroff CB, Coyle J, Charney D (eds), *Neuropsychopharmacology. The 5th Generation of Progress.* Baltimore: Lippincott Williams & Wilkins, 2002; pp. 1621–1646, with permission.

OCD patients who had recurrent streptococcal infections. This finding was not specific to OCD as it was also noted in patients with ADHD who had recurrent streptococcal infections.

Prefrontal cortex

Szeszko *et al.* [43] found bilaterally reduced orbital frontal volume in adult OCD patients versus controls. Increased opercular volume, increase in six right frontal and four left parcellation units, and a significant correlation between increased right inferior pars triangularis volume and right midfrontal cortical volumes and impaired nonverbal immediate recall testing have been reported in adult OCD patients compared with controls [20,44,45]. A significant association between impaired motor inhibition and increased cingulate grey matter has also been found in adult OCD patients and in adult unaffected relatives of OCD patients [46]. Significant associations between orbital frontal grey matter and motor inhibition and reversal learning have also been found in adult OCD patients and unaffected adult relatives [32,47].

L

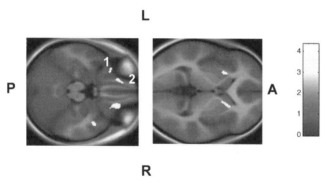

R

Figure 10.3 Regions of more gray matter in 37 psychotropic drug-naive pediatric obsessive-compulsive disorder patients compared to 26 healthy volunteers in regions predicted to differ a priori between groups ($p < 0.005$; 200 voxels, uncorrected), including the right and left orbital frontal cortex (left panel) and putamen (middle panel; right panel: color bar indicating T value). Left orbital frontal grey matter (marked region 2) positively correlated with increased OCD symptom severity in patients with predominant aggressive/checking symptoms ($r = 0.77$, d.f. = 11, $p = 0.006$). A, anterior; P, posterior; L, left; R, right. Reprinted from Szeszko P, Christian C, MacMaster F *et al.* Gray matter structural alterations in psychotropic drug-naive pediatric obsessive-compulsive disorder: An optimized voxel-based morphometry study. *Am J Psychiatry* 2008;**165**(10):1299–1307, with permission.

Increased volume of the anterior cingulate, but not the posterior cingulate or dorsolateral prefrontal cortex, has been reported in two independent paediatric samples of OCD patients compared with healthy paediatric controls [23,33]. Increased anterior cingulate volume is accounted for by increased grey but not white matter volume [33]. The normative developmental increase in anterior cingulate volume observed in healthy paediatric controls was absent in OCD patients [24]. Using VBM, Szeszko *et al.* [48] reported increased orbital frontal grey matter and reduced striatal grey matter associated with aggressive and checking subtypes of OCD, but not other subtypes, such as washing/contamination (Figure 10.3). We have also recently found (unpublished data) that pre-treatment anterior cingulate grey matter predicts both treatment response and treatment remission (Children's Yale–Brown Obsessive-Compulsive Scale score <10 after 12 weeks of treatment) in paediatric OCD patients treated with the selective serotonin reuptake inhibitors (SSRIs), paroxetine and sertraline (Figures 10.4 and 10.5).

Jenike *et al.* [20] found no significant difference in thalamic volume between adult OCD patients who had long-term illness duration and had been treated with psychotropic medication, including SSRIs, and healthy adult controls. In contrast, using VBM, Kim *et al.* [49] found increased thalamic grey matter in medication-free adult patients with OCD. Using volumetric MRI, Gilbert *et al.* [17] found significantly increased thalamic volume in 21 psychotropic-naive paediatric OCD patients and 21 age- and sex-matched healthy paediatric controls (Figure 10.6).

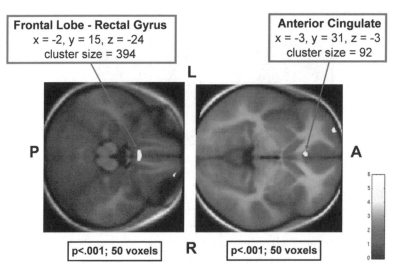

Figure 10.4 Increased anterior cingulate grey matter in paediatric obsessive-compulsive disorder (OCD) predicted treatment response to SSRI.

After 12 weeks of monodrug therapy with the SSRI paroxetine, thalamic volume decreased to levels not significantly different from healthy controls. Decrease in thalamic volume was robustly correlated with reduction in OCD symptom severity, with increased thalamic volume before treatment predicting enhanced response to SSRI (Figure 10.7). There may be some specificity of thalamic volume change with

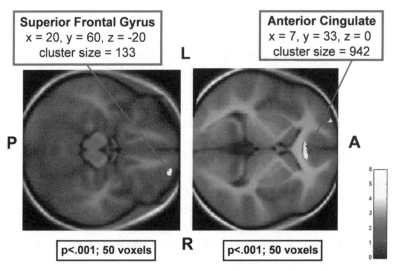

Figure 10.5 Increased anterior cingulate grey matter in paediatric obsessive-compulsive disorder (OCD) predicted symptom remission with SSRI treatment.

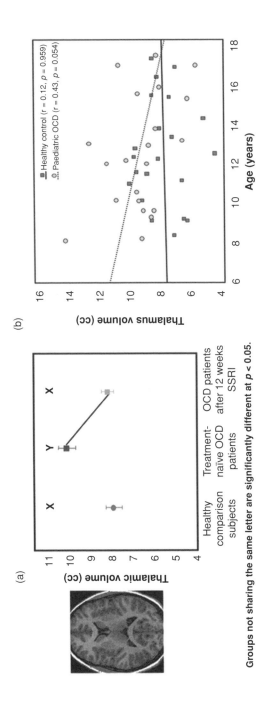

Figure 10.6 (a) Thalamic volume by diagnostic treatment condition; groups not sharing the same letter are significantly different at $p < 0.05$. (b) Thalamic volume versus age in paediatric obsessive-compulsive disorder patients and healthy comparison subjects. Adapted from Gilbert AR, Moore GJ, Keshavan MS et al. Gray matter structural alterations in psychotropic drug-naive pediatric obsessive-compulsive disorder: An optimized voxel-based morphometry study. *Arch Gen Psychiatry* 2000;**57**:449–456; and Rosenberg DR, MacMillan S. Imaging and neurocircuitry of OCD. In: Davis KL, Nemeroff CB, Coyle J, Charney D (eds), *Neuropsychopharmacology. The 5th Generation of Progress.* Baltimore: Lippincott Williams & Wilkins, 2002; pp. 1621–1646, with permission.

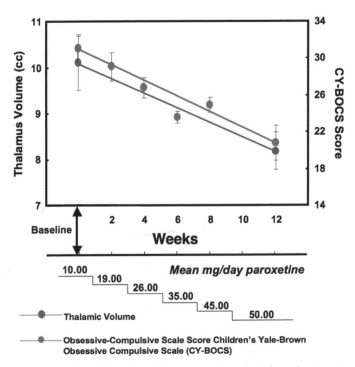

Figure 10.7 Decrease in thalamic volume associated with reduction in obsessive-compulsive score of the Children's Yale–Brown Obsessive-Compulsive Scales (CY–BOCS). Reprinted from Gilbert AR, Moore GJ, Keshavan MS *et al.* Gray matter structural alterations in psychotropic drug-naive pediatric obsessive-compulsive disorder: An optimized voxel-based morphometry study. *Arch Gen Psychiatry* 2000;**57**:449–456; and Rosenberg DR, MacMillan S. Imaging and neurocircuitry of OCD. In: Davis KL, Nemeroff CB, Coyle J, Charney D (eds), *Neuropsychopharmacology. The 5th Generation of Progress*. Baltimore: Lippincott Williams & Wilkins, 2002; pp. 1621–1646, with permission.

SSRI as no significant change in thalamic volume in psychotropic-naive paediatric OCD patients was observed before and after 12 weeks of cognitive behavioural therapy (CBT) [50].

Medial temporal-limbic cortex

Szeszko *et al.* [43] demonstrated bilateral reductions in amygdala but not hippocampal volume in adult OCD patients versus controls. Rosenberg *et al.* [23] proposed potential amygdala abnormalities in paediatric OCD, particularly given the region's rich connections to basal ganglia and prefrontal cortex [51]. Subsequently, Szeszko *et al.* [52] found increased left amygdala:right amygdala volume ratios in psychotropic-naive paediatric OCD patients compared with healthy paediatric

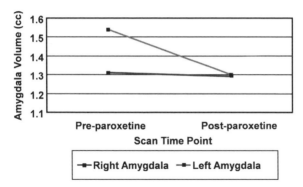

Figure 10.8 Decrease in left but not right amygdala volume after treatment with selective serotonin reuptake inhibitor (SSRI). Adapted from Szeszko PR, MacMillan S, McMeniman M *et al.* Amygdala volume reductions in pediatric patients with obsessive-compulsive disorder treated with paroxetine: Preliminary findings. *Neuropsychopharmacology* 2004;**29**:826–832, with permission.

controls. SSRI treatment resulted in a significant decrease in left but not right amygdala volume (Figure 10.8). No significant change in left or right amygdala volume was observed in an untreated healthy control group. The decrease in left amygdala volume in paediatric OCD patients was associated with a higher SSRI dose and cumulative exposure, but not with a change in OCD symptom severity.

Pituitary

MacMaster *et al.* [53] reported decreased pituitary volume associated with increased OCD symptom severity in paediatric patients with OCD versus age- and sex-matched controls (Figure 10.9). The reduction in pituitary volume was primarily accounted for by male, but not female, OCD patients. Moreover, the reduction in pituitary volume in males with OCD appeared to be specific to OCD as psychotropic-naive paediatric patients with major depression showed significantly increased pituitary volume [54], which was also noted in male, but not female, patients. A reduction in pituitary volume in paediatric OCD patients is consistent with reports of limbic-hypothalamic-pituitary-adrenal (LHPA) axis abnormalities in OCD [55–59]. This is especially intriguing since changes in endocrine function have been reported to affect pituitary morphology [60]. Combined MRI studies with neuroendocrine assessment are currently ongoing in our laboratory.

Supramarginal gyrus

The supramarginal gyrus and parietal lobe have been increasingly implicated in adult patients with OCD [61–67]. Using MRI, Fallucca *et al.* [68] recently found

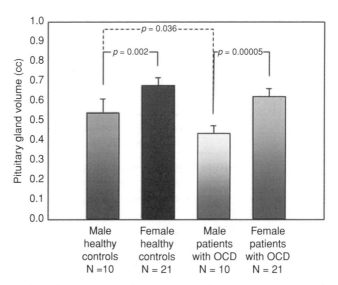

Figure 10.9 Reduced pituitary volume in psychotropic-naive paediatric patients with obsessive-compulsive disorder (OCD) compared to age- and sex-matched controls. Reprinted from MacMaster FP, Russell A, Mirza Y *et al.* Pituitary volume in pediatric obsessive-compulsive disorder. *Biol Psychiatry* 2006;**59**:252–257, with permission.

that psychotropic-naive paediatric patients with OCD had cortical thinning in the left but not right supramarginal gyrus. The supramarginal gyrus is known to play a role in set shifting, and it has been hypothesized that the repetitive, ritualistic behaviours of OCD may reflect problems in set shifting [69]. Further investigation is ongoing.

White matter

Adult OCD patients and adult first-degree relatives of OCD patients demonstrate significantly increased fractional anisotropy in the right medial frontal area as measured by DTI [46]. Certain polymorphisms for OLIG2, which regulates the development of cells that produce white matter (myelin), have been associated with OCD [71]. Associations of MOG and OLIG2 genes with white matter volume in OCD patients have been identified [10]. Rosenberg *et al.* [72] reported a larger corpus callosum area in paediatric OCD patients; an increase in white matter content may be responsible [73]. OCD patients failed to show the normative age-related increases in corpus callosum. MacMaster *et al.* [74] reported increased right but not left orbital frontal white matter in paediatric OCD patients versus healthy paediatric controls. Orbital frontal white matter increased with age in psychotropic-naive paediatric OCD patients, but not in healthy paediatric OCD controls.

FUNCTIONAL NEUROIMAGING STUDIES OF OCD

Although contradictory reports exist, functional neuroimaging studies have largely converged to demonstrate increased caudate and orbital frontal activity in OCD [75–83]. fMRI and PET studies of OCD patients undergoing symptom provocation while they were being scanned has demonstrated increased regional cerebral blood flow and brain activation in the caudate nucleus and orbitofrontal cortex [76,82,83] (Figure 10.10). Increased activation of the caudate nucleus and anterior

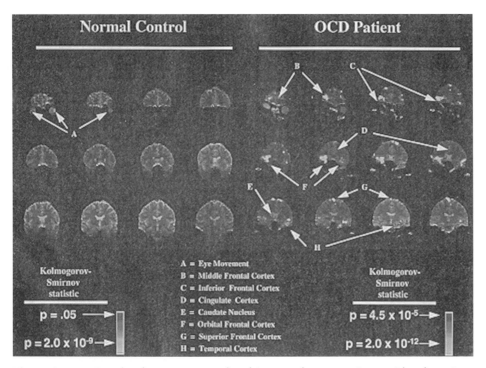

Figure 10.10 Results for one normal subject and one patient with obsessive-compulsive disorder (OCD) (normal subject 2 and patient 9 [trial B]), juxtaposed for comparison. The gradient echo functional data are shown as a $-\log(p)$ map (Kolmogorov–Smirnov statistic) in colour, superimposed over a T2-weighted high-resolution instascan image in grey tone, for anatomical reference. Twelve contiguous slices are shown for each subject. The threshold for the control subject is at a lower level to emphasize the absence of activation, while the patient's threshold is at a more stringent level ($p < 10^{-7}$, approximating Bonferroni-corrected $p < .01$). Reprinted from Breiter HC, Rauch SL, Kwong KK *et al*. Functional magnetic resonance imaging of symptom provocation in obsessive-compulsive disorder. *Arch Gen Psychiatry* 1996;**53**:595–606; and Rosenberg DR, MacMillan S. Imaging and neurocircuitry of OCD. In: Davis KL, Nemeroff CB, Coyle J, Charney D (eds), *Neuropsychopharmacology. The 5th Generation of Progress*. Baltimore: Lippincott Williams & Wilkins, 2002; pp. 1621–1646, with permission.

orbital frontal cortex appears to be specific to OCD rather than generalized to all anxiety states. Especially exciting is that specific functional/metabolic patterns pre-treatment may predict differential response, or lack thereof, to particular treatment interventions – for example, SSRI vs cognitive behavioural therapy (CBT). Comparable reductions in right caudate glucose metabolism correlated with reduction in OCD symptom severity were noted before and after 10 weeks of treatment with either fluoxetine or CBT [75,84] (Figure 10.11). Before treatment with either

Normal control compared to patient with obsessive-compulsive disorder

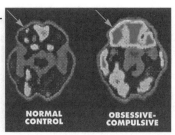

Before and after pharmacotherapy

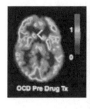 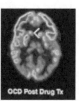

Before and after cognitive behavioral therapy

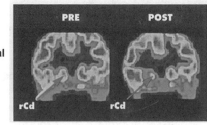

Figure 10.11 Positron emission tomography studies demonstrating increased right caudate glucose metabolism in a patient with obsessive-compulsive disorder (OCD) compared to a healthy volunteer (top). Note the significant decrease in right caudate glucose metabolism after either pharmacotherapy (middle) and cognitive behavioural therapy (bottom). rCd, right caudate. Adapted from Schwartz JM. *Brain Lock*. New York: Harper Collins Publishers Inc., 1996; and Baxter LR, Schwartz JM *et al.* Caudate glucose metabolic rate changes with both drug and behavior therapy for obsessive-compulsive disorder. *Arch Gen Psychiatry* 1992;**49**:681–689. Reprinted from Rosenberg DR, MacMillan S. Imaging and neurocircuitry of OCD. In: Davis KL, Nemeroff CB, Coyle J, Charney D (eds), *Neuropsychopharmacology. The 5th Generation of Progress*. Baltimore: Lippincott Williams & Wilkins, 2002; pp. 1621–1646, with permission.

fluoxetine or CBT, correlations among the caudate nucleus, orbital frontal cortex and thalamus were observed in OCD patients, but not in controls. After effective pharmacotherapy or CBT, there were no correlations among these regions, comparable to findings in healthy controls. OCD patients who responded to treatment with the SSRI paroxetine, demonstrated a significant reduction in glucose metabolism in the right caudate nucleus and right anterior orbital frontal cortex (Figure 10.12). Non-responders to paroxetine therapy did not exhibit a significant reduction in glucose metabolism in these regions. Overall, reduced pre-treatment glucose metabolism in left and right orbital frontal cortex of OCD patients predicted better response to paroxetine.

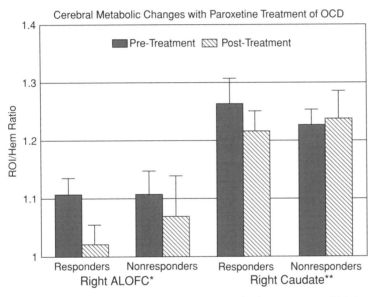

Figure 10.12 Mean pre- and post-treatment metabolic ratios ($\pm$ SD) in right anterior lateral orbital frontal cortex (ALOFC) and right caudate, normalized to ipsilateral hemisphere (ROI/Hem), in responders versus non-responders to paroxetine. There was a significant difference in the magnitude of change in right ALOFC/Hem between responders (from 1.11 ± 0.05 pre-treatment to 1.02 ± 0.05 post-treatment) and non-responders (from 1.10 ± 0.06 pre-treatment to 1.07 ± 0.08 post-treatment). Mean right Cd/Hem decreased signficantly in treatment responders (from 1.27 ± 0.06 to 1.22 ± 0.05) but not in non-responders (from 1.23 ± 0.04 to 1.24 ± 0.05). $*p = 0.04$; $**p = 0.01$. Reprinted from Saxena S, Brody AI, Maidment KM *et al.* Localized orbitofrontal and subcortical metabolic changes and predictors of response to paroxetine treatment in obsessive-compulsive disorder. *Neuropsychopharmacology* 1999;**21**:683–693; and Rosenberg DR, MacMillan S. Imaging and neurocircuitry of OCD. In: Davis KL, Nemeroff CB, Coyle J, Charney D (eds), *Neuropsychopharmacology. The 5th Generation of Progress*. Baltimore: Lippincott Williams & Wilkins, 2002; pp. 1621–1646, with permission.

NEUROCHEMISTRY

Serotonin

Serotonin's role in the pathogenesis of OCD is largely supported by clinical trials in paediatric and adult patients with OCD, which have consistently demonstrated the superiority of SSRIs versus placebo in ameliorating OCD symptoms [85,86]. As a monotherapy, SSRIs remain the only medications ever found to be superior to placebo in both paediatric and adult OCD. While contradictory reports exist, several investigations of platelets and cerebrospinal fluid (CSF) have found serotonergic alterations in patients with OCD (see Fitzgerald *et al.* [87] for review). Pharmacological challenge studies, while promising, have also been inconsistent and provide only a very peripheral window into brain function (see Fitzgerald *et al.* [87] for review). PET investigation using the probe alpha-C-11-methyl-tryptophan (AMT), an analogue of tryptophan, may be instructive and has been conducted in paediatric and adult patients with OCD. There is investigation, however, suggesting that the AMT tracer may not be reflective of serotonin synthesis, but is instead more reflective of free tryptophan [88]. The PET ligand, 18F-altanserin, may also be useful for studying OCD patients since it is a 5-HT_{2A} postsynaptic receptor antagonist. 5-HT_{2A} has been implicated in two independent populations of patients with anorexia nervosa and OCD [89]. Reduced 18F-altanserin has been reported bilaterally in orbital frontal cortex in recovered anorexic and bulimic women [90]. Some, but not all, have suggested that anorexia and bulimia nervosa share key characteristics with OCD.

N-acetyl-aspartate

N-acetyl-aspartate (NAA) is a putative neuronal marker [91] implicated in the pathogenesis of OCD. Using proton magnetic resonance spectroscopy (^{1}H MRS), Ebert *et al.* [92] found reduced NAA in the anterior cingulate cortex and striatum of adult OCD patients, with no significant differences found in parietal cortex, a region less implicated in the pathogenesis of OCD. Reduced anterior cingulate NAA was inversely correlated with increased OCD symptom severity. Bartha *et al.* [13] extended this finding in adult OCD patients by demonstrating reduced NAA in the striatum of patients with OCD versus healthy controls without volumetric changes in the striatum. They hypothesized that ^{1}H MRS may, therefore, be more sensitive and be able to detect alterations in neural circuitry with fewer patient-control pairs than conventional structural neuroimaging techniques. Fitzgerald *et al.* [93] identified reduced NAA in right and left medial thalamus, but not in right and left lateral thalamus, in psychotropic-naive paediatric OCD patients compared with age- and sex-matched controls (Figure 10.13). Neuronal dysfunction, as reflected by decreased NAA in anterior cingulate cortex, striatum and thalamus, may lead to

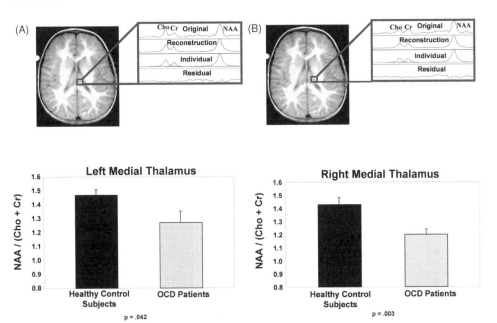

Figure 10.13 Sample spectra for voxels (top) placed in the left medial thalamus (A) and left lateral thalamus (B). Individual peaks for choline compounds (Cho), creatine/phosphocreatine (Cr) and N-acetylaspartate (NAA) were resolved from the original spectrum, leaving a residual. NAA/(Cr + Cho) metabolite ratios by group (bottom) for left (A) and right (B) medial thalamus. OCD, obsessive-compulsive disorder. Adapted from Fitzgerald KD, Moore GJ, Paulson LD *et al*. Proton spectroscopic imaging of the thalamus in treatment-naive pediatric obsessive-compulsive disorder. *Biol Psychiatry* 2000;**47**:174–182; and reprinted from Rosenberg DR, MacMillan S. Imaging and neurocircuitry of OCD. In: Davis KL, Nemeroff CB, Coyle J, Charney D (eds), *Neuropsychopharmacology. The 5th Generation of Progress*. Baltimore: Lippincott Williams & Wilkins, 2002; pp. 1621–1646, with permission.

functional hyperactivity reported in these regions resulting from increased glutamate projection [13,50,92,93]. In contrast, Russell *et al*. [94] found increased NAA concentrations in left but not right dorsolateral prefrontal cortex in psychotropic-naive paediatric OCD patients with OCD versus healthy controls (Figure 10.14). Thus, there may be region-specific abnormalities in NAA in patients with OCD.

Choline

The ^{1}H MRS choline (Cho) measure may play a critical role in signal transduction in OCD [95]. Left caudate but not occipital Cho, as measured by ^{1}H MRS, was significantly increased in 32 paediatric OCD patients versus healthy paediatric controls (Rosenberg *et al*. [96]; Benazon *et al*. [97]; combined analysis). In

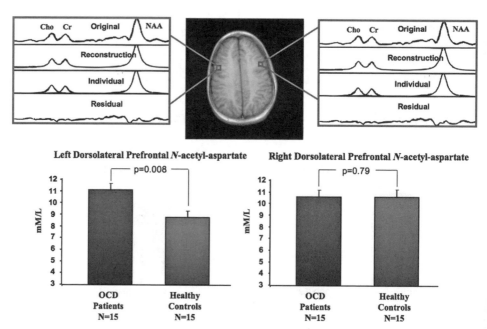

Figure 10.14 Graphs of left and right dorsolateral prefrontal cortical *N*-acetyl-aspartate (NAA) concentrations in psychotropic-naive paediatric patients with obsessive-compulsive disorder (OCD) compared to age- and sex-matched controls. mM/L, millimolar absolute metabolite concentrations. Adapted from Russell A, Cortese B, Lorch E *et al*. Localized functional neurochemical marker abnormalities in dorsolateral prefrontal cortex in pediatric obsessive-compulsive disorder. *J Child Adolesc Psychopharmacol* 2003;**13**(Suppl. 1):S31–38, with permission.

contrast, Starck *et al*. [98] did not observe right caudate Cho alterations in adult OCD patients. Treatment-naive paediatric OCD patients have been found to have increased medial, but not lateral, thalamic Cho compared with both healthy comparison subjects and psychotropic-naive paediatric patients with major depression [99] (Figure 10.15). Paediatric patients with Major Depressive Disorder (MDD) and healthy controls did not differ in medial thalamic Cho levels. Thus, medial thalamic Cho alterations may have some diagnostic specificity in distinguishing paediatric patients with OCD from paediatric patients with MDD, as well as healthy controls. Since Cho measured by ^{1}H MRS arises primarily from glycerophosphocholine and phosphocholine metabolites of phosphatidylcholine, a membrane lipid [100,101], these findings may be consistent with findings of increased thalamic volume and grey matter density [17,49]. Functional neuroimaging studies also demonstrate increased glucose metabolism in the thalamus of OCD patients [75]. It is possible that since phosphatidylcholine plays a critical role in intracellular signal transduction [102–105], alterations in signal transduction may be involved in the pathogenesis of OCD [95]. Cho alterations have been demonstrated in

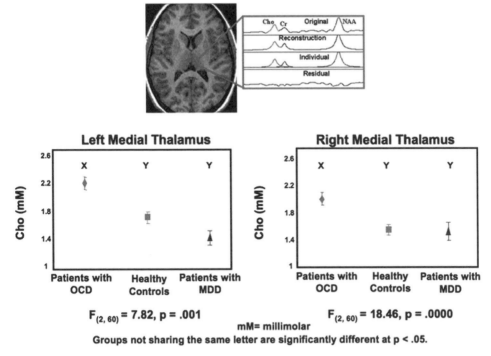

Figure 10.15 Graphs of left and right medial thalamic choline (Cho) concentrations in 27 paediatric patients with obsessive-compulsive disorder (OCD), 18 healthy control subjects, and 18 paediatric patients with major depressive disorder (MDD). Groups not sharing the same letter are significantly different at $p < 0.05$. Analysis of variance; F values are presented. Lines indicate means. mM, millimolar absolute metabolite concentrations. Adapted from Smith EA, Russell A, Lorch A *et al.* Increased medial thalamic choline found in pediatric patients with obsessive-compulsive disorder versus major depression or healthy control subjects: a magnetic resonance spectroscopy study. *Biol Psychiatry* 2003;**54**(12):1399–1405, with permission.

illnesses involving membrane metabolism, including areas of acute demyelination in multiple sclerosis [106,107] and in Alzheimer disease [108].

It is also possible that abnormalities in medial thalamic Cho in paediatric patients with OCD may result from neuroendocrine abnormalities [95]. Neuroendocrine abnormalities of the LHPA axis have been reported in paediatric patients with OCD (see Rosenberg *et al.* [95] for review). Patients with Cushing's syndrome have been found to have frontal and thalamic Cho abnormalities as measured with ^{1}H MRS [109]. Patients with hypothyroidism have been found to have increased Cho levels, which normalize after effective treatment [110]. Similarly, Cho alterations measured with ^{1}H MRS in patients with Graves disease normalize after treatment [111].

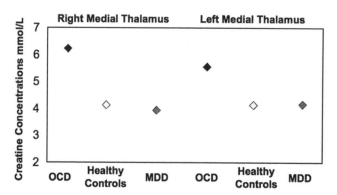

Figure 10.16 Creatine concentrations in the left and right medial thalamus of paediatric patients with obsessive-compulsive disorder (OCD), healthy controls, and major depressive disorder (MDD) patients. Adapted from Mirza Y, O'Neill J, Smith EA *et al.* Increased medial thalamic creatine-phosphocreatine found by proton magnetic resonance spectroscopy in children with obsessive-compulsive disorder versus major depression and healthy controls. *J Child Neurol* 2006;**21**(2):106–111, with permission.

Creatine/phosphocreatine

The creatine/phosphocreatine peak (Cr) consists of the high-energy phosphate, phosphocreatine and creatine as measured by ^{1}H MRS. Phosphocreatine, in particular, has high concentrations in the brain. Increased Cr has been observed in the caudate and medial thalamus of paediatric patients with OCD compared with healthy controls [50,112]. No alterations in lateral thalamic or occipital Cr were observed between paediatric patients with OCD and controls. Increased medial thalamic Cr was also found to differentiate paediatric patients with OCD from paediatric patients with MDD (Figure 10.16). Patients with MDD and healthy controls did not differ in medial thalamic Cr concentrations. Mirza *et al.* [112] hypothesized that increased caudate and medial thalamic Cr could reflect increased energy utilization in OCD patients.

Glutamate

Since Rosenberg and Keshavan [24] first hypothesized a role for glutamate in OCD, converging lines of evidence support a key role for glutamate abnormalities in the pathogenesis of OCD. Glutamate is the primary neurotransmitter within the cortico-striatal-thalamic circuit implicated in the pathogenesis of OCD [113]. Most of the axon terminals in the basal ganglia are glutamatergic [114]. Glutamate has been shown to play a key role in the anterior cingulate cortex, a key region of metabolic abnormality in OCD, with high concentrations of glutamate receptors in anterior cingulate cortex compared to other neurotransmitter binding sites [115]. Antagonists of the glutamate N-methyl-D-aspartate (NMDA) receptor result in altered anterior cingulate cortex regional cerebral blood flow [116]. Using ^{1}H MRS, Rosenberg *et al.* [96] reported increased left caudate, but not occipital, glutamatergic concentrations in psychotropic-naive paediatric OCD patients compared to controls (Figure 10.17). After 12 weeks of monodrug therapy with the SSRI paroxetine, left caudate glutamatergic levels 'normalized' to levels not significantly different from healthy paediatric controls. The decrease in left caudate glutamatergic concentrations was positively correlated with reduction in OCD symptom severity, with higher pre-treatment left caudate glutamatergic concentrations predicting better response to SSRI (Figure 10.18). In contrast, despite a significant reduction in OCD symptoms, 12 weeks of CBT did not alter left caudate Glx (glutamate/glutamine/GABA) in paediatric psychotropic-naive patients with OCD [97]. In contrast to elevated left caudate glutamatergic concentrations, Rosenberg *et al.* [117] reported decreased anterior cingulate glutamatergic concentrations in paediatric OCD patients compared to healthy paediatric controls. Yucel *et al.* [118] also found reduced anterior cingulate glutamatergic concentrations in adult patients with OCD regardless of medication status. Reduction in anterior cingulate

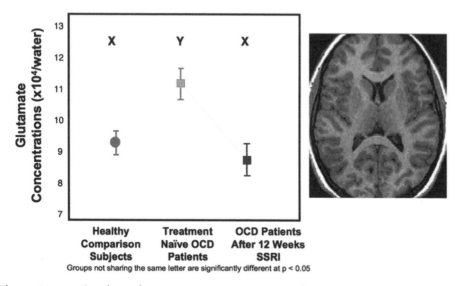

Figure 10.17 Caudate glutamatergic concentrations by diagnostic and treatment condition. Groups not sharing the same letter are significantly different at $p < 0.05$. OCD, obsessive-compulsive disorder. Adapted from Rosenberg DR, MacMaster FP, Keshavan MS. Decrease in caudate glutamatergic concentrations in pediatric obsessive-compulsive disorder patients taking paroxetine. *J Am Acad Child Adolesc Psychiatry* 2000;**39**:1096–1103, with permission.

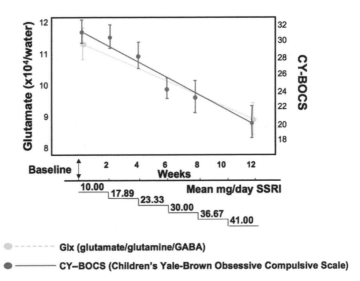

Figure 10.18 Decreases in left caudate glutamatergic concentrations associated with reduction in Obsessive-Compulsive score of the Children's Yale–Brown Obsessive-Compulsive Scales. GABA, gamma-aminobutyric acid; SSRI, selective serotonin reuptake inhibitor. Adapted from Rosenberg DR, Hanna GL. Genetic and imaging strategies in obsessive-compulsive disorder: Potential implications for treatment development. *Biol Psychiatry* 2000;**48**:1210–1222, with permission.

glutamate was inversely correlated with increased OCD symptom severity. Whiteside *et al.* [119] reported increased orbital frontal glutamatergic concentrations in adult OCD patients compared to healthy controls. Reduced anterior cingulate and increased left caudate glutamatergic concentrations in paediatric OCD patients may be consistent with prior findings of inverse correlations between increased anterior cingulate volume and reduced striatal volume in paediatric OCD patients [24]. This inverse relationship further suggests a possible tonic-phasic dysregulation of glutamate in cortico-striatal circuitry so that decreased tonic glutamate in the anterior cingulate cortex could predispose patients with OCD to phasic overactivity in the caudate and orbitofrontal cortex.

Animal model and peripheral marker studies bolster the neuroimaging studies implicating glutamate in the pathogenesis of OCD. Human models of OCD provide indirect support for glutamate involvement in OCD [120–122]. Chakrabarty *et al.* [123] measured CSF glutamate in 21 psychotropic-naive adults with OCD versus 18 healthy adult controls and found significantly elevated CSF glutamate in the OCD patients. In contrast to other psychiatric disorders where identification of consistent genetic markers has been elusive, in OCD glutamate transporter polymorphisms have been identified by three different groups in the 3' region of the glutamate transporter gene, solute carrier family 1, member 1 (*SLC1A1*), which may

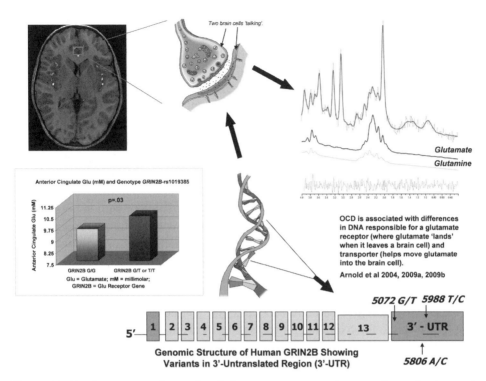

Figure 10.19 Summary schematic of the convergence of research methods used to examine the role of glutamate in obsessive-compulsive disorder. Reprinted from MacMaster FP, Rosenberg DR. Neurobiological evidence supporting glutamate's role in pediatric obsessive-compulsive disorder. *Child Adolesc Psychopharmacol News* 2010;**15**(6):6–10, 12, with permission.

contain a susceptibility allele for OCD [124–126]. In addition, the 5072T/G variant (5072G-5988T haplotype) of NMDA subunit 2B gene (*GRIN2B*) has been associated with OCD [127]. *GRIN2B* is expressed mainly in the striatum and prefrontal cortex [128], regions of hypothesized metabolic and glutamatergic abnormality in OCD. Exploiting the emerging field of combined imaging genetics, Arnold *et al.* [8] identified a significant association between the rs1019385 polymorphism of *GRIN2B* and reduced anterior cingulate glutamatergic concentrations in paediatric patients with OCD (Figure 10.19).

Perhaps most exciting of all is that, based on these converging lines of laboratory research that suggest a key role for glutamate in the pathogenesis of OCD, medications that modulate glutamate are being tested in adults and children with OCD [129–131]. Riluzole is a glutamate-modulating agent that is approved by the US Food and Drug Administration (FDA) for amyotrophic lateral sclerosis, or Lou Gehrig disease. Open label reports have found riluzole to be effective in reducing OCD symptoms in treatment-resistant paediatric and adult OCD patients [129,132,133]. These results are so promising that the National Institute of Mental Health is conducting a double-blind placebo-controlled trial of riluzole in paediatric patients with OCD. The results of this trial are not yet available. Topiramate, another glutamate-modulating agent, has also demonstrated effectiveness in treatment-resistant OCD [134–136]. However, contradictory reports exist, with case reports finding that topiramate may induce OCD behaviours [137,138]. Cognitive dulling may also be of concern in some paediatric patients treated with topiramate. The anticonvulsant medication, lamotrigine, which inhibits pathological but not normal glutamate release, may also be helpful in decreasing OCD symptoms in schizophrenic patients [139]. Additionally, Uzun [140] published a case report demonstrating that augmentation of clomipramine treatment with lamotrigine resulted in significant clinical improvement in a patient with treatment-resistant OCD. Because of the increased risk for a potentially life-threatening or permanently disfiguring skin rash, e.g., Stevens–Johnson syndrome, caution is warranted in patients under 16 years of age. N-acetylcysteine is another promising glutamate-modulating agent that has been tried in treatment-resistant OCD [141], with a marked decrease in OCD symptoms noted after N-acetylcysteine augmentation in a patient who had not responded to fluvoxamine. D-cycloserine, a partial agonist at the NMDA glutamatergic receptor, was administered in a double-blind placebo-controlled study in OCD patients 2 hours before an exposure therapy session; it decreased the number of exposure sessions needed to reduce OCD symptoms, as well as the rate of dropout [142]. The D-cycloserine group also demonstrated significantly greater reduction in OCD symptom severity after four exposure sessions than the patients treated with placebo. It should be noted, however, that the placebo group did subsequently catch up with the D-cycloserine group. Wilhelm *et al.* [143] conducted a randomized, double-blind, placebo-controlled trial of D-cycloserine augmentation of CBT and found that patients receiving D-cycloserine were more improved midway through treatment than the placebo group, but did not differ from the placebo group at the end of treatment. Thus, D-cycloserine may accelerate the effect of treatment [144]. Finally, memantine, an NMDA receptor antagonist, shows promise in treating adult and paediatric OCD. Memantine augmentation may be effective in both paediatric and adult patients with OCD [145–150].

CONCLUSION

Because the clinical phenomenology, nosology and treatment of OCD have been so well established, OCD is a particularly viable candidate for assessment of relevant biomarkers (e.g. neuroimaging, genetic). OCD is an excellent example where findings in basic neuroscience, neuroimaging and genetic laboratories are being translated into treatment development trials, for example glutamate-modulating agents. Moreover, this is a 'two-way street', where findings in the clinic further inform relevant neurobiological studies. Exciting times lie ahead in our efforts to develop novel diagnostic and treatment approaches for peadiatric OCD.

Key points

- Most structural MRI studies have focused on measurement of brain volume since volumetric measures may reflect a region's function. More recently, MRI studies have utilized (i) automated voxel-based morphometry (VBM) studies to assess for regional grey matter alterations; (ii) diffusion tensor imaging (DTI) to measure white matter tractography; and (iii) regional cortical thickness assessment.

- One of the more consistent findings in neuropsychiatry has been the identification of alterations in cortico-striatal-thalamic circuitry in adult and paediatric OCD. It should be noted, however, that recent investigation suggests that other brain regions, including the pituitary, medial temporal-limbic cortex, and supramarginal gyrus, may also be involved in the pathogenesis of OCD.

- Although contradictory reports exist, functional neuroimaging studies have largely converged to demonstrate increased activation of the caudate nucleus and anterior orbital frontal cortex in OCD [75–81,83,94], which appears to be specific to OCD rather than generalized to all anxiety states. Especially exciting is that specific functional/metabolic patterns pre-treatment may predict differential response, or lack thereof, to particular treatment interventions.

- There are several neurochemicals implicated in the pathogenesis of OCD. However, converging lines of evidence support a key role for glutamate abnormalities in the pathogenesis of OCD. Glutamate transporter polymorphisms have been identified in the 3′ region of the glutamate transporter gene, solute carrier family 1, member 1 (*SLC1A1*), which may contain a susceptibility allele for OCD [124–126]. In addition, the 5072T/G variant (5072G-5988T haplotype) of *N*-methyl-D-aspartate (NMDA) subunit 2B gene (*GRIN2B*) has been associated with OCD [127]. As a result of these converging lines of laboratory research, medications that modulate glutamate are being tested in adults and children with OCD [127,130,131].

ACKNOWLEDGEMENTS

This work was supported in part by the State of Michigan Joe F. Young Sr Psychiatric Research and Training Program, the Miriam L. Hamburger Endowed Chair of Child Psychiatry at Children's Hospital of Michigan and Wayne State University,

Detroit, MI, the Paul Strauss endowment for the integration of computer science and psychiatry, and grants from the National Institute of Mental Health (R01MH59299, R01MH65122, K24MH02037), the World Heritage Foundation, the Schutt Foundation, United Way, the National Alliance for Research on Schizophrenia and Depression (NARSAD) and the Mental Illness Research Association (MIRA).

REFERENCES

1. Rasmussen SA, Eisen JL. The epidemiology and differential diagnosis of obsessive compulsive disorder. *J Clin Psychiatry* 1994;**55**(Suppl.):5–14.
2. Robins LN, Helzer JI, Weissman MM *et al*. Lifetime prevalence of specific psychiatric disorders in three sites. *Arch Gen Psychiatry* 1984;**41**:949–958.
3. Hanna GL. Demographic and clinical features of obsessive-compulsive disorder in children and adolescents. *J Am Acad Child Adolesc Psychiatry* 1995;**34**:19–27.
4. Valleni-Basile LA, Garrison CZ, Jackson KL *et al*. Frequency of obsessive-compulsive disorder in a community sample of young adolescents. *J Am Acad Child Adolesc Psychiatry* 1994;**33**:782–791.
5. Flament MF, Whitaker A, Rapoport JL. Obsessive compulsive disorder in adolescence: An epidemiological study. *J Am Acad Child Adolesc Psychiatry* 1988;**27**:764–771.
6. Kessler RC, Berglund P, Demler O *et al*. Lifetime prevalence and age-of-onset distributions of DSM-IV disorders in the National Comorbidity Survey Replication. *Arch Gen Psychiatry* 2005;**62**:593–602.
7. Pauls DL, Alsobrook JP II, Phil M *et al*. A family study of obsessive-compulsive disorder. *Am J Psychiatry* 1995;**152**:76–84.
8. Arnold PD, Richter MA, Hanna GL *et al*. Anterior cingulate glutamatergic concentration and glutamate system genes in pediatric obsessive-compulsive disorder. *Psychiatry Res-Neuroim* 2009a;**172**:136–139.
9. Arnold PD, Richter MA, Hanna GL *et al*. Glutamate system genes associated with ventral prefrontal and thalamic volume in pediatric obsessive-compulsive disorder. *Brain Imaging Behav* 2009b;**3**:64–76.
10. Atmaca M, Onalan E, Yildirim H *et al*. The association of myelin oligodendrocyte glycoprotein gene and white matter volume in obsessive-compulsive disorder. *J Affect Disord* 2010;**124**:309–313.
11. Shenton ME, Kikinis R, Jolesz FA *et al*. Abnormalities of the left temporal lobe and thought disorder in schizophrenia. A quantitative magnetic resonance imaging study. *New Engl J Med* 1992;**327**:604–612.
12. Cendes F, Andermann F, Gloor P *et al*. MRI volumetric measurement of amygdala and hippocampus in temporal lobe epilepsy. *Neurology* 1993;**43**:719.
13. Bartha R, Stein MB, Williamson PC *et al*. A short echo 1H spectroscopy and volumetric MRI study of the corpus striatum in patients with obsessive compulsive disorder and comparison subjects. *Am J Psychiatry* 1998;**155**:1584–1591.
14. Rauch SL. Neuroimaging research and the neurobiology of obsessive-compulsive disorder: where do we go from here? *Biol Psychiatry* 2000;**47**:168–170.

15. Rosen BR, Buckner RL, Dale AM. Event-related functional MRI: Past, present, and future. *Proc Natl Acad Sci USA* 1998;**95**:773–780.

16. Liu AK, Belliveau JW, Dale AM. Spatiotemporal imaging of human brain activity using functional MRI constrained magnetoencephalography data: Monte Carlo simulations. *Proc Natl Acad Sci USA* 1998;**95**:8945–8950.

17. Gilbert AR, Moore GJ, Keshavan MS *et al.* Decrease in thalamic volumes of pediatric obsessive compulsive disorder patients taking paroxetine. *Arch Gen Psychiatry* 2000;**57**:449–456.

18. Aylward EH, Schwartz J, Machlin S *et al.* Bicaudate ratio as a measure of caudate volume on MR images. *Am J Neuroradiol* 1991;**12**:1217–1222.

19. Breiter HC, Filipek PA, Kennedy DN *et al.* Retrocallosal white matter abnormalities in patients with obsessive-compulsive disorder. *Arch Gen Psychiatry* 1994;**51**:663–664.

20. Jenike MA, Breiter HC, Baer L *et al.* Cerebral structural abnormalities in obsessive-compulsive disorder: A quantitative morphometric magnetic resonance imaging study. *Arch Gen Psychiatry* 1996;**53**:625–632.

21. Robinson D, Wu H, Munne RA *et al.* Reduced caudate nucleus volume in obsessive-compulsive disorder. *Arch Gen Psychiatry* 1995;**52**:393–398.

22. Stein DJ, Coetzer R, Lee M. Magnetic resonance brain imaging in women with obsessive-compulsive disorder and trichotillomania. *Psychiatry Res* 1997;**74**:177.

23. Rosenberg DR, Keshavan MS, O'Hearn KM *et al.* Fronto-striatal measurement of treatment-naive pediatric obsessive compulsive disorder. *Arch Gen Psychiatry* 1997;**54**:824–830.

24. Rosenberg DR, Keshavan MS. Toward a neurodevelopmental model of obsessive compulsive disorder. *Biol Psychiatry* 1998;**43**:623–640.

25. Behar D, Rapoport JL, Berg CJ *et al.* Computerized tomography and neuropsychological test measures in adolescents with obsessive-compulsive disorder. *Am J Psychiatry* 1984;**141**:363–369.

26. Insel TR, Donnelly EF, Lalakea ML *et al.* Neurological and neuropsychological studies of patients with obsessive-compulsive disorder. *Biol Psychiatry* 1983;**18**:741–751.

27. Scarone S, Colombo C, Livian S *et al.* Increased right caudate nucleus size in obsessive compulsive disorder: detection with magnetic resonance imaging. *Psychiatry Res* 1992;**45**:115–121.

28. Aylward EH, Harris GJ, Hoehn-Saric R *et al.* Normal caudate nucleus in obsessive-compulsive disorder assessed by quantitative neuroimaging. *Arch Gen Psychiatry* 1996;**53**:577–584.

29. Kellner CH, Jolley RR, Holgate RC *et al.* Brain MRI in obsessive-compulsive disorder. *Psychiatry Res* 1991;**36**:45–49.

30. Luxenberg JS, Swedo SE, Flament MF *et al.* Neuroanatomical abnormalities in obsessive-compulsive disorder determined with quantitative x-ray computed tomography. *Am J Psychiatry* 1988;**145**:1089–1093.

31. Stein DJ, Hollander E, Chan S *et al.* Computed tomography and neurological soft signs in obsessive-compulsive disorder. *Psychiatry Res-Neuroim* 1993;**50**:143–150.

32. Menzies L, Achard S, Chamberlain SR *et al.* Neurocognitive endophenotypes of obsessive-compulsive disorder. *Brain* 2007;**130**:3223–3236.

33. Szeszko PR, MacMillan S, McMeniman M *et al.* Brain structural abnormalities in psychotropic drug-naïve pediatric OCD. *Am J Psychiatry* 2004;**161**:1049–1056.

34. Peterson B, Riddle MA, Cohen DJ *et al.* Reduced basal ganglia volumes in Tourette's syndrome using three-dimensional reconstruction techniques from magnetic resonance images. *Neurology* 1993;**43**:941–949.

35. Hebebrand J, Siemon P, Lutcke A *et al.* A putaminal lesion in an adolescent with obsessive-compulsive disorder and atypical anorexia nervosa. *J Nerv Ment Dis* 1995;**181**:520–521.

36. Rothfield JM. Generalized dystonia and obsessive-compulsive disorder associated with bilateral circumscribed magnetic resonance signal changes in the putamen. *J Nerv Ment Dis* 1995;**183**:113–114.

37. Kiessling LS, Marcotte AC, Culpepper L. Antineuronal antibodies: Tics and obsessive-compulsive symptoms. *J Dev Behav Pediatr* 1994;**15**:421–425.

38. Swedo SE, Leonard HL, Garvey M *et al.* Pediatric autoimmune neuropsychiatric disorders associated with streptococcal infections: clinical description of the first 50 cases. *Am J Psychiatry* 1998;**155**:264–271.

39. Allen AJ, Leonard HL, Swedo SE. Case study: A new infection-triggered, autoimmune subtype of pediatric OCD and Tourette's syndrome. *J Am Acad Child Adolesc Psychiatry* 1995;**34**:307–311.

40. Giedd JN, Rapoport JL, Kruesi MJP *et al.* Sydenham's chorea: Magnetic-resonance-imaging of the basal ganglia. *Neurology* 1995;**45**:2199–2202.

41. Giedd JN, Rapoport JL, Garvey MA *et al.* MRI assessment of children with obsessive-compulsive disorder or tics associated with streptococcal infection. *Am J Psychiatry* 2000;**157**:281–283.

42. Peterson BS, Leckman JF, Tucker D *et al.* Preliminary findings of antistreptococcal antibody titers and basal ganglia volumes in tic, obsessive-compulsive, and attention deficit/hyperactivity disorders. *Arch Gen Psychiatry* 2000;**57**:364–372.

43. Szeszko PR, Robinson D, Alvir JM *et al.* Orbital frontal and amygdala volume reductions in obsessive-compulsive disorder. *Arch Gen Psychiatry* 1999;**56**:913–919.

44. Grachev ID, Breiter HC, Rauch SL *et al.* Structural abnormalities of frontal neocortex in obsessive-compulsive disorder. *Arch Gen Psychiatry* 1998;**55**:181–182.

45. Caviness VS Jr, Kennedy DN, Richelme C *et al.* The human brain age 7–11 years: a volumetric analysis based on magnetic resonance images. *Cereb Cortex* 1996;**6**:726–736.

46. Menzies L, Williams GB, Chamberlain SR *et al.* White matter abnormalities in patients with obsessive-compulsive disorder and their first-degree relatives. *Am J Psychiatry* 2008;**165**:1308–1315.

47. Chamberlain SR, Menzies L, Hampshire A *et al.* Orbitofrontal dysfunction in patients with obsessive-compulsive disorder and their unaffected relatives. *Science* 2008;**321**:421–422.

48. Szeszko PR, Christian C, MacMaster F *et al.* Gray matter structural alterations in psychotropic drug-naïve pediatric obsessive-compulsive disorder: An optimized voxel based morphometry study. *Am J Psychiatry* 2008;**165**:1299–1307.

49. Kim J, Lee MC, Kim J *et al.* Grey matter abnormalities in obsessive-compulsive disorder: Statistical parametric mapping of segmented magnetic resonance images. *Br J Psychiatry* 2001;**179**:330–334.

50. Rosenberg DR, Benazon NR, Gilbert AR *et al.* Thalamic volume in pediatric obsessive compulsive disorder patients before and after cognitive behavioral therapy. *Biol Psychiatry* 2000;**48**:294–300.

51. Sah P, Faber ES, Lopez De Armentia M *et al*. The amygdaloid complex: anatomy and physiology. *Physiol Rev* 2003;**83**:803–834.

52. Szeszko PR, MacMillan S, McMeniman M *et al*. Amygdala volume reductions in pediatric patients with obsessive-compulsive disorder treated with paroxetine: Preliminary findings. *Neuropsychopharmacology* 2004;**29**:826–832.

53. MacMaster FP, Russell A, Mirza Y *et al*. Pituitary volume in pediatric OCD. *Biol Psychiatry* 2006;**59**:252–257.

54. MacMaster FP, Russell A, Mirza Y *et al*. Pituitary volume in treatment-naïve pediatric major depressive disorder. *Biol Psychiatry* 2006;**60**:862–866.

55. Altemus M, Pigott T, Kalogeras KT *et al*. Abnormalities in the regulation of vasopressin and corticotrophin releasing factor secretion in obsessive-compulsive disorder. *Arch Gen Psychiatry* 1992;**49**:9–20.

56. Swedo SE, Leonard HL, Rapoport JL. Childhood-onset obsessive-compulsive disorder. *Psychiatr Clin N Am* 1992;**15**:767–775.

57. Catapano F, Monteleone P, Fuschino A *et al*. Melatonin and cortisol secretion in patients with primary obsessive-compulsive disorder. *Psychiatry Res* 1992;**44**:217–225.

58. Monteleone P, Catapano F, Tortorella A *et al*. Cortisol response to D-fenfluramine in patients with obsessive-compulsive disorder and in healthy subjects: Evidence for a gender-related effect. *Neuropsychobiology* 1997;**36**:8–12.

59. Leckman JF, Goodman WK, North WG, *et al*. (1994) The role of central oxytocin in obsessive compulsive disorder and related normal behavior. *Psychoneuroendocrinology* **19**, 723.

60. Gonzalez JG, Elizondo G, Saldivar D *et al*. Pituitary gland growth during normal pregnancy: An in vivo study using magnetic resonance imaging. *Am J Med* 1988;**85**:216–220.

61. Klauschen F, Goldman A, Barra V *et al*. Evaluation of automated brain MR image segmentation and volumetry methods. *Hum Brain Mapp* 2009;**30**:1310–1327.

62. Pantazis D, Joshi A, Jiang J *et al*. Comparison of landmark-based and automatic methods for cortical surface registration. *Neuroimage* 2010;**49**:2479–2493.

63. Zhong J, Phua DY, Qiu A. Quantitative evaluation of LDDMM, FreeSurfer, and CARET for cortical surface mapping. *Neuroimage* 2010;**52**:131–141.

64. Fonov V, Evans AC, Botteron K *et al*. Unbiased average age-appropriate atlases for pediatric studies. *Neuroimage* 2011;**54**:313–327.

65. Yoon U, Fonov V, Perusse D *et al*. The effect of template choice on morphometric analysis of pediatric brain data. *Neuroimage* 2009;**45**:769–777.

66. Krausz Y, Freedman N, Lester H *et al*. Brain SPECT study of common ground between hypothyroidism and depression. *Int J Neuropsychopharmacol* 2007;**10**:99–106.

67. Chan SW, Harmer CJ, Goodwin GM *et al*. Risk for depression is associated with neural biases in emotional categorisation. *Neuropsychologia* 2008;**46**:2896–2903.

68. Fallucca E, MacMaster FP, Haddad J et al. Regional cortical thickness distinguishes pediatric major depression from pediatric obsessive compulsive disorder and healthy pediatric controls. *Arch Gen Psychiatry* 2011 May;**68**(5):527–33.

69. Fischl B, Sereno MI, Dale AM. Cortical surface-based analysis. II: Inflation, flattening, and a surface-based coordinate system. *Neuroimage* 1999;**9**:195–207.

70. Statistical Package for the Social Sciences (v 18.0). Chicago, IL: SPSS Inc., 2010.

71. Stewart SE, Platko J, Fagerness JA *et al.* A genetic family-based association study of OLIG2 in obsessive-compulsive disorder. *Arch Gen Psychiatry* 2007;**64**:209–214.

72. Rosenberg DR, Keshavan MS, Dick EL *et al.* Corpus callosal morphology in treatment-naïve pediatric obsessive compulsive disorder. *Prog Neuropsychopharmacol Biol Psychiat* 1997;**21**:1269–1283.

73. MacMaster FP, Keshavan MS, Dick EL *et al.* Corpus callosal signal intensity in treatment-naïve pediatric obsessive compulsive disorders. *Prog Neuropsychopharmacol Biol Psychiatry* 1999;**23**:601–612.

74. MacMaster F, Vora A, Easter P *et al.* Orbital frontal cortex in treatment-naïve pediatric obsessive-compulsive disorder. *Psychiatry Res* 2010;**181**:97–100.

75. Baxter LR, Schwartz JM, Bergman KS *et al.* Caudate glucose metabolic rate changes with both drug and behavior therapy for obsessive-compulsive disorder. *Arch Gen Psychiatry* 1992;**49**:681–689.

76. Rauch SL, Jenike MA, Alpert NM *et al.* Regional cerebral blood flow measured during symptom provocation in obsessive-compulsive disorder using oxygen 15-labeled carbon dioxide and positron emission tomography. *Arch Gen Psychiatry* 1994;**51**:62–70.

77. Saxena S, Brody AL, Schwartz JM *et al.* Neuroimaging and frontal-subcortical circuitry in obsessive-compulsive disorder. *Br J Psychiatry* 1998;**173**:26–38.

78. Baxter LR, Phelps ME, Mazziotta JC *et al.* Local cerebral glucose metabolic rates in obsessive-compulsive disorder: A comparison with rates in unipolar depression and normal controls. *Arch Gen Psychiatry* 1987;**44**:211–218.

79. Baxter LR, Schwartz JM, Mazziotta JC. Cerebral glucose metabolic rates in non-depressed patients with obsessive-compulsive disorder. *Am J Psychiatry* 1988;**145**: 1560–1563.

80. Nordahl TE, Benkelfat C, Semple WE *et al.* Cerebral glucose metabolic rates in obsessive-compulsive disorder. *Neuropsychopharmacology* 1989;**2**:23–28.

81. Swerdlow NR. Serotonin, obsessive-compulsive disorder, and the basal ganglia. *Int Rev Psychiat* 1995;**7**:115–129.

82. McGuire PK, Bench CJ, Frith CD *et al.* Functional anatomy of obsessive-compulsive phenomena. *Br J Psychiatry* 1994;**164**:459–468.

83. Breiter HC, Rauch SL, Kwong KK *et al.* Functional magnetic resonance imaging of symptom provocation in obsessive compulsive disorder. *Arch Gen Psychiatry* 1996;**53**:595–606.

84. Schwartz JM, Stoessel PW, Baxter LR *et al.* Systematic changes in cerebral glucose metabolic rate after successful behavior modification treatment of obsessive-compulsive disorder. *Arch Gen Psychiatry* 1996;**53**:109–113.

85. March JS, Leonard HL. OCD in children: Research and treatment. In: Swinson R, Rachman J, Antony M, Richter M (eds), *Obsessive-Compulsive Disorder: Theory, Research and Treatment.* New York: Guilford Press, 1998; pp. 367–394.

86. Pediatric OCD Treatment Study (POTS) Team. Cognitive-behavior therapy, sertraline, and their combination for children and adolescents with obsessive-compulsive disorder: the Pediatric OCD Treatment Study (POTS) randomized controlled trial. *JAMA* 2004;**292**:1969–1976.

87. Fitzgerald KD, MacMaster FP, Paulson LD *et al.* Neurobiology of childhood obsessive-compulsive disorder. *Child Adolesc Psychiatr Clin N Am* 1999;**8**:533–575.

88. Shoaf SE, Carson R, Hommer D *et al.* Brain serotonin synthesis rates in rhesus monkeys determined by [11C] alpha-methyl-L-tryptophan and positron emission tomography compared to CSF 5-hydroxyindole-3-acetic acid concentrations. *Neuropsychopharmacology* 1998;**19**:345–353.

89. Enoch MA, Kaye, W, Rotondo, A *et al.* 5-HT$_{2A}$ promoter polymorphism −1438G/A, anorexia nervosa, and obsessive-compulsive disorder. *The Lancet* 1998;**351**:1785–1786.

90. Goldman D, Enoch MA, Rotondo A *et al.* The 5-HT2a-1438G: A polymorphism in anorexia nervosa and obsessive-compulsive disorder. *Biol Psychiatry* 1999;**45**:174S.

91. Birken DL, Oldendorf WH. N-acetyl-L-aspartic acid: A literature review of a compound prominent in 1H-NMR spectroscopic studies of brain. *Neurosci Biobehavior Rev* 1989;**13**:23–31.

92. Ebert D, Speck O, Konig A *et al.* 1H magnetic resonance spectroscopy in obsessive-compulsive disorder: Evidence for neuronal loss in the cingulate gyrus and the right striatum. *Psychiatry Res* 1997;**74**:173–176.

93. Fitzgerald KD, Moore GJ, Paulson LD *et al.* Priority Communication: Proton spectroscopic imaging of the thalamus in treatment naïve pediatric OCD. *Biol Psychiatry* 2000;**47**:174–182.

94. Russell A, Cortese B, Lorch E *et al.* Localized functional neurochemical marker alterations in dorsolateral prefrontal cortex in pediatric OCD. *J Child Adolesc Psychopharmacol* 2003;**13**:31–38.

95. Rosenberg DR, Amponsah A, Sullivan A *et al.* Increased medial thalamic choline in pediatric obsessive compulsive disorder as detected by quantitative in vivo spectroscopic imaging. *J Child Neurology* 2001;**16**:636–641.

96. Rosenberg DR, MacMaster FP, Keshavan MS *et al.* Decrease in caudate glutamatergic concentrations in pediatric obsessive-compulsive disorder patients taking paroxetine. *J Am Acad Adolesc Psychiatry* 2000;**39**:1096–1103.

97. Benazon NR, Moore GJ, Rosenberg DR. Neurochemical analyses in pediatric obsessive-compulsive disorder in patients treated with cognitive-behavioral therapy. *J Am Acad Child Adolesc Psychiatry* 2003;**42**:1279–1285.

98. Starck G, Ljungberg M, Nilsson M *et al.* A 1H magnetic resonance spectroscopy study in adults with obsessive-compulsive disorder: Relationship between metabolite concentrations and symptom severity. *J Neural Transm* 2008;**115**:1051–1062.

99. Smith E, Russell A, Lorch E *et al.* Increased medial thalamic choline found in pediatric patients with OCD vs. major depression or healthy controls: An MRS study. *Biol Psychiatry* 2003;**54**:1399–1405.

100. Barker PB, Breiter SN, Soher BJ *et al.* Quantitative proton spectroscopy of canine brain: In vivo and in vitro correlations. *Magn Reson Med* 1994;**32**:157–163.

101. Miller BL, Chang L, Booth R *et al.* In vivo 1H MRS choline: Correlation with in vitro chemistry/histology. *Life Sci* 1996;**58**:1929–1935.

102. Loffelholz K. Receptor regulation of choline phospholipids hydrolysis: A novel source of diacylglycerol and phosphatidic acid. *Biochem Pharmacol* 1989;**38**:1543–1549.

103. Exton JH. Signaling through phosphatidycholine breakdown. *Biol Chem* 1990;**265**:1–4.

104. Exton JH. Phosphatidylcholine breakdown and signal transduction. *Biochim Biophys Acta* 1994;**1212**:26–42.

105. Zeisel SH. Choline phospholipids: signal transduction and carcinogenesis. *FASEB J* 1993;**7**:551–557.
106. Ross B, Michaelis T. Clinical applications of magnetic resonance spectroscopy. *Magn Reson Q* 1994;**10**:191–247.
107. Vion-Dury J, Confort-Gouny S, Nicoli F *et al*. Localized brain proton MRS metabolic patterns in HIV-related encephalophathies. *C R Acad Sci III* 1994;**317**:833–840.
108. Kato T, Inubushi T, Kato N. Magnetic resonance spectroscopy in affective disorder. *J Neuropsychiatry Clin Neurosci* 1998;**10**:133–147.
109. Khiat A, Bard C, Lacroix A *et al*. Brain metabolic alterations in Cushing's syndrome as monitored by proton magnetic resonance spectroscopy. *NMR Biomed* 1999; **12**:357–363.
110. Gupta RK, Bhatia V, Poptani H *et al*. Brain metabolite changes on in vivo proton magnetic resonance spectroscopy in children with congenital hypothyroidism. *J Pediatr* 1995;**126**:389–392.
111. Bhatara VS, Tripathi RP, Sankar R *et al*. Frontal lobe proton magnetic-resonance spectroscopy in Graves' disease: A pilot study. *Psychoneuroendocrinology* 1998;**23**: 605–612.
112. Mirza Y, O'Neill J, Smith EA *et al*. Increased medial thalamic creatine/phosphocreatine found by proton magnetic resonance spectroscopy in children with OCD versus major depression and healthy controls. *J Child Neurol* 2006;**21**:106–111.
113. Bronstein Y, Cummings J. Neurochemistry of fronto-subcortical circuits. In: Lichter D, Cummings J (eds), *Fronto-Subcortical Circuits in Psychiatric and Neurologic Disorders*. New York: Guilford Press, 2001; pp. 59–91.
114. Parent A, Cicchetti F, Beach TG. Calretinin-immunoreactive neurons in the human striatum. *Brain Res* 1995;**674**:347–351.
115. Bozkurt A, Zilles K, Schleicher A *et al*. Distributions of transmitter receptors in the macaque cingulate cortex. *Neuroimage* 2005;**25**:219–229.
116. Toyoda H, Zhao MG, Zhuo M. Roles of NMDA receptor NR2A and NR2B subtypes for long-term depression in the anterior cingulate cortex. *Eur J Neurosci* 2005;**22**:485–494.
117. Rosenberg DR, Mirza Y, Russell A *et al*. Reduced anterior cingulate glutamatergic concentrations in childhood OCD and major depression versus healthy controls. *J Am Acad Child Adolesc Psychiatry* 2004;**43**:1146–1153.
118. Yucel M, Wood SJ, Wellard RM *et al*. Anterior cingulate glutamate-glutamine levels predict symptom severity in women with obsessive-compulsive disorder. *Aust N Z J Psychiatry* 2008;**42**:467–477.
119. Whiteside SP, Port JD, Deacon BJ *et al*. A magnetic resonance spectroscopy investigation of obsessive-compulsive disorder and anxiety. *Psychiatry Res* 2006;**146**: 137–147.
120. Nordstrom EJ, Burton FH. A transgenic model of comorbid Tourette's syndrome and obsessive-compulsive disorder circuitry. *Mol Psychiatry* 2002;**7**:617–625.
121. Welch JM, Lu J, Rodriguiz RM *et al*. Cortico-striatal synaptic defects and OCD-like behaviours in Sapap3-mutant mice. *Nature* 2007;**448**:894–900.
122. Presti MF, Gibney BC, Lewis MH. Effects of intrastriatal administration of selective dopaminergic ligands on spontaneous stereotypy in mice. *Physiol Behav* 2004;**80**:433–439.

123. Chakrabarty K, Bhattacharyya S, Christopher R *et al.* Glutamatergic dysfunction in OCD. *Neuropsychopharmacology* 2005;**30**:1735–1740.

124. Arnold PD, Sicard T, Burroughs E *et al.* Glutamate transporter gene SLC1A1 associated with obsessive-compulsive disorder. *Arch Gen Psychiatry* 2006;**63**:769–776.

125. Dickel DE, Veenstra-VanderWeele J, Cox NJ *et al.* Association testing of the positional and functional candidate gene SLC1A1/EAAC1 in early-onset obsessive-compulsive disorder. *Arch Gen Psychiatry* 2006;**63**:778–785.

126. Stewart SE, Fagerness JA, Platko J *et al.* Association of the SLC1A1 glutamate transporter gene and obsessive-compulsive disorder. *Am J Med Genet B Neuropsychiatr Genet* 2007;**144**:1027–1033.

127. Arnold PD, Rosenberg DR, Mundo E *et al.* Association of a glutamate (NMDA) subunit receptor gene (GRIN2B) with obsessive-compulsive disorder: A preliminary study. *Psychopharmacology (Berl)* 2004;**174**:530–538.

128. Loftis JM, Janowsky A. The N-methyl-D-aspartate receptor subunit NR2B: Localization, functional properties, regulation, and clinical implications. *Pharmacol Ther* 2003;**97**:55–85.

129. Grant P, Lougee L, Hirschtritt M *et al.* An open-label trial of riluzole, a glutamate antagonist, in children with treatment-resistant obsessive-compulsive disorder. *J Child Adolesc Psychopharmacol* 2007;**17**:761–767.

130. Stewart SE, Stack DE, Tsilker S *et al.* Long-term outcome following intensive residential treatment of obsessive-compulsive disorder. *J Psychiatr Res* 2009;**43**:1118–1123.

131. Pittenger C, Krystal JH, Coric V. Glutamate-modulating drugs as novel pharmacotherapeuticagents in the treatment of obsessive-compulsive disorder. *NeuroRx* 2006;**3**:69–81.

132. Coric V, Milanovic S, Wasylink S *et al.* Beneficial effects of the antiglutamatergic agent riluzole in a patient diagnosed with obsessive-compulsive disorder and major depressive disorder. *Psychopharmacology (Berl)* 2003;**167**:219–220.

133. Coric V, Taskiran S, Pittenger C *et al.* Riluzole augmentation in treatment-resistant obsessive-compulsive disorder: an open-label trial. *Biol Psychiatry* 2005;**58**:424–428.

134. Hollander E, Dell'Osso B. Topiramate plus paroxetine in treatment-resistant obsessive-compulsive disorder. *Int Clin Psychopharmacol* 2006;**21**:189–191.

135. Rubio G, Jiménez-Arriero MA, Martínez-Gras I *et al.* The effects of topiramate adjunctive treatment added to antidepressants in patients with resistant obsessive-compulsive disorder. *J Clin Psychopharmacol* 2006;**26**:341–344.

136. Van Ameringen M, Mancini C, Patterson B *et al.* Topiramate augmentation in treatment-resistant obsessive-compulsive disorder: a retrospective, open-label case series. *Depress Anxiety* 2006;**23**:1–5.

137. Ozkara C, Ozmen M, Erdogan A *et al.* Topiramate related obsessive-compulsive disorder. *Eur Psychiatry* 2005;**20**:78–79.

138. Thuile J, Even C, Guelfi JD. Topiramate may induce obsessive-compulsive disorder. *Psychiatry Clin Neurosci* 2006;**60**:394.

139. Poyurovsky M, Glick I, Koran LM. Lamotrigine augmentation in schizophrenia and schizoaffective patients with obsessive-compulsive symptoms. *J Psychopharmacol* 2010;**24**:861–866.

140. Uzun O. Lamotrigine as an augmentation agent in treatment-resistant obsessive-compulsive disorder: a case report. *J Psychopharmacol* 2010;**24**:425–427.

141. Lafleur DL, Pittenger C, Kelmendi B *et al*. N-acetylcysteine augmentation in serotonin reuptake inhibitor refractory obsessive-compulsive disorder. *Psychopharmacology (Berl)* 2006;**184**:254–256.

142. Kushner MG, Kim SW, Donahue C *et al*. D-cycloserine augmented exposure therapy for obsessive-compulsive disorder. *Biol Psychiatry* 2007;**62**:835–838.

143. Wilhelm S, Buhlmann U, Tolin DF *et al*. Augmentation of behavior therapy with D-cycloserine for obsessive-compulsive disorder. *Am J Psychiatry* 2008;**165**:335–341.

144. Chasson GS, Buhlmann U, Tolin DF *et al*. Need for speed: evaluating slopes of OCD recovery in behavior therapy enhanced with d-cycloserine. *Behav Res Ther* 2010;**48**:675–679.

145. Poyurovsky M, Weizman R, Weizman A *et al*. Memantine for treatment-resistant OCD. *Am J Psychiatry* 2005;**162**:2191–2192.

146. Hezel DM, Beattie K, Stewart SE. Memantine as an augmenting agent for severe pediatric OCD. *Am J Psychiatry* 2009;**166**:237.

147. Pasquini M, Biondi M. Memantine augmentation for refractory obsessive-compulsive disorder. *Prog Neuropsychopharmacol Biol Psychiatry* 2006;**30**:1173–1175.

148. Aboujaoude E, Barry JJ, Gamel N. Memantine augmentation in treatment-resistant obsessive-compulsive disorder: an open-label trial. *J Clin Psychopharmacol* 2009;**29**:51–55.

149. Feusner JD, Kerwin L, Saxena S *et al*. Differential efficacy of memantine for obsessive-compulsive disorder vs. generalized anxiety disorder: an open-label trial. *Psychopharmacol Bull* 2009;**42**:81–93.

150. Stewart SE, Jenike EEA, Hezel DM *et al*. A single-blinded case-control study of memantine in severe obsessive-compulsive disorder. *J Clin Psychopharmacol* 2010;**30**:34–39.

CHAPTER 11

The Genetics of Obsessive-Compulsive Disorder: Current Status

David L. Pauls

Psychiatric and Neurodevelopmental Genetics Unit, Center for Human Genetic Research, Massachusetts General Hospital, Harvard Medical School, Boston, USA

INTRODUCTION

Obsessive-compulsive disorder (OCD) is characterized by disabling obsessions (intrusive unwanted thoughts and/or images) and/or compulsions (ritualized repetitive behaviours) [1]. Both children and adults suffer with OCD. Originally thought to be rare, current estimates of lifetime prevalence range between 1% and 3% worldwide [2,3]. Thus, OCD is one of the more common and serious mental conditions [4].

Supporting results from twin and family studies, neuroimaging studies, treatment studies and molecular genetic studies suggest that biochemical, biological and genetic factors are all important for the development of OCD. The author has previously reviewed these data [5]. In this chapter, the historic evidence is again summarized and updated with recent results. Thus, sections of this manuscript will be similar to those previously published reviews

TWIN STUDIES

Twin studies can help to determine if genetic factors are important for the manifestation of complex disorders. The heritability (i.e. the amount of phenotypic variance that can be accounted for by genetic factors) can be estimated by comparing the concordance rates between monozygotic (MZ) and dizygotic twins (DZ).

A number of twin studies for OCD have been published; many are case reports or concern only a few twin pairs so are not summarized here (for a complete

Obsessive-Compulsive Disorder: Current Science and Clinical Practice, First Edition. Edited by Joseph Zohar.
© 2012 John Wiley & Sons, Ltd. Published 2012 by John Wiley & Sons, Ltd.

Table 11.1 Twin studies of obsessive-compulsive disorder (OCD) with sample size greater than 30 twin pairs.

Study type	No. of twin pairs	MZ concordance	DZ concordance
DSM-III/DSM-III-R OCD			
Carey and Gottesman [7]	30	13/15	7/15
Andrews et al. [8]	48	0/18	0/30
DSM-IV		MZ Tetrachoric r	DZ Tetrachoric r
Bolton et al. [9]	854	0.57 (0.24–0.80)	0.22 (−0.02–0.43)
		h^2	
Tambs et al. [10]	2801	0.29	
OC behaviours		h^2	
Young et al. [11]	32	0	
Torgersen [12]	99	0.18 (men)	
		0.23 (women)	
Clifford et al. [13]	419	0.44 (traits)	
		0.47 (symptoms)	
Jonnal et al. [14]	527	0.33 (obsessions)	
		0.26 (compulsions)	
Eley et al. [15]	4564	0.65 (OC behaviour)	
Hudziak et al. [16]	4246	0.45–0.61	

Modified from Pauls [5].
DSM-III-R, *Diagnostic and Statistical Manual of Mental Disorders, Third Edition, Text Revision*; DZ, dizygotic; MZ, monozygotic.

review see ref. [6]). van Grootheest and colleagues [6] summarized the results of all twin studies from 1929 through 2005. As noted by these authors, the results from the early studies have serious limitations and should be interpreted with these in mind. These limitations include small sample sizes and differing diagnostic criteria. Furthermore, in almost all studies, the investigator assessing the co-twin was not blind to the diagnosis of the index twin (Table 11.1).

It should also be noted that of the six studies with adequate sample sizes (at least 100 twin pairs) five of the studies estimated the heritability of obsessive-compulsive symptoms, not OCD. Only two studies [9,10] were able to estimate the heritability of OCD as determined by *Diagnostic and Statistical Manual of Mental Disorders* (DSM) diagnostic criteria.

In the first study [9], 854 six-year-old twins identified as having OCD in a community sample were included in the study. The mothers of these twins were then interviewed and these data were used to assign DSM-IV criteria. This study is the first with a large enough sample size to more accurately estimate the influence of genetic factors on OCD rather that evaluating the heritability of obsessive-compulsive symptoms in twins from a population sample. The results reported by

Bolton and colleagues [9] are consistent with the studies with sufficient sample sizes (see Table 11.1). They demonstrated that genetic factors play an important role in the manifestation of obsessive-compulsive behaviours as well as OCD.

It is notable that these investigators also examined the genetic relationship between OCD and two common comorbid disorders, tic disorder and anxiety disorders. Their reports are consistent with the hypothesis that there are shared genetic factors for OCD and tics as well as for OCD and other anxiety disorders, and support the hypothesis that there are subtypes of OCD that may have unique aetiological risk factors [17–21].

In a study published in 2009 [10], Tambs and colleagues assessed 2801 young-adult Norwegian twins using the Composite International Diagnostic Interview (CIDI). In this study the heritability was estimated for five anxiety disorders (generalized anxiety disorder, panic disorder, phobias, obsessive-compulsive disorder and post-traumatic stress disorder). Of the 2801 twins, reliable anxiety data were available for only 1385 twin pairs. Of those 1385 there were only 57 pairs where one twin was diagnosed with OCD. To increase the sample size, twins where one met criteria for subthreshold OCD were included. There were 165 twin pairs where at least one had a diagnosis of OCD or subthreshold OCD. The heritability estimated from this sample was 29%. However, 55% of this heritability appeared to be due to a common factor shared by all five anxiety disorders and 45% appeared to be due to specific factors for OCD.

In summary, it is evident that genetic factors play a role in the aetiology of OCD. In their comprehensive review of studies published prior to 2006, van Grootheest and colleagues [6] concluded that 'in children, obsessive-compulsive (OC) symptoms are heritable, with genetic influences in the range of 45% to 65%. In adults, studies are suggestive for a genetic influence on OC symptoms, ranging from 27% to 47%'. Results reported in the two recent studies [9,10] are remarkably similar when co-twins with subthreshold OCD were included. In both studies, additive genetic effects accounted for 29% of the variance for OCD and subclinical OCD. Furthermore, Bolton and colleagues [9] reported that 47% of the phenotypic variance could be explained by the familial aggregation due to combined additive genetic and shared environmental factors. Unfortunately, these investigators were unable to estimate the separate effects of additive genetic and shared environmental factors [9].

FAMILY STUDIES

Many family studies examining the familial aggregation of OCD and obsessional neurosis have been published since 1930. In the majority of these studies the results demonstrate that at least some forms of OCD are familial. Given the results of the twin studies summarized above, it is clear that genetic factors play some role in this familiality, However, the findings from Bolton and colleagues [9] also demonstrate that non-genetic factors influence obsessive-compulsive behaviours and are also familial [9]. Environmental (i.e. non-genetic factors) are clearly important in the aetiology of obsessive-compulsive behaviours since the concordance rates for MZ twins for OCD and obsessive-compulsive behaviours are always less than 1.0. Understanding the impact of these environmental/cultural factors will be crucial for eventual identification of factors that increase the risk of OCD. Nevertheless, even if genetic factors alone cannot explain all of the observed inheritance of OCD, demonstrating that OCD and related behaviours are familial is important for the ultimate determination of genetic factors that increase the risk for OCD.

Family history studies

Prior to 1987, all studies of the familial aggregation of obsessive-compulsive illness and/or obsessive-compulsive features relied on family history data (i.e. studies in which all information about OCD and OC behaviours in family members is obtained from one or possibly two informants). Family history data generally result in underestimates of the true rates of illness within families [22,23]. Thus, it is important to note that data from these early family history studies show that, for the most part, obsessive-compulsive illness and/or obsessive-compulsive features are familial [24–31]. One caveat of these early studies is that no control samples were obtained so it is difficult to interpret these findings since the population prevalence of OCD could not be reliably estimated.

Family interview studies

All family studies completed after 1986 attempted to collect direct interviews from as many relatives as possible in the family. All available relatives were directly interviewed, except in one study [32]. In this study all adult family members completed the Leyton Obsessional Inventory (LOI), and only those who scored high were interviewed directly. Only one of the relatives who were interviewed met criteria for obsessive-compulsive neurosis, suggesting that the OCD may not be familial.

It is likely that some relatives with OCD may not have been identified with this ascertainment scheme. Individuals with OCD who have only a few obsessions and/or compulsions that consume significant time and cause considerable distress and result in a diagnosis may score low on the LOI. Thus, it is possible that some non-interviewed relatives who scored low on the LOI might have been diagnosed with OCD had they been interviewed. It is important to note that an increased rate of mental illness was observed among the relatives of these OCD probands.

All of the other published family studies of OCD directly interviewed all available first-degree relatives with structured psychiatric interviews [18,20,21,32–45].

Table 11.2 Family studies of obsessive-compulsive disorder (OCD): frequencies of these conditions among first-degree relatives.

	Cases		Controls	
	OCD	Subclinical OCD	OCD	Subclinical OCD
Studies of families ascertained through adults with OCD				
McKeon and Murray [32]	0.007	–	0.007	
Bellodi et al. [33]	0.034	–	–	–
Black et al. [34]	0.025	0.156	0.023	0.029
Nicolini et al. [35]	0.049	–	–	–
Pauls et al. [18]	0.103	0.079	0.019	0.020
Nestadt et al. [36]	0.117	0.046	0.027	0.030
Albert et al. [37]	0.035	–	–	–
Fyer et al. [38]	0.062	0.084	0	0
Lipsitz et al. [39]	0.026	0.057	0.013	0.013
Grabe et al. [40]	0.064	0.055	0.012	0.030
Studies of families ascertained through children/adolescents with OCD				
Lenane et al. [41]	0.170	–	–	–
Riddle et al. [42]	0.095	–	–	–
Leonard et al. [43]	0.130	–	–	–
Reddy et al. [44]	0.050	–	0	–
Chabane et al. [45]	0.170	–	–	–
Hanna et al. [20]	0.225	–	0.026	–
Rosario-Campos et al. [21]	0.227	0.065	0.009	0.015

Modified from Pauls [5].

In some studies, relatives were interviewed not only about themselves, but also about all of their first-degree relatives regarding the presence of other psychiatric disorders, including OCD. Best estimate diagnoses were then made using both direct interview and family history data for all of the family members.

The majority of the more recent studies yielded data that demonstrate that some forms of OCD are familial. Seven of these studies examined relatives of children and/or adolescents with OCD, and in the remaining eight studies, relatives of adults with OCD were studied (Table 11.2).

Studies of families of children/adolescents with OCD

Recurrence rates of OCD and subclinical OCD were significantly higher in families ascertained through children and/or adolescents with OCD [20,21,41–45], when compared to the rates among controls or estimates of population prevalence. While the prevalence of OCD and subclinical OCD varied within families across studies, the overall conclusion was that OCD and subclinical OCD are familial. Significantly, the occurrence of OCD and subclinical OCD within these families was noticeably higher than the observed prevalence in families ascertained through adults (see below). The prevalence of OCD in families ascertained through adults with OCD was approximately two times that among controls. In contrast, the frequency of OCD among families ascertained through children and adolescents with OCD was approximately 10-fold higher than controls and/or the population prevalence.

Studies of families of adults with OCD

The findings among family studies of adults with OCD were more variable than those summarized above for families of children/adolescents with OCD. As noted earlier, McKeon and Murray [32] did not observe an increased rate of OCD among relatives of adult OCD probands. In the first controlled study of OCD in which all relatives were directly interviewed, Black and colleagues [34] examined 120 first-degree relatives of 32 adult OCD probands and 129 relatives of 33 psychiatrically age-matched normal controls. All interviewers were blind to the diagnostic status of the proband. Diagnoses were assigned using DSM-III criteria. Only data from the direct interviews were used to assign diagnoses. It should be noted that family history data had been obtained from all interviewed relatives about other first-degree relatives, but that information was not available to the diagnosticians. The age-corrected rate of DSM-III OCD was 2.5% among relatives of individuals with OCD compared to 2.3% in controls, suggesting that OCD is not familial. However, the rate of a more broadly defined OCD was 15.6% among parents of the OCD probands compared to only 2.9% among the parents of controls. Of note, is the increased rate of other non-OCD anxiety disorders among the relatives of OCD probands.

One possible explanation for the low rates in the study by Black *et al.* is that only data from direct interviews were used to assign diagnoses. Lipsitz and colleagues [39] examined whether using data from an informant could affect the recurrence risk estimates. In the majority of family studies of OCD, diagnoses were made using both direct interview of the individual and family history data about the individuals collected from other individuals in the family. When only data from the direct interviews were used to assign diagnoses, the rate of OCD and subclinical OCD was 5.4% compared to 1.7% among controls ($p = 0.17$). In contrast, when all available data were used to assign diagnoses, the rate of OCD and subclinical OCD was 8.9% among relatives of individuals with OCD compared to only 1.7% among controls ($p = 0.02$). These investigators concluded that 'evidence of familial transmission of OCD was found only when diagnoses were made using information from the proband about the relative'. Lipsitz and colleagues proffered that since individuals with OCD can be quite secretive about their symptoms, it is possible that they might deny OC symptomatology when being interviewed. This might be especially important when the individual has never sought treatment for their obsessive-compulsive symptoms. However, it is also possible that an affected individual who has been treated for OCD could 'over-report' obsessive-compulsive symptoms in their relatives. Lipsitz and colleagues [39] only collected family history information from the affected probands, all of whom had sought treatment. Thus, it is possible that the reporter was 'projecting' their own behaviours onto their relatives, which would result in an overestimate of the affected status among relatives. This is unlikely, since in other studies where family history data were collected from all interviewed relatives [18,36], both affected and unaffected relatives were interviewed and one would expect that it would be less likely that these relatives would over-report OC symptomatology. Similar to the findings in the Black et al. study, Lipsitz and colleagues [39] also observed an increased rate of other non-OCD anxiety disorders among the relatives. Of interest is that Black and colleagues did report that a number of family members indicated that other relatives did have OC symptomatology. Thus, it is possible that the recurrence risk estimates reported by these investigators could be lower than the true risks.

In all of the remaining studies of families ascertained through adult individuals with OCD, the estimated prevalence among first-degree relatives provided evidence that OCD is a familial disorder [38,46–51]. In all studies, the frequency of OCD among relatives of individuals with OCD was significantly higher when compared to the population prevalence or the rate among controls. In contrast to earlier studies, Grabe and colleagues [40] studied families ascertained through affected individuals from both a clinic and a population sample. A significant increase in frequency was observed in both relatives of individuals who were ascertained through a clinic and individuals who were identified from the general population. This study was the first controlled study of OCD in Europe and replicated the results of the studies done in the United States [16,36] in families ascertained from OCD clinics. The finding of Grabe and colleagues is particularly significant. As the authors nicely summarize, 'the finding of a comparable familial aggregation of definite OCD and a higher familial aggregation of subclinical OCD in relatives of never treated persons with OCD from the community strongly supports the impact of familial-genetic factors in OCD.'

Associated conditions

Several investigators have used family data to examine whether other disorders were significantly increased among relatives of OCD probands [52,53]. Bienvenu and colleagues[52] analyzed data from an earlier family study [36] to determine whether the frequency of OCD-spectrum disorders was significantly higher among relatives of adults with OCD. They reported significantly higher rates of body dysmorphic disorder (BDD; odds ratio (OR) = 5.4), somatoform disorders (OR = 3.9), grooming disorders (OR = 1.8) and all spectrum disorders combined (OR = 2.7). Similarly, Grados and colleagues [53] reported an increased prevalence of tic disorders among relatives of adults with OCD when compared with controls. In addition, these investigators reported an association between earlier age of OCD onset and tic prevalence, which is consistent with findings from earlier studies [9,20,21]. Taken together, these data support the hypothesis that there may be at least three different types of OCD: (i) one that is related to tic disorder (TD) and is familial; (ii) one that is familial but not related to TD (but possibly related to anxiety); and (iii) one that does not aggregate in families.

In sum, these studies provide compelling evidence that risk factors for at least some forms of OCD are inherited. These findings are consistent with the results of a meta-analysis of five OCD family studies published before 2001 and involving 1209 first degree relatives [54]. While these data are consistent with a hypothesis that genetic factors increase the risk for OCD, alone they demonstrate only that OCD is familial. However, taken together with the results of twin studies summarized above, there is strong evidence that genetic factors are important risk factors for some types of OCD.

SEGREGATION ANALYSES

Given that OCD is familial and that results from twins provide evidence that this familiality is in part due to genetic factors, several research groups performed segregation analyses to evaluate whether the pattern of transmission in these families could be explained by specific genetic models. Complex segregation analyses provide a way to compare the 'goodness-of-fit' of the pattern of transmission expected for a specific genetic model with that of the observed patterns of transmission within families. The results from complex segregation analyses cannot prove the existence of genes, but they can provide estimates of an underlying genetic model that could be helpful in future molecular genetic studies.

Four complex segregation analyses of OCD transmission in families have been reported [55–58]. In all studies the results are consistent with models of genetic transmission. However, the specific genetic model that best fits the transmission within families differed across studies. These findings are not surprising given the high likelihood that OCD is genetically heterogeneous. Nevertheless, there was some consistency in the reports in that all groups hypothesized some genes of major effect important for the manifestation of OCD

Together with advances in our understanding regarding the genetic risk factors that probably are important for the manifestation of OCD, our understanding of the phenotype of OCD has increased dramatically over the last decades.

Arguably, the most important advances relevant to genetic research are new ways to assess the dimensions of the OCD phenotype rather than relying on the traditional categorical diagnostic classifications. Findings from a number of independent studies have consistently demonstrated that specific OCD symptoms occur together more often than expected by chance, and that these clusters together comprise the OCD phenotype [46–49]. Furthermore, these clusters appear to be heritable [46,50]. Thus it is highly likely that there are several different genetic risk factors that might contribute to the manifestation of these different components of OCD.

CANDIDATE GENE STUDIES

Over 80 candidate gene studies have been published over the last decade (Table 11.3). Most of these investigations have studied genes in the serotonergic, dopaminergic, glutamatergic and opioid systems based on the current understanding of the pathophysiology and pharmacology of OCD [51,59]. None of the reported findings have been replicated in large enough samples to achieve genome-wide significance (i.e. 5×10^{-8}). One possible exception may be the glutamate transporter gene *SLCL1A1* [51,59,61,62]; however, one recent study [63], in which the investigators conducted a capillary electrophoresis single-strand conformation polymorphism (CE-SSCP) screen in 378 OCD affected individuals for all 12 identified exons of *SLC1A1*, including all coding regions and approximately 50 bp of flanking introns, found no statistical differences in genotype and allele frequencies of common coding SNPs (cSNPs) in *SLC1A1* between the OCD cases and controls . Finally, in addition to undertaking candidate gene studies, investigators have begun to examine the function of some of the genes being studied. Early findings suggest that this may be a promising approach [64]. However, it is too early to reach any definite conclusions, since none of these studies have so far been replicated.

Given the heterogeneity of OCD, both phenotypically and genetically, it is highly unlikely that any one candidate gene will be a unique risk factor for all cases of OCD. Although a gene or genes may be associated with the time of onset, or the severity or persistence of OCD symptoms, it will be highly unlikely to increase the risk for all types of OCD. What is most probable is that other risk genes will be involved. Nevertheless, since many of the effective pharmacological agents target the serotonergic and dopaminergic systems, it is possible that some of the genes in those systems could be important in mediating response to treatment. Identifying genes that impact treatment response would represent a significant advance in how individuals with OCD are treated. However, these genes would not necessarily be important in the aetiology of OCD. Genes important for treatment response might not be involved in the aetiology of a disorder.

Table 11.3 Candidate gene studies of obsessive-compulsive disorder (OCD).

Candidate gene	Investigator	Study design	Sample size			Significance	Associated allele
			Cases	Controls	Families		
Serotonin transporter	McDougle et al. [65]	FB	–	–	35	$p < 0.03$	L allele
	Bengel et al. [66]	CC	75	397	–	$p = 0.023$	LL genotype
	Frisch et al. [67]	CC	75	172	–	ns	–
	Kinnear et al. [68]	CC	54	82	–	ns	–
	Denys et al. [69]	CC	156	134	–	ns	–
	Dickel et al. [70]	FB	–	–	54	ns	–
	Saiz et al. [71]	CC	99	420	–	ns	–
	Wendland et al. [64]	CC	347	749	–	ns	–
	Wendland et al. [72]	CC	295	657	–	$p < 0.018$	Three marker haplotype
Serotonin transporter promoter	Kinnear et al. [73]	CC	129	479	–	ns	–
	Camarena et al. [74]	CC/FB	115	136	43	ns	–
	Cavallini et al. [75]	CC	180	112	–	ns	–
	Walitza et al. [76]	FB	–	–	63	ns	–
	Meira-Lima et al [77]	CC	79	202	–	ns	–
	Chabane et al. [78]	CC/FB	106	171	86	ns	–
Serotonin receptor 2A	Nicolini et al. [79]	CC	67	54	–	ns	–
	Enoch et al. [80]	CC	62	144	–	$p < 0.05$	A allele
	Enoch et al. [81]	CC	101	138	–	$p = 0.015$	A allele
	Frisch et al. [67]	CC	75	172	–	ns	–
	Walitza et al. [82]	CC	55	223	–	ns	–
	Hemmings et al. [83]	CC	71	129	–	ns	–
	Tot et al. [84]	CC	??	??	–	ns	–
	Hemmings et al. [85]	CC	58	83	–	ns	–

Meira-Lima et al. [77]	CC	79	202	–	$p < 0.00007$	C allele
Denys et al. [69]	CC	156	134	–	ns	–
Dickel et al. [70]	FB	–	–	54	ns	–
Saiz et al. [71]	CC	99	420	–	$p = 0.02$	–
Serotonin receptor 2C						
Cavallini et al. [86]	CC	109	107	–	ns	–
Frisch et al. [67]	CC	75	172	–	ns	–
Meira-Lima et al. [77]	CC	79	202	–	ns	–
Serotonin receptor 2C						
Cavallini et al. [86]	CC	109	107	–	ns	–
Frisch et al. [67]	CC	75	172	–	ns	–
Meira-Lima et al. [77]	CC	79	202	–	ns	–
Serotonin receptor 1B (1Dβ)						
Mundo et al. [87]	FB	–	–	32	$p < 0.006$	G allele
Mundo et al. [88]	FB	–	–	121	$p = 0.023$	G allele
DiBella et al. [89]	FB	–	–	48	ns	–
Hemmings et al. [83]	CC	77	129	–	ns	–
Camarena et al. [90]	FB	–	–	47	ns	–
Walitza et al. [76]	FB	–	–	63	ns	–
Denys et al. [69]	CC	156	134	–	ns	–
Dickel et al. [70]	FB	–	–	54	ns	–
Tryptophan hydroxylase						
Frisch et al. [67]	CC	75	172	–	ns	–
Walitza et al. [76]	FB	–	–	63	ns	–
Mössner et al. [91]	FB	–	–	71	$p = 0.035$	G-C haplotype
Dopamine receptor 4						
Cruz et al. [92]	CC	12	49	–	$p = 0.018$	7 allele less frequent
Billet et al. [93]	CC	118	118	–	$p = 0.021$	–
Frisch et al. [67]	CC	75	172	–	$p = 0.04$	–
Millet et al. [94]	CC/FB	49	63	34	$p = 0.03$	2 allele protective
Hemmings et al. [83]	CC	71	129	–	ns	–
Hemmings et al. [85]	CC	95	85	–	$p = 0.013$	Early vs late onset

(Continued)

Table 11.3 Candidate gene studies of obsessive-compulsive disorder (OCD). (Continued)

Candidate gene	Investigator	Study design	Sample size			Significance	Associated allele
			Cases	Controls	Families		
Dopamine receptor 2	Nicolini et al. [79]	CC	67	54	–	ns	–
	Billet et al. [93]	CC	110	110	–	p = 0.014	CC genotype
Dopamine receptor 3	Catalano et al. [95]	CC	97	97	–	ns	–
	Nicolini et al. [79]	CC	67	54	–	ns	–
	Billet et al. [93]	CC	103	103	–	ns	–
Dopamine transporter	Billet et al. [93]	CC	103	103	–	ns	–
	Frisch et al. [67]	CC	75	172	–	ns	–
	Hemmings et al. [83]	CC	71	129	–	ns	–
Monamine oxidase A	Karayiorgou et al. [96]	FB	–	–	110	p = 0.019 (males	G allele
	Camarena et al. [74]	CC/FB	122	124	51	CC: p = 0.024 FB: p = 0.022	T allele
Catechol O-methyltransferase	Hemmings et al. [83]	CC	71	129	–	ns	–
	Karayiorgou et al. [97]	CC	73	148	–	p = 0.0002	L allele in males
	Karayiorgou et al. [96]	FB	–	–	110	p = 0.0079	L allele
	Schindler et al. [98]	FB	–	–	67	p = 0.006	L allele
	Niehaus et al. [99]	CC	54	54	–	p = 0.0017	HL genotype
	Alsobrook et al. [100]	FB	–	–	56	p = 0.048	L allele in females
	Ohara et al. [101]	CC	17	35	–	ns	–
	Erdal et al. [102]	CC	59	114	–	ns	–
	Azzam et al. [103]	CC	144	337	–	ns	–
	Meira-Lima et al. [77]	CC	79	202	–	ns	–
	Katerberg et al. [104]	CC	373	462	–	ns	–
Glutamate receptor subtype 2B	Arnold et al. [105]	FB	–	–	130	p = 0.002	5072G-5988T haplotype

Protein	Reference	CC/FB				p	
Kainite glutamate receptor 2	Delorme et al. [106]		156	156	141	CC: ns FB: p = 0.03	8671 allele under-transmitted
Gamma-aminobutyric acid type B receptor 1	Zai et al. [107]	FB	–	–	159	p = 0.006	A-7265G
Brain-derived neurotrophic factor	Hall et al. [108]	FB	–	–	164	p < 0.020	Multiple SNPs
	Dickel et al. [70]	FB	–	–	54	ns	–
	Wendland et al. [72]	CC	347	749	–	ns	–
Myelin oligodendrocyte	Zai et al. [109]	FB	–	–	160	p = 0.022	MOG4 2-repeat allele
Glutamate transporter	Arnold et al. [60]	FB	–	–	157	p = 0.006	2 marker haplotype (males)
	Dickel et al. [51]	FB	–	–	71	p = 0.030	2 marker haplotype (males)
	Stewart et al. [61]	FB	–	–	66	p = 0.0015	3 marker haplotype
	Wendland et al. [62]	CC	325	662	–	p < 0.001	3 marker haplotype
	Wang et al. [63]	CC	378	281	–	ns	–
Oligodendrocyte lineage transcription factor 2	Stewart et al. [110]	FB	–	–	66	p = 0.004	5 marker haplotype
Neurotrophin-3 receptor gene (NTRK3)[a]	Muiños-Gimeno et al. [111]	CC	153	324	–	p = 0.005	–
Extraneuronal monoamine transporter, EMT (SLC22A3),	Lazar et al. [112]	CC	84	204	–	ns	–
SAPAP3	Boardman et al. [113]	CC	172	153	–	p = 0.036	4 marker haplotype with early-onset OCD

Adapted from Pauls [5] and Hemmings and Stein [114] and updated through 3/2011.
[a] Association with the hoarding phenotype.

GENETIC LINKAGE STUDIES

To date, only three genome-wide linkage studies of OCD have been completed [20,115,116]. None of the findings reached genome-wide significance; however, all studies identified chromosomal regions that should be explored in future research. Hanna and colleagues [20] completed a genome scan on seven families ascertained through children with OCD. Sixty-five of 66 relatives were evaluated using structured psychiatric interviews. Thirty-two met criteria for a diagnosis of OCD.

All individuals in these families were genotyped with 349 microsatellite markers. An additional 24 markers were genotyped for the fine-mapping done after the initial genome scan. Possible linkage was observed for marker D9S288 on chromosome 9p (LOD=2.25). However, after the additional 24 markers were genotyped in the region on 9p the log odds (LOD) score dropped to 1.97. LOD scores greater than 3.6 are needed for genome-wide significance for these types of linkage studies.

Willour and colleagues [117] attempted to replicate these results in 50 OCD pedigrees. Most of these families comprised two affected siblings and their parents. These researchers reported LOD scores of over 2.0 for markers D9S1792 and D9S1813. Markers D9S1813 and D9S1792 are within 350 kb of marker D9S288, the marker which had the highest LOD score in the Hanna study [20].

The second genome-wide linkage study genotyped individuals in 219 families. These families consisted of nuclear families with at least two affected siblings and multigenerational families [115]. Suggestive linkage was observed for markers on chromosomes 3q, 7p, 1q, 15q and 6q. The strongest evidence for linkage was obtained for markers on chromosome 3q27-28 when both definite and probable cases of OCD were included in the analyses. The maximum LOD score calculated using a method developed by Kong and Cox was 2.67 for markers D3S1262 ($p = 0.0003$) and D3S2398 ($p = 0.0004$) on 3q. This method estimates the degree of allele sharing between affected individuals within a family. It provides additional evidence for the significance of the markers since if there is no linkage there should be no allele sharing greater than expected by chance.

Samuels and colleagues [118] reanalyzed these families to evaluate whether compulsive hoarding behaviour might be linked to other markers across the genome. Interestingly, they observed suggestive evidence for linkage of marker D14S588 (Kong and Cox LOD = 2.9) on chromosome 14. When the analyses were repeated for families where there were two or more hoarding relatives, the Kong and Cox LODall score increased to 3.7.

Hanna and colleagues reported the results of another genome-wide linkage study [116]. This study included 26 multigenerational families with 121 individuals. All family members were genotyped with markers with an average spacing of 10 centimorgans (cM). (A centimorgan is defined as the distance on a chromosome in which 1% crossing-over occurs. Given the completion of the Human Genome Project and the sequencing of the entire human genome, this metric is no longer commonly reported since one can now determine precisely how many base pairs there are between specific markers.) Again, all relatives were evaluated using semi-structured psychiatric interviews. Lifetime psychiatric diagnoses were assigned using these interview data as well as data from other sources when available (e.g. medical records). The highest LOD score of 2.43 was observed for markers on chromosome 10p15. When these investigators combined the data from this study with their earlier study, the maximum LOD score decreased to 1.79 in this region on chromosome 10p.

A follow-up family-based association study was conducted on these families in which 35 single nucleotide polymorphisms (SNPs) were genotyped in this 10p15 region. Notably, an association was detected for three adjacent SNPs in this region, including an amino acid variant rs2271275 in the 3′ region of the adenosine deaminase acting on RNA 3 (*ADAR3*) gene (p < 0.05).

A caveat for all of these studies is that all consisted of relatively small samples. It is noteworthy, however, that in the study reported by Willour and colleagues [117] suggestive linkage was observed in the same 9p chromosome region that was reported by Hanna *et al*. Furthermore, as discussed above, four independent studies have reported an association of OCD and the glutamate transporter, a gene located in this 9p region. Unfortunately, in the study reported by Shugart *et al*. [115] there was no evidence for linkage at 9p. Even so, the region at 9p is still of interest; the data from the Shugart study simply indicate that it is not a gene with major effect in all cases of OCD.

FUTURE WORK

It is clear from twin and family studies that genetic risk factors are important for at least some forms of OCD. However, the linkage and association studies provide only suggestive evidence for risk genes that have a moderate effect on expression of OCD. Thus, genome-wide association studies (GWAS) or whole-genome sequencing studies of OCD are warranted as the next step in our effort to identify risk genes for this condition. These types of studies are preferred over linkage studies or candidate gene studies because they can yield data that have more power to help identify risk genes of relatively small effect. The primary difference between genome-wide linkage studies and genome-wide association or whole-genome sequencing studies is that in linkage studies co-transmission of a specific DNA marker within a family is examined, while in these other whole-genome studies it is possible to examine many markers/genes across the entire genome at one time. Linkage studies have been very successful in identifying genes that have a major effect on a specific disorder; usually these are disorders caused by a single gene. Whole-genome association and sequencing studies are advantageous when trying to identify genes of relatively small effect. These new generation studies allow the examination of both common and rare markers, enabling the identification of different types of risk genes. It is becoming evident that complex disorders such as OCD may be 'caused' either by rare genes of major effect or several common genes acting together.

Genome-wide association studies or whole-genome sequencing studies with an adequate sample size are the most promising approaches for the elucidation of OCD risk genes. Candidate gene studies with small samples do little to advance our knowledge of the specific risk genes important for the expression of OCD.

The findings from both family and twin studies clearly suggest that OCD is aetiologically heterogeneous. Consequently, large samples of affected individuals are needed so that phenotypically homogeneous subgroups can be identified from the larger population – these subgroups are more likely to be aetiologically homogeneous [119,120]. Large enough samples can only be achieved when there is collaboration between researchers at different centres. Two collaborative efforts of this type – the International OCD Foundation Genetics Collaborative (IOCDFGC) and the Obsessive Compulsive Genetic Association Study, led by investigators at Johns Hopkins University – are currently conducting genome-wide association studies of OCD. The IOCDFGC study includes over 3000 samples contributed from 21 different research sites around the world. Hopefully, these studies will yield findings that will help in advancing our understanding of the aetiology of this debilitating disorder.

ACKNOWLEDGEMENTS

This work was supported in part by NIH grants NS-016648, NS-040024, MH079489 and the David Judah Foundation.

REFERENCES

1. Calvocoressi L, Libman D, Vegso SJ *et al*. Global functioning of inpatients with obsessive-compulsive disorder, schizophrenia, and major depression. *Psychiatric Services* 1998;**49**:379–381.
2. Karno M, Golding JM, Sorenson SB *et al*. The epidemiology of obsessive-compulsive disorder in five U.S. communities. *Arch Gen Psychiatry* 1988;**45**:1084–1099.
3. Weissman MM, Bland RC, Canino GJ *et al*. The cross national epidemiology of obsessive compulsive disorder. *J Clin Psychiatry* 1994;**55**:5–10.
4. Eaton WW, Martins SS, Nestadt G *et al*. The burden of mental disorders. *Epidemiol Rev* 2008;**30**:1–14.
5. Pauls DL. The genetics of Obsessive Compulsive Disorder: A review. *Dialogues Clin Neurosci* 2010;**12**:149–163.
6. van Grootheest DS, Cath DC, Beekman AT, Boomsma DI. Twin studies on obsessive-compulsive disorder: a review. *Twin Res Hum Genet* 2005;**8**:450–458.

7. Carey G, Gottesman II. Twin and family studies of anxiety, phobic, and obsessive disorders. In: Klein DF, Rabkin J (eds), *Anxiety: New Research and Changing Concepts.* New York: Raven Press, 1981; pp. 117–136.

8. Andrews G, Stewart G, Allen R, Henderson AS. The genetics of six neurotic disorders: A twin study. *J Aff Disord* 1990;**19**:23–29.

9. Bolton D, Rijsdijk F, O'Connor TG *et al.* Obsessive-compulsive disorder, tics and anxiety in 6-year-old twins. *Psychol Med* 2007;**37**:39–48.

10. Tambs K, Czajkowsky N, Røysamb E *et al.* Structure of genetic and environmental risk factors for dimensional representations of DSM-IV anxiety disorders. *Br J Psychiatry* 2009;**195**:301–307.

11. Young JP, Fenton, GW, Lader MH. The inheritance of neurotic traits: A twin study of the Middlesex Hospital Questionnaire. *Br J Psychiatry* 1971;**119**:393–398.

12. Torgersen S. The oral, obsessive, and hysterical personality syndromes. A study of hereditary and environmental factors by means of the twin method. *Arch Gen Psychiatry* 1980;**37**:1272–1277.

13. Clifford CA, Murray RM, Fulker DW. Genetic and environmental influences on obsessional traits and symptoms. *Psychol Med* 1984;**14**:791–800.

14. Jonnal AH, Gardner CO, Prescott CA, Kendler KS. Obsessive and compulsive symptoms in a general population sample of female twins. *Am J Med Genet* 2000;**96**:791–796.

15. Eley TC, Bolton D, O'Connor TG *et al.* A twin study of anxiety related behaviours in pre-school children. *J Child Psych Psychiat Allied Dis* 2003;**44**:945–960.

16. Hudziak JJ, van Beijsterveldt CEM, Althoff RR *et al.* Genetic and environmental contributions to the Child Behavior Checklist Obsessive-Compulsive Scale: A cross-cultural twin study. *Arch Gen Psychiatry* 2004;**61**:608–616.

17. Pauls DL, Raymond CL, Stevenson JM, Leckman JF. A family study of Gilles de la Tourette syndrome. *Am J Hum Genet* 1991;**48**:154–163.

18. Pauls DL, Alsobrook J 2nd, Goodman W *et al.* A family study of obsessive compulsive disorder. *Am J Psychiatry* 1995;**152**:76–84.

19. Grados MA, Riddle MA, Samuels JF *et al.* The familial phenotype of obsessive-compulsive disorder in relation to tic disorders: the Hopkins OCD family study. *Biol Psych* 2001;**50**:559–565.

20. Hanna GL, Veenstra-VanderWeele J, Cox NJ *et al.* Genome-wide linkage analysis of families with obsessive-compulsive disorder ascertained through pediatric probands. *Am J Med Genet (Neuropsych Genet)* 2002;**114**:541–552.

21. do Rosario-Campos MC, Leckman JF, Curi M *et al.* A family study of early-onset obsessive-compulsive disorder. *Am J Med Genet (Neuropsych Genet)* 2005;**136**:92–97.

22. Thompson WD, Weissman MM. Quantifying lifetime risk of psychiatric disorder. *J Psychiatr Res* 1981;**16**:113–126.

23. Gershon ES, Guroff JJ. Information from relatives. Diagnosis of affective disorders. *Arch Gen Psychiatry* 1984;**41**:173–180.

24. Luxenburger H. Heredität und Familientypus der Zwangsneurotiker. *Arch Psychiatr* 1930;**91**:590–594.

25. Lewis A. Problems of obsessional illness. *Proc R Soc Med* 1936;**29**:325–336.

26. Brown FW. Heredity in the psychoneuroses. Paper presented at the Royal Society of Medicine, 1942.

27. Rüdin E. Beitrag zur Frage der Zwangskrankheit, insbesondere ihrer hereditaren Beziehungen. *Arch Psychiatr Nervenkrankh* 1953;**191**:14–54.

28. Kringlen E. Obsessional neurotics: a long term follow-up. *Br J Psychiatry* 1965;**111**:709–722.

29. Rosenberg CM. Familial aspects of obsessional neurosis. *Br J Psychiatry* 1967;**113**:405–413.

30. Insel T, Hoover C, Murphy DL. Parents of patient with obsessive-compulsive disorder. *Psychol Med* 1983;**13**:807–811.

31. Rasmussen SA, Tsuang MT. Clinical characteristics and family history in DSM-III obsessive-compulsive disorder. *Am J Psychiatry* 1986;**143**:317–322.

32. McKeon P, Murray R. Familial aspects of obsessive-compulsive neurosis. *Br J Psychiatry* 1987;**151**:528–534.

33. Bellodi L, Sciuto G, Diaferia G. Psychiatric disorders in the families of patients with obsessive-compulsive disorder. *Psychiat Res* 1982;**42**:111–120.

34. Black DW, Noyes R Jr, Goldstein RB, Blum N. A family study of obsessive-compulsive disorder. *Arch Gen Psychiatry* 1992;**49**:362–368.

35. Nicolini H, Weissbecker K, Mejia JM *et al.* Family study of obsessive-compulsive disorder in a Mexican population. *Arch Med Res* 1993;**24**:193–198.

36. Nestadt G, Samuels J, Riddle MA *et al.* A family study of obsessive-compulsive disorder. *Arch Gen Psychiatry* 2000;**57**:358–363.

37. Albert U, Maina G, Ravizza L, Bogetto F. An exploratory study on obsessive-compulsive disorder with and without a familial component: are there any phenomenological differences? *Psychopathology* 2002;**35**:8–16.

38. Fyer AJ, Lipsitz JD, Mannuzza S *et al.* A direct interview family study of obsessive-compulsive disorder I. *Psychol Med* 2005;**35**:1611–1621.

39. Lipsitz JD, Manuzza S, Chapman TF *et al.* A direct interview family study of obsessive-compulsive disorder. II. Contribution of proband informant information. *Psychol Med* 2005;**35**:1623–1631.

40. Grabe HJ, Ruhrmann S, Ettelt S *et al.* Familiality of obsessive-compulsive disorder in nonclinical and clinical subjects. *Am J Psychiatry* 2006;**163**:1986–1992.

41. Lenane MC, Swedo SE, Leonard H *et al.* Psychiatric disorders in first degree relatives of children and adolescents with obsessive-compulsive disorder. *J Am Acad Child Adolesc Psychiat* 1990;**29**:407–412.

42. Riddle MA, Scahill L, King R *et al.* Obsessive compulsive disorder in children and adolescents: phenomenology and family history. *J Am Acad Child Adolesc Psychiat* 1990;**29**:766–772.

43. Leonard H, Lenane MC, Swedo SE *et al.* Tics and Tourette's disorder: a 2- to 7-year follow-up of 54 obsessive-compulsive children. *Am J Psychiatry* 1992;**149**:1244–1251.

44. Reddy PS, Reddy YC, Srinath S *et al.* A family study of juvenile obsessive-compulsive disorder. *Can J Psychiat* 2001;**46**:346–351.

45. Chabane N, Delorme R, Millet B *et al.* Early-onset obsessive-compulsive disorder: a subgroup with a specific clinical and familial pattern? *J Child Psychol Psychiat* 2005;**46**:881–887.

46. Leckman JF, Grice DE, Boardman J *et al.* Symptoms of obsessive-compulsive disorder. *Am J Psychiatry* 1997;**154**:911–917.

47. Stewart SE, Rosario MC, Brown TA *et al.* Principal components analysis of obsessive-compulsive disorder symptoms in children and adolescents. *Biol Psych* 2007;**61**:285–291.

48. Hasler G, Pinto A, Greenberg BD, *et al.* Familiality of factor analysis-derived YBOCS dimensions in OCD-affected sibling pairs from the OCD Collaborative Genetics Study. *Biol Psychiat* 2007;**61**:617–625.

49. Pinto A, Greenberg BD, Grados MA *et al.* Further development of YBOCS dimensions in the OCD Collaborative Genetics study: symptoms vs. categories. *Psychiat Res* 2008;**160**:83–93.

50. Arnold PD, Richter MA, Mundo E *et al.* Quantitative and qualitative traits in obsessive-compulsive disorder: association with a glutamate receptor gene. *Int J Neuropsychopharmacol* 2002;**5**(S1):S116.

51. Dickel, DE, Veenstra-VanderWeele J, Cox NJ *et al.* Association testing of the positional and functional candidate gene SLC1A1/EAAC1 in early-onset obsessive-compulsive disorder. *Arch Gen Psychiatry* 2006;**63**:778–785.

52. Bienvenu OJ, Samuels JF, Riddle MA, *et al.* (2000) The relationship of obsessive–compulsive disorder to possible spectrum disorders: results from a family study. *Biol Psychiat* **48**, 287–293.

53. Grados MA, Riddle MA, Samuels JF, *et al.* (2001) The familial phenotype of obsessive–compulsive disorder in relation to tic disorders: the Hopkins OCD family study. *Biol Psych* **50**, 559–565.

54. Hettema JM, Neale MC, Kendler KS. (2001) A review and meta–analysis of the genetic epidemiology of anxiety disorders. *Am J Psychiat* **158**, 1568–1578.

55. Nicolini H, Hanna GL, Baxter L *et al.* (1991) Segregation analysis of obsessive compulsive disorders. Preliminary results. *Ursus Medicus.* **1**, 25–28.

56. Alsobrook JP, II, Leckman JF, Goodman WK *et al.* (1999) Segregation analysis of obsessive–compulsive disorder using symptom–based factor scores. *Am J Med Genet* **88**, 669–675.

57. Cavallini MC, Bertelli S, Chiapparino D *et al.* (2000) Complex segregation analysis of obsessive–compulsive disorder in 141 families of eating disorder probands, with and without obsessive–compulsive disorder. *Am J Med Genet (Neuropsych Genet)* **96**, 384–391.

58. Nestadt G, Lan T, Samuels J, *et al.* (2000) Complex segregation analysis provides compelling evidence for a major gene underlying obsessive–compulsive disorder and for heterogeneity by sex. *Amn J Hum Genet* **67**, 1611–1616.

59. Summerfeldt LJ, Richter MA, Antony MM, Swinson RP. Symptom structure in obsessive-compulsive disorder: a confirmatory factor-analytic study. *Behav Res Therapy* 1999;**37**:297–311.

60. Arnold PD, Sicard T, Burroughs E, Richter MA, Kennedy JL. Glutamate transporter gene SLC1A1 associated with obsessive-compulsive disorder. *Arch Gen Psychiatry* 2006;**63**:769–776.

61. Stewart SE, Fagerness JA, Platko J *et al.* Association of the SLC1A1 glutamate transporter gene and obsessive-compulsive disorder. *Am J Med Genet (Neuropsychiatr Genet)* 2007;**144**:1027–1033.

62. Wendland JR, Moya PR, Timpano KR *et al.* A haplotype containing quantitative trait loci for SLC1A1 gene expression and its association with obsessive-compulsive disorder. *Arch Gen Psychiatry* 2009;66:408–416.

63. Wang Y, Adamczyk A, Shugart YY *et al.* A screen of SLC1A1 for OCD-related alleles. *Am J Med Genet B Neuropsychiatr Genet* 2010;**153B**:675–679.

64. Wendland JR, Moya PR, Kruse MR *et al.* A novel, putative gain-of-function haplotype at SLC6A4 associates with obsessive-compulsive disorder. *Hum Mol Genet* 2008;**17**:717–723.

65. McDougle CJ, Epperson CN, Price LH *et al.* Evidence for linkage disequilibrium between serotonin transporter protein gene (SLC6A4) and obsessive compulsive disorder. *Mol Psychiatry* 1998;**3**:270–273.

66. Bengel D, Greenberg BD, Cora-Locatelli G *et al.* Association of the serotonin transporter promoter regulatory region polymorphism and obsessive-compulsive disorder. *Mol Psychiatry* 1999;**4**:463–466.

67. Frisch A, Michaelovsky E, Rockah R *et al.* Association between obsessive-compulsive disorder and polymorphisms of genes encoding components of the serotonergic and dopaminergic pathways. *Eur Neuropsychopharmacol* 2000;**10**:205–209.

68. Kinnear CJ, Niehaus DJ, Moolman-Smook JC *et al.* Obsessive-compulsive disorder and the promoter region polymorphism (5-HTTLPR) in the serotonin transporter gene (SLC6A4): a negative association study in the Afrikaner population. *Int J Neuropsychopharmacol* 2000;**3**:327–331.

69. Denys D, Van Nieuwerburgh F, Deforce D, Westenberg HGM. Association between serotonergic candidate genes and specific phenotypes of obsessive compulsive disorder. *J Aff Disord* 2006;**91**:39–70.

70. Dickel DE, Veenstra-VanderWeele J, Bivens NC *et al.* Association studies of serotonin system candidate genes in early-onset obsessive-compulsive disorder. *Biol Psychiatry* 2007;**61**:322–329.

71. Saiz PA, Garcia-Portilla MP, Arango C *et al.* Association study between obsessive-compulsive disorder and serotonergic candidate genes. *Prog in Neuro-Psychopharmacol Biol Psychiatry* 2008;**32**:765–770.

72. Wendland JR, Kruse MR, Cromer KC, Murphy DL. A large case-control study of common functional SLC6A4 and BDNF variants in obsessive-compulsive disorder. *Neuropsychopharmacol* 2007;**32**:2543–2551.

73. Kinnear CJ, Niehaus DJ, Moolman-Smook JC *et al.* Obsessive-compulsive disorder and the promoter region polymorphism (5-HTTLPR) in the serotonin transporter gene (SLC6A4): a negative association study in the Afrikaner population. *Int J Neuropsychopharmacol* 2000;**3**:327–331.

74. Camarena B, Rinetti G, Cruz C *et al.* Association study of the serotonin transporter gene polymorphism in obsessive-compulsive disorder. *Int J Neuropsychopharmacol* 2001;**4**:269–272.

75. Cavallini MC, Di Bella D, Siliprandi F *et al.* Exploratory factor analysis of obsessive-compulsive patients and association with 5-HTTLPR polymorphism. *Am J Med Genet* 2002;**114**:347–353.

76. Walitza S, Wewetzer C, Gerlach M *et al.* Transmission disequilibrium studies in children and adolescents with obsessive-compulsive disorders pertaining to polymorphisms of genes of the serotonergic pathway. *J Neural Transm* 2004;**111**:817–825.

77. Meira-Lima I, Shavitt RG, Miguita K *et al*. Association analysis of the catechol-O-methyltransferase (COMT), serotonin transporter (5-HTT) and serotonin 2A receptor (5HT2A) gene polymorphisms with obsessive-compulsive disorder. *Genes Brain Behav* 2004;**3**:75–79.

78. Chabane N, Millet B, Delorme R *et al*. Lack of evidence for association between serotonin transporter gene (5-HTTLPR) and obsessive-compulsive disorder by case control and family association study in humans. *Neurosci Lett* 2004;**363**:154–156.

79. Nicolini H, Cruz C, Camarena B *et al*. DRD2, DRD3and 5HT2A receptor genes polymorphisms in obsessive-compulsive disorder. *Mol Psychiatry* 1996;**1**:461–465.

80. Enoch MA, Kaye WH, Rotondo A *et al*. 5-HT2A promoter polymorphism –1438G/A, anorexia nervosa, and obsessive-compulsive disorder. *Lancet* 1998;**351**:1785–1786.

81. Enoch MA, Greenberg BD, Murphy DL *et al*. Sexually dysmorphic relationship of a 5-HT2A promoter polymorphism with obsessive-compulsive disorder. *Biol Psychiatry* 2001;**49**:385–388.

82. Walitza S, Wewetzer C, Warnke A *et al*. 5-HT2A promoter polymorphism –1438G/A in children and adolescents with obsessive-compulsive disorders. *Mol Psychiatry* 2002;**7**:1054–1057.

83. Hemmings SM, Kinnear CJ, Niehaus DJ *et al*. Investigating the role of dopaminergic and serotonergic candidate genes in obsessive-compulsive disorder. *Eur Neuropsychopharmacol* 2003;**13**:93–98.

84. Tot S, Erdal ME, Yazici K *et al*. T102C and –1438 G/A polymorphisms of the 5-HT2A receptor gene in Turkish patients with obsessive-compulsive disorder. *Eur Psychiatry* 2003;**18**:249–254.

85. Hemmings SM, Kinnear CJ, Lochner C *et al*. Early- versus late-onset obsessive-compulsive disorder: investigating genetic and clinical correlates. *Psychiatry Res* 2004;**128**:175–182.

86. Cavallini MC, Di Bella D, Pasquale L *et al*. 5HT2C CYS23/SER23 polymorphism is not associated with obsessive-compulsive disorder. *Psychiatry Res* 1998;**77**:97–104.

87. Mundo E, Richter MA, Sam F *et al*. Is the 5-HT(1Dbeta) receptor gene implicated in the pathogenesis of obsessive-compulsive disorder? *Am J Psychiatry* 2000;**157**:1160–1161.

88. Mundo E, Richter MA, Zai G *et al*. 5HT1Dbeta receptor gene implicated in the pathogenesis of obsessive-compulsive disorder: further evidence from a family-based association study. *Mol Psychiatry* 2002;**7**:805–809.

89. Di Bella D, Cavallini MC, Bellodi L. No association between obsessive-compulsive disorder and the 5-HT(1Dbeta) receptor gene. *Am J Psychiatry* 2002;**159**:1783–1785.

90. Camarena B, Aguilar A, Loyzaga C *et al*. A family-based association study of the 5-HT-1Dbeta receptor gene in obsessive-compulsive disorder. *Int J Neuropsychopharmacol* 2004;**7**:49–53.

91. Mössner R, Walitza S, Geller F *et al*. Transmission disequilibrium of polymorphic variants in the tryptophan hydroxylase-2 gene in children and adolescents with obsessive-compulsive disorder. *Int J Neuropsychopharmacol* 2005;**9**:1–6.

92. Cruz C, Camarena B, King N *et al*. Increased prevalence of the seven-repeat variant of the dopamine D4 receptor gene in patients with obsessive-compulsive disorder with tics. *Neurosci Lett* 1997;**231**:1–4.

93. Billet EA, Richter MA, Sam F *et al*. Investigation of dopamine system genes in obsessive compulsive disorder. *Psychiatr Genet* 1998;**8**:163–169.

94. Millet B, Chabane N, Delorme R *et al*. Association between the dopamine receptor D4 (DRD4) gene and obsessive-compulsive disorder. *Am J Med Genet* 2003;**116**: 55–59.

95. Catalano M, Sciuto G, Di Bella D *et al*. Lack of association between obsessive-compulsive disorder and the dopamine D3 receptor gene: some preliminary considerations. *Am J Med Genet* 1994;**54**:253–255.

96. Karayiorgou M, Altemus M, Galke BL *et al*. Genotype determining low catechol-O-methyltransferase activity as a risk factor for obsessive-compulsive disorder. *Proc Natl Acad Sci USA* 1997;**94**:4572–4575.

97. Karayiorgou M, Sobin C, Blundell ML *et al*. Family-based association studies support a sexually dimorphic effect of COMT and MAOA on genetic susceptibility to obsessive compulsive disorder. *Biol Psychiatry* 1999;**45**:1178–1189.

98. Schindler KM, Richter MA, Kennedy JL, *et al*. Association between homozygosity at the COMT gene locus and obsessive compulsive disorder. *Am J Med Genet* 2000;**96**:721–724.

99. Niehaus DJ, Kinnear CJ, Corfield VA *et al*. Association between a catechol-O-methyltransferase polymorphism and obsessive-compulsive disorder in the Afrikaner population. *J Affect Disord* 2001;**65**:61–65.

100. Alsobrook JP, Zohar AH, Leboyer M *et al*. Association between the COMT locus and obsessive-compulsive disorder in females but not males. *Am J Med Genet* 2002;**114**:116–120.

101. Ohara K, Nagai M, Suzuki Y *et al*. No association between anxiety disorders and catechol-O-methyltransferase polymorphism. *Psychiatry Res* 1998;**80**:145–148.

102. Erdal ME, Tot S, Yazici K *et al*. Lack of association of catechol-O-methyltransferase gene polymorphism in obsessive-compulsive disorder. *Depress Anxiety* 2003;**18**:41–45.

103. Azzam A, Mathews CA. Meta-analysis of the association between the catecholamine-O-methyltransferase gene and obsessive-compulsive disorder. *Am J Med Genet* 2003;**123B**:64–69.

104. Katerberg H, Cath D, Denys D *et al*. An association study of the COMT Val[158]Met genotype with factor-analysed Y-BOCS symptom category scores: preliminary findings. *Am J Med Genet B* 2010;**153B**:167–176.

105. Arnold PD, Rosenberg DR, Mundo E *et al*. Association of a glutamate (NMDA) subunit receptor gene (GRIN2B) with obsessive-compulsive disorder: a preliminary study. *Psychopharmacology (Berl)* 2004;**174**:530–538.

106. Delorme R, Krebs MO, Chabane N *et al*. Frequency and transmission of glutamate receptors GRIK2 and GRIK3 polymorphisms in patients with obsessive compulsive disorder. *Neuroreport* 2004;**15**:699–702.

107. Zai G, Arnold P, Burroughs E *et al*. Evidence for the gamma-amino-butyric acid type B receptor 1 (GABBR1) gene as a susceptibility factor in obsessive-compulsive disorder. *Am J Med Genet* 2005;**134B**:25–29.

108. Hall D, Dhilla A, Charalambous A *et al*. Sequence variants of the brain-derived neurotrophic factor (BDNF) gene are strongly associated with obsessive-compulsive disorder. *Am J Hum Genet* 2003;**73**:370–376.

109. Zai G, Bezchlibnyk YB, Richter MA *et al*. Myelin oligodendrocyte glycoprotein (MOG) gene is associated with obsessive-compulsive disorder. *Am J Med Genet* 2004;**129B**:64–68.

110. Stewart SE, Platko J, Fagerness J *et al*. A genetic family-based association study of OLIG2 in obsessive-compulsive disorder. *Arch Gen Psychiatry* 2007;**64**:209–214.

111. Muiños-Gimeno M, Guidi M, Kagerbauer B *et al*. Allele variants in functional microRNA target sites of the neurotrophin-3 receptor gene (NTRK3) as susceptibility factors for anxiety disorders. *Hum Mutat* 2009;**30**:1062–1071.

112. Lazar A, Walitza S, Jetter A *et al*. Novel mutations of the extraneuronal monoamine transporter gene in children and adolescents with obsessive-compulsive disorder. *Int J Neuropsychopharmacol* 2008;**11**:35–48.

113. Boardman L, van der Merwe L, Lochner C *et al*. Investigating SAPAP3 variants in the etiology of obsessive-compulsive disorder and trichotillomania in the South African white population. *Compr Psychiatry* 2011;**52**:181–187.

114. Hemmings SM, Stein DJ. The current status of association studies in obsessive-compulsive disorder. *Psychiat Clinics North Am* 2006;**29**:411–444 .

115. Shugart YY, Samuels J, Willour VL *et al*. Genome wide linkage scan for obsessive-compulsive disorder: evidence for susceptibility loci on chromosomes 3q, 7p, 1q, 15q, and 6q. *Mol Psychiatry* 2006;**11**:763–770.

116. Hanna GL, Veenstra-Vanderweele J, Cox NJ *et al*. Evidence for a susceptibility locus on chromosome 10p15 in early-onset obsessive-compulsive disorder. *Biol Psychiatry* 2007;**62**:856–862.

117. Willour VL, Yao Shugart Y, Samuels J *et al*. Replication study supports evidence for linkage to 9p24 in obsessive-compulsive disorder. *Am J Hum Genet* 2004;**75**:508–513.

118. Samuels J, Shugart YY, Grados MA *et al*. Significant linkage to compulsive hoarding on chromosome 14 in families with obsessive-compulsive disorder: results from the OCD Collaborative Genetics Study. *Am J Psychiatry* 2007;**164**:493–499.

119. Greenberg DA, Abreu P, Hodge SE. The power to detect linkage in complex disease by means of simple LOD-score analyses. *Am J Hum Genet* 1998;**63**:870–879.

120. Leboyer M, Bellivier F, Nosten-Bertrand M *et al*. Psychiatric genetics: search for phenotypes. *Trends Neurosci* 1998;**21**:102–105.

CHAPTER 12

Neurocognitive Angle: The Search for Endophenotypes

Samuel R. Chamberlain and Lara Menzies

Department of Psychiatry, University of Cambridge, Box 189,
Addenbrooke's Hospital, Cambridge, CB2 0QQ, UK

INTRODUCTION

Obsessive-compulsive disorder (OCD) is a prevalent neuropsychiatric disorder characterized by maladaptive perseverative patterns of thought and behaviour, which suggest underlying dysregulation of cognitive processes and their affiliated brain substrates and neurochemical systems [1,2]. Despite considerable research, the aetiology of OCD, as with many complex Axis-I psychiatric disorders, remains far from clear. This is unfortunate given that the lifetime prevalence of OCD is estimated at 2–3% [3], and that OCD mediates a considerable burden in terms of deleterious effects on quality of life and everyday functioning [4]. From an economic perspective, OCD is also damaging: annual impact on the US economy has been estimated at 8 billion USD or greater [5]. Similar proportions of males and females are affected, and OCD typically initiates in late adolescence or early adulthood, often following a chronic course into older age [6].

There has been a shift in recent years towards considering OCD from the point of view of neural circuitry within the brain [1,7]. This chapter considers OCD from the 'neurocognitive angle', by which is meant that OCD be considered from the point of view of the underlying neurobiology. Central to this approach, as will be outlined, is the notion of hierarchical models of the disorder and the search for intermediate brain-based markers that occupy a position on the chain of pathogenesis between 'bottom level' genetic factors, and the overt 'top level' manifestation of OCD symptoms, that is, the obsessions and/or compulsions. Rather than studying OCD from a phenomenological perspective, we encourage dissection of the underlying cognitive problems and ask whether such problems might indeed predispose towards the development of the condition. Another important feature of

Obsessive-Compulsive Disorder: Current Science and Clinical Practice, First Edition. Edited by Joseph Zohar.
© 2012 John Wiley & Sons, Ltd. Published 2012 by John Wiley & Sons, Ltd.

this approach is the use of translational medicine: by modelling aspects of OCD and its neurocognitive sequelae across species, considerable light can be shed on the underlying implicated brain regions and neurotransmitter systems [8–10]. It is worth noting here that intermediate cognitive markers of OCD may be easier to model than OCD symptoms per se across species: the recurrent intrusive thoughts characteristic of OCD are not amenable to this approach at all; and while compulsions can be modelled in animals, they often bear limited face validity in relation to those symptoms manifested in patients. In contrast, specific neurocognitive tests tapping aspects of inhibitory control and cognitive flexibility have been applied across species and have in some cases been shown to have comparable neural substrates [10–13].

In this chapter, we begin by outlining the heritability of OCD and use this as a springboard for introducing the concept of endophenotypes in psychiatry and in medicine more broadly, and provide examples of their utility. We then provide a hierarchical model of OCD and identify key areas that may be fruitful in the search for intermediate brain-based markers of disease. Findings from OCD endophenotyping studies to date are surveyed and summarized, alongside their limitations. We discuss the implications of these results and unanswered questions and how these may be addressed in future work.

HERITABILITY OF OCD

With regard to the aetiology of OCD, the disorder has been shown to be of moderate heritability (see Chapter 11 for in-depth discussion). This is a complex field, with studies indicating that OCD has multifactorial roots, with both environmental and genetic contributions. Twin and family studies have provided logical starting points for the investigation of the role of genetics in OCD pathophysiology and were being conducted as long ago as the 1920s (for comprehensive review see refs [14,15]).

Family studies of OCD have found there to be an increased risk of obsessive-compulsive symptoms in first-degree relatives of an affected individual or 'proband'; results from 22 family studies have been recently reviewed and indicate that OCD is familial [15]. For example, this first-degree relative risk has been estimated at between 8.2% and 11.7% compared with a background population risk of 2% in control relatives [16–18]. An intrinsic caveat to such studies must, however, be noted; family studies cannot control for joint environmental influences on both relative and proband. The information they produce can therefore only provide evidence for familiality as opposed to confirmed heritability of obsessive-compulsive symptoms.

Twin studies have probed the heritability of OCD further, making use of their unique opportunity to control for shared environmental factors. Twin studies have indicated monozygotic concordance rates as high as 87% for obsessive symptoms or features, compared to dizygotic rates of 47% [19]. Of note, many of the older twin studies, whilst at least sparking interest in a genetic aetiology, attract criticism due to: (i) unclear methods of zygosity determination; (ii) lack of blinding procedures; (iii) heterogeneity in terms of diagnostic and symptomatic categorization (e.g. in terms of distinguishing between OCD vs obsessive-compulsive personality traits); and (iv) lack of exclusion of individuals with other psychiatric comorbidities.

More recent twin studies, using more robust inclusion criteria in combination with sophisticated modelling techniques such as structural equation modelling (SEM) to assess multivariate genotypic and environmental effects on phenotype, have been regarded as more convincing. For example, Hudziak *et al.* used a SEM twin study approach, finding a genetic influence of 55% on obsessional behaviour in children, as compared to 45% for environmental factors [20]. The findings of twin studies regarding OCD have been comprehensively reviewed by van Grootheest *et al.*, who concluded that obsessive-compulsive symptoms are heritable, with a genetic influence of 45–65% in children, and 27–47% in adults [14].

Once reasonable evidence has been amassed to indicate the at least partial genetic basis of a disorder, a logical progression is to search for specific genetic models that can account for family transmission and phenotypic variation, that is, to hunt for specific chromosomal loci at which genetic variance significantly impacts upon phenotypic variation. Two genetic linkage studies (involving initially seven families and then 50 pedigrees) suggested a susceptibility locus on chromosome 9 at the locus 9p24 [21,22]. This finding has generated significant interest since a neuronal glutamate transporter entitled SLC1A1 is encoded by a gene at this locus; several groups have gone on to identify an association with OCD for a number of single nucleotide polymorphisms (SNPs) within this gene [23–25].

However, the linkage findings to chromosome 9 were not replicated in a subsequent larger (219 families) genome-wide linkage study, which found loci on chromosomes 1, 3, 6, 7, 15 and 16, with the strongest evidence for a region on chromosome 3 [26]. These rather variable results are frustrating for the field; however, it must be remembered that the clinical criteria currently used for assigning a diagnosis of OCD are somewhat subjective and likely subtended by a heterogeneous group of pathologies at the biological level and contributed to by a number of genetic and environmental factors. There have also now been over 80 candidate gene studies, which, except for the glutamate transporter gene discussed above, have not been replicated [27]. Again this is likely to reflect a need to more precisely define the phenotype with which we are looking for association. The endophenotype concept is designed to facilitate this process and so will be discussed further below.

THE CONCEPT OF AN ENDOPHENOTYPE

The term 'endophenotype' was first coined in the 1960s, and can be broadly defined as an objectively measurable component that cannot be seen by the unaided eye, which occupies a location on the pathway between distal genotype and disease [28–30]. It will be seen that, implicit in this definition, is the notion that technology will likely be required for discerning such a measure. Since its introduction, this term has attracted considerable scientific interest, especially in neuropsychiatry where illnesses are often polygenic, involving multiple subtle gene × environment interactions [31]. Such research was also driven in part by frustration at attempts to correlate subjectively assessed overt symptoms with genetic polymorphisms.

The notion of an endophenotype has evolved and today is held to represent a heritable quantitative trait associated with increased risk of disease and therefore present at unexpectedly high rates not only in patients with a given disorder but also in unaffected first-degree relatives of such patients [32]. Critically, the presence of an endophenotype does not automatically lead to the manifestation of clinical disease. Rather, it may be viewed as a heritable predisposing risk factor. The effects of such risk factors may be small individually, but cumulatively can contribute to the disorder, as per multifactorial threshold models of disease, which hold that many factors (genetic and environmental) contribute cumulatively.

In the study of complex polygenic disorders, epigenetic and pleiotropic mechanisms may also play a role. Epigenetic processes affect the phenotype without changing the underlying DNA sequence – for example, imprinting, X chromosome inactivation and DNA methylation. Such epigenetic processes have been implicated in schizophrenia but may also be important in OCD [33]. Pleiotropy refers to a single gene exhibiting multiple defects in different cell types over time, such that a single genetic variation can subtend overarching and profound effects on the organism in question. For example, transcription factors can mediate a variety of effects across cell lines through complex roles in gene expression/regulation. Therefore, pleiotropic transcription factor mutations could contribute to the heterogeneous nature of the symptoms of neuropsychiatric disorders.

The utility of endophenotyping has been demonstrated in multiple non-psychiatric contexts. For example, certain people are predisposed to a cardiac syndrome that includes dysrhythmias and sudden cardiac death. Research has identified unduly prolonged QT intervals on electrocardiograms in affected individuals with this cardiac syndrome and in their asymptomatic close relatives. Linkage and association studies used prolonged QT intervals as an effective intermediate marker to identify a susceptibility locus on chromosome 11. Initially, it was thought that the Harvey-ras-1 gene was important [34] but subsequent work suggested that the implicated gene was *LVKQT1*, a gene coding for voltage-gated potassium channels [35]. Thus, genetic factors were identified by means of an intermediate marker or candidate endophenotype.

The potential value of endophenotypes has been explored in the context of several psychiatric conditions, but perhaps most convincingly in the context of schizophrenia, a highly heritable condition associated with abnormalities of cognition and perception [36]. We provide here, in brief, an example of an endophenotype that has generated significant advances in schizophrenia research.

Difficulties filtering out extraneous stimuli have long been implicated in the pathophysiology of the disorder. One paradigm used to explore sensory gating defects in schizophrenia is the P50 model [37]. In brief, subjects hear a series of pairs of loud clicks and the brain responses are recorded using EEG. The P50 wave is a positive wave recorded at the top of the head 50 milliseconds after the occurrence of a given click. In health, the P50 amplitude to the second click is diminished relative to the first click (i.e., low test:conditioning amplitude ratio) due to neuronal inhibition/filtering mechanisms (see, e.g., ref. [37]). In initial work, impaired P50 gating (increased test:conditioning amplitude ratios) was reported in patients with schizophrenia, and in their unaffected first-degree relatives, versus controls [38]. The neurobiological mechanism of P50 inhibition was subsequently explored using translational modelling in rats and in humans, which suggested involvement of the hippocampal pyramidal neurons and the alpha7-nicotinic cholinergic receptor subunit [39,40]. In a genetic linkage study, Freedman and colleagues then found evidence linking impaired P50 inhibition to a polymorphism at chromosome 15q13-14 – the site of the gene encoding the above-named nicotinic subreceptor, suggesting that this gene may account for the inheritance of this candidate endophenotype [39]. Follow-up studies supported this proposition [41], and contributed to the recent exploration of nicotinic-modulating drugs in the treatment of schizophrenia and cognitive deficits therein [42]. In sum, the initial identification of a physiological-cognitive candidate endophenotype for schizophrenia spurred several decades of exciting research with implications for understanding the neurobiology of the disorder and its pharmacological treatment [43,44].

Why might the endophenotype construct be valuable in the study of OCD? As with other Axis-I disorders, the study of the genetic basis of OCD has met with limited success [15], probably for several reasons. It is recognized that OCD is a heterogeneous disorder and that the definition of the disorder itself, as described in the *International Classification of Diseases, Tenth Revision* (ICD-10) or the *Diagnostic and Statistical Manual of Mental Disorders, Fourth Edition* (DSM-IV), is relatively subjective and arbitrary. It is probable that broad phenotypes such as ICD-10/DSM-IV OCD encompass much heterogeneity, with several different genetic factors impacting different levels of the organism, yet with these specific and differing influences being indistinguishable at the level of the phenotype. The diagnosis of OCD itself is dependent on subjective interpretation of clinical criteria. Dissecting these underlying factors and understanding the interplay between them could thus be valuable and yield more objective diagnostic criteria for this and other disorders [45]. Another issue is the complexity of the human brain, as opposed – for example – to other organs within the body. The human brain contains approximately 20 billion neocortical neurons, each of which has around 7000 synaptic connections [46]. The endophenotype strategy may help to break down this organ and its machinations into more tractable and comprehensible markers whose relationship with genes can then be explored.

Endophenotypes may thus be valuable in dissecting complex polygenic disorders such as OCD. Candidate markers may be (*inter alia*) symptom-derived, personality-derived, physiological, biochemical, endocrinological, neuroanatomical/functional or cognitive in nature. As will be described, markers can even combine several of these domains. It is hoped that the validation of objective, reliable traits would lead to improved diagnostic precision, improved neurobiological models, and reduction of the inherent heterogeneity subtended at the level of clinical diagnosis.

APPLYING THE ENDOPHENOTYPE CONSTRUCT TO OCD

Complex polygenetic disorders like OCD and other neuropsychiatric disorders such as schizophrenia, depression and attention-deficit disorder, known to have a multifactorial aetiology, provide a difficult challenge when it comes to deciphering their pathophysiology. The endophenotype concept, outlined above, can be invoked to help deconstruct this complexity into more manageable elements. In order to do this, it is necessary to form a hierarchical disease model that considers the steps between genotype and phenotype, and the potential impact of environmental factors at each level (Figure 12.1). For example, it is well established that our genotype modulates protein composition and structure, which may therefore impact on both that protein's function and subsequently the function of the cell in which that protein has been translated. Various cell types working in synergy will lead to effects at what can be considered a systems-based level within a tissue or organ. This can generate changes in our behaviours, for example cognition, and ultimately affect the phenotype, which can be considered the final step in the hierarchy.

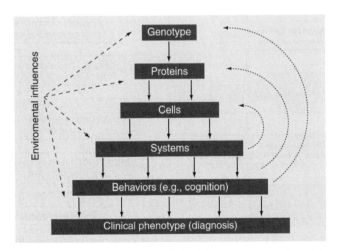

Figure 12.1   The generic hierarchical model of disease. Reproduced from Chamberlain SR, Menzies L. *Expert Rev Neurother* 2009;**9**(8):1133–1146, with permission of Expert Reviews Ltd.

An important consideration is that environmental factors can also impact upon function at all of the levels discussed. To consider a simple example, change in temperature could directly lead to modifications at the level of gene expression, protein function (consider enzymes) and behaviour (essentially thermoregulation). A further complexity to such a model are the notions of epigenetics and pleiotropy. As discussed earlier, these phenomena can provide an alternative explanation other than classical gene inheritance for potentially phenotypic changes.

With regard to OCD, the hierarchical model can be conceived as displayed in Figure 12.2; changes in genotype may impact upon protein function, which therefore affects neuronal development and function. This is likely therefore to influence how both neural networks and the brain as a whole operate at a systems level, ultimately leading to changes in cognitive behaviour and the complex phenotype of clinically observed OCD. Key evidence for this model comes from the finding that brain structure is known to be highly heritable [47–49]; our understanding of how brain structure impacts upon brain function and cognition is currently fairly limited, but has been advancing rapidly as a result of the availability of neuroimaging such as positron emission tomography (PET) and functional magnetic resonance imaging (fMRI), together with neurocognitive testing facilities.

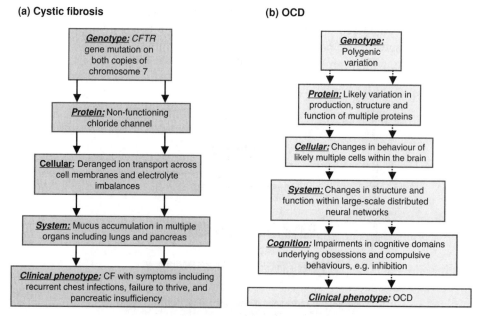

Figure 12.2 Applying the hierarchical model (a) to an example of a monogenic disorder, cystic fibrosis, the disease mechanism of which is well-elucidated (continuous arrows); and (b) to obsessive-compulsive disorder (OCD) as a hypothesis for level-based investigation (dotted arrows).

The situation with OCD is of course complicated by our understanding of OCD as a polygenic disorder; whereas the direct impact of genotype at each hierarchical level is well understood for monogenic diseases with a simple mendelian inheritance pattern such as cystic fibrosis (see Figure 12.2), the impact of multiple genes and resulting interactions at each level is not straightforward. Currently, with the existing heterogeneous and clinically based criteria for phenotypic classification, compounded by a polygenic aetiology with considerable influence from environmental factors, the search for specific genes involved in obsessive-compulsive phenotypes is extremely challenging. The aim of endophenotypes is to reduce that complexity by identifying 'intermediate phenotypes' of obsessive-compulsive behaviours. By virtue of their position more proximal to genotype than is the clinical phenotype, it is postulated that these 'intermediate phenotypes' will be more directly related to genetic function.

DOMAINS OF INTEREST IN HIERARCHICAL MODELLING OF OCD

Cognition

Over the past 20 years, many studies have investigated cognitive functions in patients with OCD compared to healthy volunteers and, in some instances, other clinical groups (for reviews see, e.g., refs [2,50]). Results are inconsistent, reflecting factors such as presence of comorbidities (e.g. depression, which is itself associated with cognitive dysfunction), treatment history (psychological and pharmacological) and the different tasks deployed (which varied in their likely neural and neurochemical substrates, and psychometric properties). Researchers have focused on several broad domains: memory (given that the repetitive symptoms of OCD could suggest mnemonic failures), motor inhibitory control (since repetitive behaviours that are difficult to suppress suggest dysfunction in this ability), decision-making (OCD has been conceptualized by some as a condition characterized by dysfunctional decision-making mechanisms) and cognitive flexibility (repetitive behaviours suggest problems with flexibly altering behaviour in light of changing environmental feedback). Indeed, it is these domains that may be useful in the search for cognitive endophenotypes of OCD. A focus on these functions also has support from knowledge of the implicated fronto-striatal brain circuitry (discussed later). Here, we consider an initial study that provided the groundwork for subsequent endophenotyping work, which assessed two cognitive functions using translational paradigms in patients with OCD.

We assessed response inhibition and cognitive flexibility in 20 patients with OCD (washers/checkers), 17 patients with trichotillomania (pathological hair pulling) and 20 healthy controls [51]. Response inhibition was quantified using the stop-signal test (SST), which requires volunteers to make rapid responses to a series of directional arrows appearing one at a time on a computer screen [52,53]. Appearance of a left arrow necessitates a left button response and vice versa. On a subset of SST trials, a 'stop signal' occurs in the form of an auditory beep, which signals to the volunteer that they should attempt to suppress the response for that one trial. By varying the time between presentation of the go cue and the stop signal dynamically, the SST quantifies inhibitory control in terms of the stop-signal reaction time (SSRT), with longer SSRTs corresponding to poorer motor inhibitory control.

This cognitive function is dependent on distributed neural circuitry including the right inferior frontal gyrus [54,55] and appears to be dependent on noradrenergic and possibly dopaminergic transmission across species [56–61]. Cognitive flexibility was assessed using the Intra-dimensional/Extra-dimensional (IDED) set-shift task from the Cambridge Neuropsychological Test Automated Battery (CANTAB). On the IDED task, subjects attempt to select the 'correct' picture from a choice of two presented on-screen by a computer; there is an underlying rule governing which of the two pictures is correct at any time. Through trial and error ('correct' or 'incorrect' appearing on-screen), subjects learn this rule. One learning criterion is obtained, the computer alters the rule, and the subject must show cognitive flexibility. Essentially this task decomposes several aspects of rule learning and flexibility and is derived from the Wisconsin Card Sorting Test of frontal lobe integrity. Extra-Dimensional (ED) shifting is dependent on neural circuitry including the ventrolateral prefrontal cortices across species [62,63].

It was found that patients with OCD and patients with trichotillomania showed impaired response inhibition on the SST, compared to controls. In contrast, only patients with OCD showed cognitive inflexibility on the IDED task, making more errors before succeeding in shifting their attention between stimulus dimensions (ED shifting). These findings suggested overlapping problems with motor inhibition between these two putatively related disorders, but that cognitive problems in OCD extended to other domains that are spared in trichotillomania, such as the ability to inhibit and shift attention away from one aspect of the environment to another. We can infer from these data more specific neural dysfunction in trichotillomania, perhaps limited to the right frontal gyrus, anterior cingulate cortex and connections, with more generalized dysfunction in OCD, extending to more lateral aspects of the prefrontal cortices.

Neuroimaging

The 1980s heralded the start of brain imaging in the field of OCD. This was an exciting era since it highlighted a role for organic dysfunction in OCD, greatly strengthening neurobiological models of this disorder. The initial studies used PET and were functional metabolic protocols that used radiographic labelling of glucose to investigate metabolic activity in the brains of people with OCD compared to healthy controls, either at rest or following symptom provocation [64–70]. Findings from these studies suggested fairly consistently that there was increased metabolic activity in bilateral orbitofrontal cortex in patients compared to controls. Striatal regions were also implicated in a number of studies, but with variable findings as to whether metabolism was increased or decreased. Explanations for variation in study findings could include (i) variation in study design (i.e. whether the study was performed at rest or during a specific behavioural paradigm); (ii) the frequent inclusion of individuals suffering from psychiatric comorbidities; and (iii) variation in whether or not patients were taking medication (there is some evidence to indicate medication effects on brain metabolism in patients with OCD [71]).

The results from these initial PET studies helped to formulate the 'orbito-fronto-striatal' cortical loop hypothesis of OCD. This relied upon a concept developed predominantly from animal studies, which suggested that there are a number of relatively discrete fronto-striatal circuits operating in the mammalian brain, involving parallel connections between somewhat functionally segregated areas of frontal cortex and basal ganglia (Figure 12.3) [72]. This body of research provided evidence to suggest the existence of a lateral orbitofrontal circuit that included

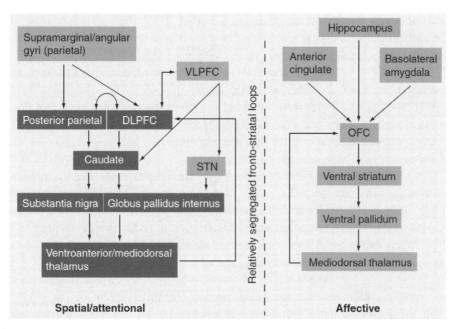

Figure 12.3 Fronto-striatal loop circuitry implicated in the pathophysiology of obsessive-compulsive disorder (OCD). OFC, orbitofrontal cortex; VLPFC, ventro-lateral prefrontal cortex; DLPFC, dorsolateral prefrontal cortex; STN, subthalamic nucleus. Reproduced from Chamberlain SR, Menzies L. *Expert Rev Neurother* 2009;**9**(8):1133–1146, with permission of Expert Reviews Ltd.

projections from the orbitofrontal and cingulate cortex to the ventral striatum and ventral pallidum, and then back to orbitofrontal regions via the mediodorsal nucleus of the thalamus. Connections between the hippocampus and amygdala and the ventral striatum were also included in this circuit, and, based on knowledge of the effects of damage to these brain regions, an affective function was ascribed to the circuit.

The OCD hypothesis suggested that there was metabolic overactivity in the orbitofronto-striatal 'affective' circuit leading to the emergence of emotionally distressing obsessions, coupled with repetitive and compulsive behaviours aiming to relieve the patient from these obsessions. This anatomical targeting of symptoms paved the way for structural neuroimaging studies of OCD, using MRI to probe the implicated areas further. A number of structural MRI studies of OCD then appeared fairly rapidly in the literature; however, a number of difficulties were present when interpreting these [73–80]. In addition to variation in screening for subject comorbidities and medications, MRI imaging methodology was also rather problematic.

At that time, the technology available for MRI brain imaging relied upon a 'region-of-interest' (ROI) approach. This relies on researchers having an *a priori* hypothesis that predetermines a small number of brain regions to focus upon. These must then be precisely defined by identifying region boundaries, and the information concerning the rest of the brain is discarded. This approach has a number of inherent difficulties: firstly, the manually intensive method of ROI identification meant that only small sample sizes were considered feasible; secondly, regions not included in the *a priori* hypothesis may be overlooked; and thirdly, there is no universal agreement as to the exact boundaries of specific brain regions. Finally, even when numerous ROIs were included in a given analysis, the impact of this on statistical significance was often not considered, so generating errors of multiple comparisons when correction for this was not applied.

Consequently, a large number of different regions were potentially implicated in OCD, with both increased and decreased grey matter reported, leading to a rather confused picture. See Menzies *et al.* [81] for a comprehensive review of these studies. Of note, it is at least reassuring to see that despite these caveats, probably the most consistent finding in these ROI studies is reduction of volume of the orbitofrontal cortex in patients with OCD, a finding compatible with the original hypothesis. Another important feature of neuroimaging studies of OCD is that despite the initial hypothesis focusing on the orbito-fronto-striatal disease model, more recent evidence has emerged to support the involvement of an additional circuit, the dorsolateral prefrontal-parietal loop, thought to be responsible for spatial and attentional abilities [81]. This is also corroborated by cognitive studies of OCD, as discussed above.

Relatively recently, more statistically powerful imaging techniques have been developed. These rely on computational morphometry, an analysis that considers changes across the whole brain; it is thereby not subject to bias from an *a priori* hypothesis, and corrects appropriately for the multiple comparisons entailed (for further details see refs [82,83]). These voxel-based morphometry (VBM) studies, of which there are now 10 concerning OCD, have been comprehensively reviewed and incorporated into a formal meta-analysis [84]. Results from this meta-analysis provide strong evidence for reductions in grey matter density in OCD patients in both orbitofrontal and dorsolateral prefrontal cortex, together with parietal regions, and increased grey matter density in the basal ganglia. This now increasingly well-consolidated area of research provides strong evidence for systems-level dysfunction in large-scale neurocognitive brain circuits, supporting the hierarchical model of OCD proposed above.

Functional MRI has also played an important part in our understanding of the brain basis of OCD, and has helped to integrate changes in cognitive behaviour with changes in brain structure, providing a link between these hierarchical levels. Numerous functional paradigms have been used, considering both symptom provocation and cognitive tasks (including working memory, response inhibition and attentional domains). Formal meta-analysis of such studies has again provided evidence for changes in widely distributed large-scale neural networks in OCD [81] and the circuits thought to be affected are brought together in Figure 12.3.

A more appropriate method of investigating changes in a number of brain regions thought to be both structurally and functionally connected (and therefore behaving non-independently) is to use a multivariate analysis method, rather than traditional VBM, which involves multiple independent univariate analyses and is therefore limited by the necessary correction for multiple comparisons. A study evaluating both a univariate and multivariate analysis technique to investigate PET changes in OCD similarly concluded that a multivariate approach was preferable in studying OCD given its likely well-distributed circuit abnormalities [85]. Such studies have provided further evidence of broad network dysfunction in regions contributing to both the affective and spatial/attentional fronto-striatal circuits [86]. We have also employed a multivariate neuroimaging analysis technique known as partial least squares (PLS) to identify systems-level changes in brain structure in patients with OCD (for further details see ref. [87]). This study also included investigation of a cohort of the patients' first-degree relatives, in order to identify putative endophenotypes of OCD, and is therefore discussed later herein.

SEARCHING FOR ENDOPHENOTYPES OF OCD

Cognition

Having identified cognitive deficits in patients using objective translational tests, the logical 'next step' in the search for OCD endophenotypes is to explore whether such deficits also exist in close relatives of patients who are them-selves not afflicted with the disease. By definition, endophenotypes occur at higher rates in patients with the disorder of interest and their unaffected relatives than people with no known family history of the disorder of interest [29,30]. This section reviews all available cognitive studies to date that have included such unaffected relatives.

The first relevant study, conducted by our group, followed up the previous study [88] that identified impaired response inhibition and ED shifting in patients with OCD compared to controls. We used a paired relative-proband design, in which each patient with OCD took part in the study along with an unaffected first-degree relative (by preference a same sex and similarly aged sibling) [89]. Patients had no Axis-I comorbidities while relatives were free from OCD and other Axis-I disorders. Controls were recruited on the basis of being free from Axis-I disorders and of there being no known family history of OCD itself. The sample size was 20 subjects per group. Intriguingly, compared to controls, both patients with OCD and their unaffected relatives showed impaired response inhibition and impaired ED shifting (cognitive flexibility). The magnitude of deficit did not differ significantly between patients and their clinically unaffected relatives.

In a study of unaffected first-degree relatives of patients with OCD, unaffected first-degree relatives of patients with autism, and healthy controls (approximately 50 subjects per group), cognition was assessed using verbal fluency, design fluency, trail-making and Tower of London tests [90]. Relatives of patients with OCD and relatives of patients with autism showed impaired executive planning on the Tower of London task compared to the controls.

Several studies in patient relatives have subsequently been conducted using a variety of tests. Viswanath *et al.* measured cognition in 25 unaffected siblings of OCD patients with familial OCD, and 25 healthy controls [91], using a variety of paradigms. The authors identified deficits in unaffected siblings of OCD patients, versus the controls, on the Iowa Gambling and Delayed Alternation tests, which are thought to be dependent upon orbitofrontal circuitry. Cavedini and colleagues re-cruited 35 pairs of OCD patients and unaffected first-degree relatives, along with 31 pairs of healthy control subjects and their first-degree relatives [92]. Cognition was assessed using the Iowa Gambling, Tower of Hanoi, and Wisconsin Card Sorting tasks. OCD patients and their unaffected relatives showed deficits across these tasks compared to the controls, suggestive of a shared dysfunctional executive profile thought to be independent of the clinical expression of OCD. Concordance anal-yses suggested that decision-making and planning deficits aggregated in families and might be a heritable component of the disorder.

In summary, the available cognitive endophenotyping studies of OCD provide compelling evidence for the existence of cognitive dysfunction in at least a pro-portion of relatives of patients with OCD, even in the absence of clinical symp-toms. There is tentative evidence that these deficits may be somewhat heritable.

Impairments on tests of decision-making, reversal, flexibility and inhibition suggest disseminated dysfunction of both orbitofrontal circuitry and also more dorsolateral circuitry. We now turn to neuroimaging studies, which more directly assess the underlying status of neuroanatomical circuitry.

Neuroimaging

Following the work described above showing cognitive impairment in both patients with OCD and their first-degree relatives, we explored whether this effect was also evident at a systems level, that is, whether it was also present in brain structure and function, in order to further strengthen the endophenotype model.

In a sample of 93 subjects, comprising patients with OCD, their (healthy) first-degree relatives and unrelated, matched healthy controls, we employed the multivariate technique of partial least squares, discussed above [93]. This allowed us to identify two distinct large-scale brain systems in which variation in grey matter density was associated with variation in performance on the stop-signal task of motor inhibition (SSRT) described above.

The first system (Figure 12.4), comprising bilateral orbitofrontal, inferior frontal and temporal cortices, displayed a pattern of reduced grey matter density in the individuals with the poorest performance on the motor inhibition task (i.e. those with longer SSRTs). Conversely, a second group of regions (Figure 12.4), including parieto-occipital and cingulate cortices, was found to have increased grey matter density in those individuals with the poorest motor inhibition (i.e. longer SSRTs).

Behavioural performance on the motor inhibition task, and grey matter density in the two brain systems identified above, were significantly different between the three groups. This was due to both patients and their relatives performing significantly more poorly on the stop signal task (impaired motor inhibition) compared to controls, and in association with this, having significantly higher grey matter density in the parieto-cingulo-striatal system, and significantly lower grey matter density in the fronto-temporal system. The strongest between-group differences in brain structure occurred in the orbitofrontal/inferior frontal cortex (reduced grey matter density in both patients and relatives compared to controls) and in parieto-occipital cortex (increased grey matter density in patient and relatives compared to controls).

These results suggest that there are familial, and potentially genetic, influences on large-scale, widely distributed neural systems, and that variation in the grey matter density in these systems is associated with both cognitive performance (in inhibition) and phenotype: (i) healthy with low risk of OCD; (ii) healthy with high familial risk of OCD; and (iii) OCD proband. Interestingly, there were no differences in motor inhibition or grey matter density between patients and their

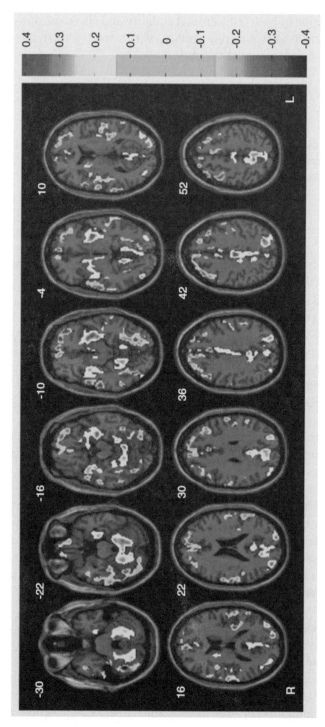

Figure 12.4 Regions in which impaired response inhibition was associated with increased grey matter (yellow/red) and reduced grey matter (blue) in an endophenotyping study of OCD. Reprinted with permission from Menzies L, Achard S, Chamberlain SR, Fineberg NA, Chen CH, del Campo N et al. Neurocognitive endophenotypes of obsessive-compulsive disorder. *Brain* 2007;**130**(12):3223–3236. Copyright Oxford University Press.

unaffected relatives, suggesting that both these parameters may be driven by familial (possibly genetic) factors. These characteristics lend strong support to the notion that these cognitive markers and brain system patterns represent endophenotypes (markers of genetic risk) for OCD.

To further explore the familial aspects of motor inhibition and brain structure, we used both correlation analysis and permutation testing. These analyses indicated that grey matter density within these structural maps was more tightly regulated by familial influences than was the cognitive marker (the SSRT). This adds further strength to the hierarchical model of OCD, providing evidence that measures at levels located more proximally to genotype are more strongly influenced by familial (and likely genetic) factors.

In a second study, we used diffusion-weighted imaging to explore differences in white matter between OCD patients and relatives compared with unrelated healthy controls [94]. Diffusion-weighted imaging measures the diffusion of water molecules through a given medium [95]. This diffusivity is affected by tissue structure; when structure is highly directional, such as in white matter where myelin-lined axons run in parallel, the extent to which water molecules can diffuse is highly dependent on direction and will be highly anisotropic. This is in contrast to grey matter, in which diffusion occurs to approximately the same extent in all orientations and is described as isotropic [96,97]. Fractional anisotropy (FA) is a measure of the extent to which diffusion is affected by direction. We found differences in FA between patients and controls, and relatives and controls, but not between patients and their relatives, again suggesting potential endophenotypes. These regions of differential FA occurred in right parietal white matter (reduced FA in patients and relatives) and right medial frontal white matter (increased FA in patients and relatives). Of note, these regions are close to areas of grey matter that were found to be different in patients and their relatives compared to controls, suggesting that there is large-scale dysconnectivity between fronto-parietal regions in individuals at risk of OCD.

Given the emerging evidence for both cognitive and brain structure endophenotypic differences in OCD, it is intriguing to consider whether the gap between these hierarchical levels can be bridged by functional MRI. We used a cognitive flexibility paradigm that allowed us to fractionate specific aspects of the task such as association learning and reversal learning [98]. All subjects were pre-trained in the task to avoid performance-related confounds of activation. Strikingly, during both encoding and reversal learning, both patients with OCD and their first-degree relatives showed reduced activation in orbitofrontal, prefrontal and parietal regions, suggesting that dysfunction of these regions is a key endophenotype for OCD (Figure 12.5).

In summary, there is emerging evidence that objective biological markers of familial risk for obsessive-compulsive symptoms exist at levels of widely distributed patterns in brain structure, brain function and cognition. These will likely be helpful in the search for underlying genetic contributions.

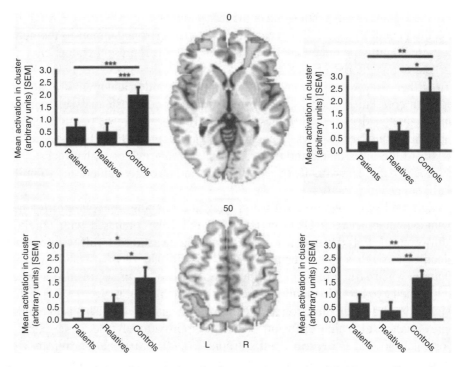

Figure 12.5 Functional imaging endophenotyping study of OCD. In yellow, clusters where there was significant brain activation irrespective of group. In blue, regions of underactivation during reversal in patients with OCD and their unaffected relatives, versus controls (also indicated in peripheral graphs). Reprinted with permission from Chamberlain SR, Menzies LA, Hampshire A, Fineberg NA, del Campo N, Craig K, Aitken M, Owen AM, Bullmore ET, Robbins TW, Sahakian BJ. Orbitofrontal dysfunction in patients with obsessive-compulsive disorder and their unaffected relatives. *Science* 2008 July 18;**321**(5887):421–422. Copyright American Association for the Advancement of Science (AAAS).

Other potential endophenotypes

Though we have focused here on cognitive and imaging markers of OCD, personality traits are also worth considering as possible endophenotypes. Patients with OCD exhibit increased rates of Cluster C personality traits including obsessive-compulsive personality disorder (OCPD). In a retrospective analysis of cognitive data, we found that the magnitude of cognitive inflexibility was greater in OCD patients with comorbid OCPD than in those without [99].

Elsewhere, Rector and colleagues explored obsessive beliefs using the Obsessive Beliefs Questionnaire (OBQ) in 24 patients with OCD and their unaffected first-degree relatives, versus controls [100]. It was found that relatives of patients (as with OCD patients themselves) manifested significantly greater obsessive beliefs relating to inflated responsibility and overestimation of threat compared to controls.

Hur investigated personality traits (Neuroticism and Extraversion from the Eysenck Personality Scale) in 524 monozygotic and 228 dizygotic pairs of adolescents/young adults from the South Korean Twin Registry [101]. Recruits also undertook the Maudsley Obsessive Compulsive Inventory (MOCI), which comprises 30 true/false items designed to measure aspects of obsessive-compulsive symptoms. Using multivariate modelling, it was found that additive genetic correlations in the model of best fit were 0.51 between Neuroticism and MOCI scores and −0.17 between Extraversion and MOCI scores. Though conducted in generic recruits rather than subjects known to meet OCD diagnostic criteria, these findings suggest an association between obsessive-compulsive symptoms and high neuroticism (and, to a lesser degree, between obsessive-compulsive symptoms and intraversion) in the general population that are mediated in part by genetic factors.

These preliminary studies hint at personality traits as another fruitful avenue in the search for candidate endophenotypes. That said, personality-based endophenotypes would in some instances be difficult to relate to specific brain processes when contrasted to these other types of marker, and difficult to use in translational models. It may be possible in future to link together personality traits (e.g. rigidity, perfectionism) with cognitive measures (e.g. cognitive inflexibility, slowed responses on tasks requiring perfect solutions).

SUMMARY

This chapter has addressed a concept initially introduced in the 1960s but only recently applied to the study of OCD, namely the notion of endophenotypes. To an extent, it has taken time for technology to 'catch up' with the concept – researchers and clinicians now have at their disposal a variety of techniques from the neurosciences to explore the neuropsychiatry of OCD and candidate endophenotypes, including objective translational cognitive tests, and a variety of imaging methods (e.g. structural and functional MRI, PET and, more recently, receptor/reuptake transporter specific radioligands). We have seen that OCD is a heritable condition underpinned by dysfunction of orbitofronto-striatal and dorsolateral prefronto-parieto-striatal circuitry [81], along with corresponding deficits in aspects of cognition relating to flexible responding, impulse control, and executive planning [32]. This work concords well with early imaging work identifying orbitofrontal abnormalities in OCD, but also builds significantly upon it, by also implicating dorsolateral and parietal dysfunction.

The next step in developing such research avenues is to consider using such endophenotypes to inform gene-searching strategies, for example using brain structure endophenotypes rather than clinical constructs when conducting genome-wide associations (GWA) and searching for chromosome loci and SNPs associated with OCD. It would be hypothesized that these objective biomarkers, lying more proximally to genotype than clinical diagnosis, might allow increased power when searching for gene associations. Taking GWA, for example, although there is little experience using indices of human brain structure or function as quantitative traits to identify associated genetic polymorphisms, proof of concept of this technique has been shown in mouse models where measures of cortical and subcortical grey matter have been used to identify genetic markers [102].

Ideally, in order for human endophenotypes to be helpful in this scenario, they should be confirmed as being heritable, rather than just familial; the studies discussed above using proband-relative pairs have focused upon the latter of these, leaving open the possibility that findings could be explained by shared environmental influences in addition to shared genes. Encouragingly, in a recent paper, the heritabilities of 12 candidate endophenotypes for schizophrenia were investigated, yielding estimates of 24–55% [103]. In other contexts also (e.g. alcoholism) endophenotypes have also been found to be heritable [104], supporting their use in this context in future research.

The finding of cognitive deficits and structural/functional brain abnormalities in unaffected first-degree relatives of people with OCD has profound implications. These studies suggest that certain of the abnormalities previously found in patients with OCD were not attributable to the symptoms themselves or directly affiliated with them; rather they were candidate vulnerability markers that predated symptoms and rendered one susceptible to the development of rigid thinking patterns and compulsive patterns of behaviour. Some discrepancies in the prior literature may stem from failure to account for prevalence of Axis-I disorders, especially OCD, in control subjects' relatives. It is probable but has yet to be demonstrated that cognitive problems in patients with OCD and their relatives have deleterious effects on activities of daily living and occupational function; this will need to be studied in future work. If this is the case, it will be apt to consider whether specific psychotherapies and/or treatment with cognitive-enhancing agents can mitigate such effects.

Despite pilot studies, several critical questions remain in the context of OCD endophenotypes. If relatives of people with OCD exhibit cognitive abnormalities, why do only a proportion of these people ultimately develop OCD? Little is known regarding the interaction between clinical phenotypes, intermediate phenotypes, environmental factors and genetics. It will be important to study not only precipitating factors but also protective (i.e. resilience) factors. Also, there may well be some measurable markers that exist in patients (like the symptoms) but not in patient relatives, which may help to account for the development of symptoms. We speculate that endophenotypes may overlap between OCD and related Axis-I disorders and help to account for their comorbid overlap.

Key points

- OCD and other neuropsychiatric disorders can be conceptualized hierarchically.
- A hierarchical model considers 'knock-on' effects of dysfunction at multiple levels from genotype to 'systems-level' brain networks and circuitry through to cognition, leading finally to a complex behavioural phenotype.
- A key difficulty in understanding the neurobiology of OCD is the current (necessary) use of a clinical diagnostic classification that is likely to subtend considerable heterogeneity at the genotype level.
- Endophenotypes are objective 'biomarkers' located more proximally along the pathway from genotype to phenotype, which could help to deconstruct the clinical phenotype of OCD, thereby facilitating understanding of its genetic basis and modes of transmission.
- OCD is associated with abnormal structure and function within large-scale neurocognitive networks that predominantly involve orbitofronto-striatal and dorsolateral prefrontal-parieto-striatal circuitry.
- Putative endophenotypes of OCD have been identified in both the cognitive and neuroimaging domains; indeed, most fruitfully where both domains have been combined.
- Identification and validation of OCD endophenotypes has the potential to improve diagnostic classification systems, understanding of disease vulnerability (and resilience), and to facilitate early detection of those at risk.
- Future research should explore relationships between putative endophenotypes identified here and underlying genetic factors; and whether the presence or absence of particular endophenotypes can predict treatment response.

ACKNOWLEDGEMENTS AND DISCLOSURES

Dr Chamberlain consults for Cambridge Cognition, Shire and P1Vital. Dr Menzies has received financial compensation resulting from the transfer of a technology not relating to the subject matter of this article between Cambridge Enterprise Limited, University of Cambridge, Cambridge, UK, and Cypress Bioscience, Inc., San Diego. This work was supported in part by a Wellcome Trust Programme Grant (076274/Z/04/Z) to Dr Robbins, Dr Sahakian, BJ Everitt and AC Roberts. The Behavioural and Clinical Neuroscience Institute is supported by a joint award from the Medical Research Council (MRC) and Wellcome Trust (G001354). Support also comes from the National Alliance for Research on Schizophrenia and Depression

(RG37920 Distinguished Investigator Award to Dr Bullmore), the Harnett Fund and James Baird Fund (University of Cambridge) and the University of Cambridge School of Clinical Medicine, (previous MB/PhD studentship to Dr Menzies), and the Medical Research Council (previous MB/PhD studentship to Dr Chamberlain).

REFERENCES

1. Stein DJ. Neurobiology of the obsessive-compulsive spectrum disorders. *Biol Psychiatry* 2000;**47**:296–304.
2. Chamberlain SR, Blackwell AD, Fineberg NA, Robbins TW, Sahakian BJ. The neuropsychology of obsessive compulsive disorder: the importance of failures in cognitive and behavioural inhibition as candidate endophenotypic markers. *Neurosci Biobehav Rev.* 2005;**29**:399–419.
3. Fontenelle LF, Mendlowicz MV, Versiani M. The descriptive epidemiology of obsessive-compulsive disorder. *Prog Neuropsychopharmacol Biol Psychiatry* 2006;**30**:327–337.
4. Hollander E, Kwon JH, Stein DJ, Broatch J, Rowland CT, Himelein CA. Obsessive-compulsive and spectrum disorders: overview and quality of life issues. *J Clin Psychiatry* 1996;**57**(Suppl. 8):3–6.
5. DuPont RL, Rice DP, Shiraki S, Rowland CR. Economic costs of obsessive-compulsive disorder. *Med Interface* 1995;**8**:102–109.
6. Rasmussen SA, Tsuang MT. The epidemiology of obsessive compulsive disorder. *J Clin Psychiatry* 1984;**45**): 450–457.
7. Westenberg HG, Fineberg NA, Denys D. Neurobiology of obsessive-compulsive disorder: serotonin and beyond. *CNS Spectr* 2007;**12**(2 Suppl. 3):14–27.
8. Welch JM, Lu J, Rodriguiz RM *et al.* Cortico-striatal synaptic defects and OCD-like behaviours in Sapap3-mutant mice. *Nature* 2007;**448**:894–900.
9. Boulougouris V, Chamberlain SR, Robbins TW. Cross-species models of OCD spectrum disorders. *Psychiatry Res* 2009;**170**:15–21.
10. Fineberg NA, Potenza MN, Chamberlain SR *et al.* Probing compulsive and impulsive behaviors, from animal models to endophenotypes: a narrative review. *Neuropsychopharmacology* 2010;**35**:591–604.
11. Aron AR, Robbins TW, Poldrack RA. Inhibition and the right inferior frontal cortex. *Trends Cogn Sci* 2004;**8**:170–177.
12. Chamberlain SR, Sahakian BJ. The neuropsychiatry of impulsivity. *Curr Opin Psychiatry* 2007;**20**:255–261.
13. Kehagia AA, Murray GK, Robbins TW. Learning and cognitive flexibility: frontostriatal function and monoaminergic modulation. *Curr Opin Neurobiol* 2010;**20**:199–204.
14. van Grootheest DS, Cath DC, Beekman AT, Boomsma DI. Twin studies on obsessive-compulsive disorder: a review. *Twin Res Hum Genet* 2005;**8**:450–458.
15. Pauls DL. The genetics of obsessive compulsive disorder: a review of the evidence. *Am J Med Genet C Semin Med Genet* 2008;**148**:133–139.

16. Pauls DL, Alsobrook JP 2nd, Goodman W, Rasmussen S, Leckman JF. A family study of obsessive-compulsive disorder. *Am J Psychiatry* 1995;**152**:76–84.

17. Nestadt G, Samuels J, Riddle M *et al.* A family study of obsessive-compulsive disorder. *Arch Gen Psychiatry* 2000;**57**:358–363.

18. Hettema JM, Neale MC, Kendler KS. A review and meta-analysis of the genetic epidemiology of anxiety disorders. *Am J Psychiatry* 2001;**158**:1568–1578.

19. Carey G, Gottesman II. Twin and family studies of anxiety, phobic and obsessive disorders. In: Klein D, Radkin J (eds), *Anxiety; New Research and Changing Concepts*. New York: Raven Press, 1981, pp. 117–136.

20. Hudziak JJ, Van Beijsterveldt CE, Althoff RR *et al.* Genetic and environmental contributions to the Child Behavior Checklist Obsessive-Compulsive Scale: a cross-cultural twin study. *Arch Gen Psychiatry* 2004;**61**:608–616.

21. Hanna GL, Veenstra-VanderWeele J, Cox NJ *et al.* Genome-wide linkage analysis of families with obsessive-compulsive disorder ascertained through pediatric probands. *Am J Med Genet* 2002;**114**:541–552.

22. Willour VL, Yao Shugart Y, Samuels J *et al.* Replication study supports evidence for linkage to 9p24 in obsessive-compulsive disorder. *Am J Hum Genet* 2004;**75**:508–513.

23. Dickel DE, Veenstra-VanderWeele J, Cox NJ *et al.* Association testing of the positional and functional candidate gene SLC1A1/EAAC1 in early-onset obsessive-compulsive disorder. *Arch Gen Psychiatry* 2006;**63**:778–785.

24. Arnold PD, Sicard T, Burroughs E, Richter MA, Kennedy JL. Glutamate transporter gene SLC1A1 associated with obsessive-compulsive disorder. *Arch Gen Psychiatry* 2006;**63**:769–776.

25. Shugart YY, Wang Y, Samuels JF *et al.* A family-based association study of the glutamate transporter gene SLC1A1 in obsessive-compulsive disorder in 378 families. *Am J Med Genet B Neuropsychiatr Genet* 2009;**150B**:886–892.

26. Shugart YY, Samuels J, Willour VL *et al.* Genomewide linkage scan for obsessive-compulsive disorder: evidence for susceptibility loci on chromosomes 3q, 7p, 1q, 15q, and 6q. *Mol Psychiatry* 2006;**11**:763–770.

27. Pauls DL. The genetics of obsessive-compulsive disorder: a review. *Dialogues Clin Neurosci* 2010;**12**:149–163.

28. Hasler G, Drevets WC, Gould TD, Gottesman, II, Manji HK. Toward constructing an endophenotype strategy for bipolar disorders. *Biol Psychiatry* 2006;**60**:93–105.

29. Gould TD, Gottesman II. Psychiatric endophenotypes and the development of valid animal models. *Genes Brain Behav* 2006;**5**:113–119.

30. Gottesman II, Gould TD. The endophenotype concept in psychiatry: etymology and strategic intentions. *Am J Psychiatry* 2003;**160**:636–645.

31. Insel TR, Collins FS. Psychiatry in the genomics era. *Am J Psychiatry* 2003;**160**:616–620.

32. Chamberlain SR, Menzies L. Endophenotypes of obsessive-compulsive disorder: rationale, evidence and future potential. *Expert Rev Neurother* 2009;**9**:1133–1146.

33. Oh G, Petronis A. Environmental studies of schizophrenia through the prism of epigenetics. *Schizophr Bull* 2008;**34**:1122–1129.

34. Roy N, Kahlem P, Dausse E *et al.* Exclusion of HRAS from long QT locus. *Nat Genet* 1994;**8**:113–114.

35. Wang Q, Curran ME, Splawski I *et al.* Positional cloning of a novel potassium channel gene: KVLQT1 mutations cause cardiac arrhythmias. *Nat Genet* 1996;**12**:17–23.

36. Aukes MF, Alizadeh BZ, Sitskoorn MM, Kemner C, Ophoff RA, Kahn RS. Genetic overlap among intelligence and other candidate endophenotypes for schizophrenia. *Biol Psychiatry* 2009;**65**:527–534.

37. Freedman R, Adler LE, Baker N, Waldo M, Mizner G. Candidate for inherited neurobiological dysfunction in schizophrenia. *Somat Cell Mol Genet* 1987;**13**:479–484.

38. Siegel C, Waldo M, Mizner G, Adler LE, Freedman R. Deficits in sensory gating in schizophrenic patients and their relatives. Evidence obtained with auditory evoked responses. *Arch Gen Psychiatry* 1984;**41**:607–612.

39. Freedman R, Coon H, Myles-Worsley M *et al.* Linkage of a neurophysiological deficit in schizophrenia to a chromosome 15 locus. *Proc Natl Acad Sci U S A* 1997;**94**:587–592.

40. Leonard S, Adams C, Breese CR *et al.* Nicotinic receptor function in schizophrenia. *Schizophr Bull* 1996;**22**:431–445.

41. Leonard S, Gault J, Hopkins J *et al.* Association of promoter variants in the alpha7 nicotinic acetylcholine receptor subunit gene with an inhibitory deficit found in schizophrenia. *Arch Gen Psychiatry* 2002;**59**:1085–1096.

42. Leiser SC, Bowlby MR, Comery TA, Dunlop J. A cog in cognition: how the alpha 7 nicotinic acetylcholine receptor is geared towards improving cognitive deficits. *Pharmacol Ther* 2009;**122**:302–311.

43. Olincy A, Braff DL, Adler LE *et al.* Inhibition of the P50 cerebral evoked response to repeated auditory stimuli: results from the Consortium on Genetics of Schizophrenia. *Schizophr Res* 2010;**119**:175–182.

44. Tregellas JR, Olincy A, Johnson L *et al.* Functional magnetic resonance imaging of effects of a nicotinic agonist in schizophrenia. *Neuropsychopharmacology* 2010;**35**:938–942.

45. Hollander E, Kim S, Khanna S, Pallanti S. Obsessive-compulsive disorder and obsessive-compulsive spectrum disorders: diagnostic and dimensional issues. *CNS Spectr* 2007;**12**(2 Suppl. 3):5–13.

46. Drachman DA. Do we have brain to spare? *Neurology* 2005;**64**:2004–2005.

47. Thompson PM, Cannon TD, Narr KL *et al.* Genetic influences on brain structure. *Nat Neurosci* 2001;**4**:1253–1258.

48. Wright IC, Sham P, Murray RM, Weinberger DR, Bullmore ET. Genetic contributions to regional variability in human brain structure: methods and preliminary results. *Neuroimage* 2002;**17**:256–271.

49. Toga AW, Thompson PM. Genetics of brain structure and intelligence. *Annu Rev Neurosci* 2005;**28**:1–23.

50. Greisberg S, McKay D. Neuropsychology of obsessive-compulsive disorder: a review and treatment implications. *Clin Psychol Rev* 2003;**23**:95–117.

51. Chamberlain SR, Fineberg NA, Blackwell AD, Robbins TW, Sahakian BJ. Motor inhibition and cognitive flexibility in obsessive-compulsive disorder and trichotillomania. *Am J Psychiatry* 2006;**163**:1282–1284.

52. Logan GD, Cowan WB, Davis KA. On the ability to inhibit simple and choice reaction time responses: a model and a method. *J Exp Psychol Hum Percept Perform* 1984;**10**:276–291.

53. Aron AR, Fletcher PC, Bullmore ET, Sahakian BJ, Robbins TW. Stop-signal inhibition disrupted by damage to right inferior frontal gyrus in humans. *Nat Neurosci* 2003;**6**:115–116.

54. Rubia K, Smith AB, Brammer MJ, Taylor E. Right inferior prefrontal cortex mediates response inhibition while mesial prefrontal cortex is responsible for error detection. *Neuroimage* 2003;**20**:351–358.

55. Hampshire A, Chamberlain SR, Monti MM, Duncan J, Owen AM. The role of the right inferior frontal gyrus: inhibition and attentional control. *Neuroimage* 2010;**50**:1313–1319.

56. Bari A, Eagle DM, Mar AC, Robinson ES, Robbins TW. Dissociable effects of noradrenaline, dopamine, and serotonin uptake blockade on stop task performance in rats. *Psychopharmacology (Berl)* 2009;**205**:273–283.

57. Robbins TW, Arnsten AF. The neuropsychopharmacology of fronto-executive function: monoaminergic modulation. *Annu Rev Neurosci* 2009;**32**:267–287.

58. Chamberlain SR, Hampshire A, Müller U *et al*. Atomoxetine modulates right inferior frontal activation during inhibitory control: a pharmacological functional magnetic resonance imaging study. *Biol Psychiatry* 2009;**65**:550–555.

59. Robinson ES, Eagle DM, Mar AC *et al*. Similar effects of the selective noradrenaline reuptake inhibitor atomoxetine on three distinct forms of impulsivity in the rat. *Neuropsychopharmacology* 2008;**33**:1028–1037.

60. Chamberlain SR, Del Campo N, Dowson J *et al*. Atomoxetine improved response inhibition in adults with attention deficit/hyperactivity disorder. *Biol Psychiatry* 2007;**62**:977–984.

61. Chamberlain SR, Müller U, Blackwell AD, Clark L, Robbins TW, Sahakian BJ. Neurochemical modulation of response inhibition and probabilistic learning in humans. *Science* 2006;**311**:861–863.

62. Owen AM, Roberts AC, Polkey CE, Sahakian BJ, Robbins TW. Extra-dimensional versus intra-dimensional set shifting performance following frontal lobe excisions, temporal lobe excisions or amygdalo-hippocampectomy in man. *Neuropsychologia* 1991;**29**:993–1006.

63. Hampshire A, Owen AM. Fractionating attentional control using event-related fMRI. *Cereb Cortex* 2006;**16**:1679–1689.

64. Baxter LR Jr, Phelps ME, Mazziotta JC, Guze BH, Schwartz JM, Selin CE. Local cerebral glucose metabolic rates in obsessive-compulsive disorder. A comparison with rates in unipolar depression and in normal controls. *Arch Gen Psychiatry* 1987;**44**:211–218.

65. Swedo SE, Schapiro MB, Grady CL *et al*. Cerebral glucose metabolism in childhood-onset obsessive-compulsive disorder. *Arch Gen Psychiatry* 1989;**46**:518–523.

66. Baxter LR Jr, Schwartz JM, Mazziotta JC *et al*. Cerebral glucose metabolic rates in nondepressed patients with obsessive-compulsive disorder. *Am J Psychiatry* 1988;**145**:1560–1563.

67. Nordahl TE, Benkelfat C, Semple WE, Gross M, King AC, Cohen RM. Cerebral glucose metabolic rates in obsessive compulsive disorder. *Neuropsychopharmacology* 1989;**2**:23–28.

68. McGuire PK, Bench CJ, Frith CD, Marks IM, Frackowiak RS, Dolan RJ. Functional anatomy of obsessive-compulsive phenomena. *Br J Psychiatry* 1994;**164**:459–468.

69. Rauch SL, Jenike MA, Alpert NM *et al.* Regional cerebral blood flow measured during symptom provocation in obsessive-compulsive disorder using oxygen 15-labeled carbon dioxide and positron emission tomography. *Arch Gen Psychiatry* 1994;**51**:62–70.

70. Cottraux J, Gerard D, Cinotti L *et al.* A controlled positron emission tomography study of obsessive and neutral auditory stimulation in obsessive-compulsive disorder with checking rituals. *Psychiatry Res* 1996;**60**:101–112.

71. Perani D, Colombo C, Bressi S *et al.* [18F]FDG PET study in obsessive-compulsive disorder. A clinical/metabolic correlation study after treatment. *Br J Psychiatry* 1995;**166**:244–250.

72. Alexander GE, DeLong MR, Strick PL. Parallel organization of functionally segregated circuits linking basal ganglia and cortex. *Annu Rev Neurosci* 1986;**9**:357–381.

73. Szeszko PR, Robinson D, Alvir JM *et al.* Orbital frontal and amygdala volume reductions in obsessive-compulsive disorder. *Arch Gen Psychiatry* 1999;**56**:913–919.

74. Choi JS, Kang DH, Kim JJ *et al.* Left anterior subregion of orbitofrontal cortex volume reduction and impaired organizational strategies in obsessive-compulsive disorder. *J Psychiatr Res* 2004;**38**:193–199.

75. Kang DH, Kim JJ, Choi JS *et al.* Volumetric investigation of the frontal-subcortical circuitry in patients with obsessive-compulsive disorder. *J Neuropsychiatry Clin Neurosci* 2004;**16**:342–349.

76. Atmaca M, Yildirim BH, Ozdemir BH, Aydin BA, Tezcan AE, Ozler AS. Volumetric MRI assessment of brain regions in patients with refractory obsessive-compulsive disorder. *Prog Neuropsychopharmacol Biol Psychiatry* 2006;**30**:1051–1057.

77. Atmaca M, Yildirim H, Ozdemir H, Tezcan E, Poyraz AK. Volumetric MRI study of key brain regions implicated in obsessive-compulsive disorder. *Prog Neuropsychopharmacol Biol Psychiatry* 2007;**31**:46–52.

78. Robinson D, Wu H, Munne RA *et al.* Reduced caudate nucleus volume in obsessive-compulsive disorder. *Arch Gen Psychiatry* 1995;**52**:393–398.

79. Rosenberg DR, Keshavan MS, O'Hearn KM *et al.* Frontostriatal measurement in treatment-naive children with obsessive-compulsive disorder. *Arch Gen Psychiatry* 1997;**54**:824–830.

80. Szeszko PR, MacMillan S, McMeniman M *et al.* Brain structural abnormalities in psychotropic drug-naive pediatric patients with obsessive-compulsive disorder. *Am J Psychiatry* 2004;**161**:1049–1056.

81. Menzies L, Chamberlain SR, Laird AR, Thelen SM, Sahakian BJ, Bullmore ET. Integrating evidence from neuroimaging and neuropsychological studies of obsessive-compulsive disorder: The orbitofronto-striatal model revisited. *Neurosci Biobehav Rev* 2008;**32**:525–549.

82. Bullmore ET, Suckling J, Overmeyer S, Rabe-Hesketh S, Taylor E, Brammer MJ. Global, voxel, and cluster tests, by theory and permutation, for a difference between two groups of structural MR images of the brain. *IEEE Trans Med Imaging* 1999;**18**:32–42.

83. Ashburner J, Friston KJ. Voxel-based morphometry – the methods. *Neuroimage* 2000;**11**:805–821.

84. Rotge JY, Langbour N, Guehl D *et al*. Gray matter alterations in obsessive-compulsive disorder: an anatomic likelihood estimation meta-analysis. *Neuropsychopharmacology* 2010;**35**:686–691.

85. Harrison BJ, Yucel M, Shaw M *et al*. Evaluating brain activity in obsessive-compulsive disorder: preliminary insights from a multivariate analysis. *Psychiatry Res* 2006;**147**:227–231.

86. Soriano-Mas C, Pujol J, Alonso P *et al*. Identifying patients with obsessive-compulsive disorder using whole-brain anatomy. *Neuroimage* 2007;**35**:1028–1037.

87. McIntosh AR, Lobaugh NJ. Partial least squares analysis of neuroimaging data: applications and advances. *Neuroimage* 2004;**23**(Suppl. 1):S250–263.

88. Odlaug BL, Chamberlain SR, Grant JE. Motor inhibition and cognitive flexibility in pathologic skin picking. *Prog Neuropsychopharmacol Biol Psychiatry* 2010;**34**:208–211.

89. Chamberlain SR, Blackwell AD, Fineberg NA, Robbins TW, Sahakian BJ. Impaired cognitive flexibility and motor inhibition in unaffected first-degree relatives of OCD patients: on the trail of endophenotypes. *Am J Psychiatry* 2007;**164**:335–338.

90. Delorme R, Gousse V, Roy I *et al*. Shared executive dysfunctions in unaffected relatives of patients with autism and obsessive-compulsive disorder. *Eur Psychiatry* 2007;**22**:32–38.

91. Viswanath B, Janardhan Reddy YC, Kumar KJ, Kandavel T, Chandrashekar CR. Cognitive endophenotypes in OCD: a study of unaffected siblings of probands with familial OCD. *Prog Neuropsychopharmacol Biol Psychiatry* 2009;**33**:610–615.

92. Cavedini P, Zorzi C, Piccinni M, Cavallini MC, Bellodi L. Executive dysfunctions in obsessive-compulsive patients and unaffected relatives: searching for a new intermediate phenotype. *Biol Psychiatry* 2010;**67**:1178–1184.

93. Menzies L, Achard S, Chamberlain SR *et al*. Neurocognitive endophenotypes of obsessive-compulsive disorder. *Brain* 2007;**130**:3223–3236.

94. Menzies L, Williams GB, Chamberlain SR *et al*. White matter abnormalities in patients with obsessive-compulsive disorder and their first-degree relatives. *Am J Psychiatry* 2008;**165**:1308–1315.

95. Le Bihan D, Mangin JF, Poupon C *et al*. Diffusion tensor imaging: concepts and applications. *J Magn Reson Imaging* 2001;**13**:534–546.

96. Basser PJ, Pierpaoli C. Microstructural and physiological features of tissues elucidated by quantitative-diffusion-tensor MRI. *J Magn Reson B* 1996;**111**:209–219.

97. Beaulieu C. The basis of anisotropic water diffusion in the nervous system – a technical review. *NMR Biomed* 2002;**15**:435–455.

98. Chamberlain SR, Menzies L, Hampshire A *et al*. Orbitofrontal dysfunction in patients with obsessive-compulsive disorder and their unaffected relatives. *Science* 2008;**321**:421–422.

99. Fineberg NA, Sharma P, Sivakumaran T, Sahakian B, Chamberlain SR. Does obsessive-compulsive personality disorder belong within the obsessive-compulsive spectrum? *CNS Spectr* 2007;**12**:467–482.

100. Rector NA, Cassin SE, Richter MA, Burroughs E. Obsessive beliefs in first-degree relatives of patients with OCD: a test of the cognitive vulnerability model. *J Anxiety Disord* 2009;**23**:145–149.

101. Hur YM. Genetic and environmental covariations among obsessive-compulsive symptoms, neuroticism, and extraversion in South Korean adolescent and young adult twins. *Twin Res Hum Genet* 2009;**12**:142–148.
102. Beatty J, Laughlin RE. Genomic regulation of natural variation in cortical and non-cortical brain volume. *BMC Neurosci* 2006;**7**:16.
103. Greenwood TA, Braff DL, Light GA *et al*. Initial heritability analyses of endophenotypic measures for schizophrenia: the consortium on the genetics of schizophrenia. *Arch Gen Psychiatry* 2007;**64**:1242–1250.
104. Dick DM, Jones K, Saccone N *et al*. Endophenotypes successfully lead to gene identification: results from the collaborative study on the genetics of alcoholism. *Behav Genet* 2006;**36**:112–126.

CHAPTER 13

Conclusion and Future Directions

Joseph Zohar

Division of Psychiatry, Chaim Sheba Medical Center, Tel Hashomer, Israel

This book celebrates 25 years of research in obsessive-compulsive disorder (OCD). In 1987 Tom Insel and I published the first double-blind prospective study that demonstrated the specific efficacy of serotonergic medication (clomipramine in this study), in comparison to the lack of efficacy of noradrenergic medication (desipramine) [1]. This line of research paved the way for clomipramine to merit a specific indication for OCD [2]. This later opened the door for the specific OCD indication for the SSRIs, from the early 1990s on.

In parallel, groundbreaking epidemiological and biological studies have started to generate exciting data. A seminal epidemiological study clearly demonstrated that OCD is quite prevalent – about 2% in the general population [3]. It was also found that not only does OCD affect males and females equally, but it is also distributed equally in developed as well as developing countries [4].

Capitalizing on the specific response to 5-HT (serotonin), careful exploration of the 5-HT hypothesis took place [5–7], lending further support for a unique role of 5-HT not only in the pharmacotherapy of OCD, but also as a pathological base for the disorder.

To the busy and rapidly evolving scheme of OCD, brain imaging experts, equipped with exciting modern functional tools – e.g. positron emission tomography (PET), functional magnetic resonance imaging (fMRI) – joined in. They managed to achieve another breakthrough with the unfolding of the brain circuitry of OCD [8,9], along with further exploration of the 5-HT hypothesis of OCD [5–7,10,11].

Very exciting progress also took place in the psychological therapeutic arena. A generic, not well-defined psychological intervention with strong psychodynamic concepts [12] has been replaced with a specific manual of interventions, based on a cognitive behavioural approach [12], and focusing on exposure coupled with response prevention.

This volume summarizes this impressive progress. Harnessing the advanced technologies in brain imaging, genetics, neurocognition, clinical research methodology, psychological interventions and neuropsychopharmacological tools, the OCD field has broadened and deepened.

What is the major lesson? It could probably be summarized by the multifactorial concept, by the integration message. It is becoming clear that the key to success, the avenue for progress, the platform for moving forward, lies in the appreciation of the complexity of behavioural brain disorders like OCD. Placing together, in an individualized fashion, the interplay of genetic vulnerability, traumatic life events, current family interactions and contemporary cultural backgrounds might be the way, not only to understand the clinical presentation, but also to grasp the biological heterogeneity and consequently to offer adequate personalized treatment strategies. In this intricate mosaic of OCD there are some important parts that are missing, that need to be further explored. These include the glutaminergic component, the opioid input and the white/grey matter connectivity. The key to these and other fundamental questions is related to a proper diagnostic system. For example, questions regarding OCD and behavioural addiction (e.g. pathological gambling, internet addiction, etc.) are pending, awaiting better answers.

Only when we can identify the true OCD patients will it be possible to reach valid answers. As long as we mix the core OCD phenomenon with OCD epiphenomena, the signal may be confusing. Neurocognitive tools, along with modern brain imaging techniques and genetic input, *together* with quantified and qualified environmental factors, may provide the ingredients for progress. The answer will probably not come by a single breakthrough, but by an orchestrated combination of the different technologies, personally adjusted for a given patient and in a more dimensional (rather than categorical) diagnostic scheme.

More sophisticated technologies, state-of-the-art mapping and cutting-edge neuropharmacology must be integrated with basic, fundamental insights in order to attain meaningful scientific progress. An integrative approach is also called for on the practical therapeutic front: for example, if the family interaction maintains (or, even worse, supports) the obsessive-compulsive loop, even the most brilliant neuropsychopharmacology or physical stereotactic brain intervention will not help. Hence, along these lines of twenty-first century progress the twentieth century insights on therapeutic alliance, patient motivation and family intervention should be preserved and practised.

The future for OCD patients is brighter. Whether new technologies like H-coil transcranial magnetic stimulation (TMS) (coined as deep TMS) or deep brain stimulation (DBS) will be significant additions to our clinical armamentarium is yet to be seen. However, the greatest progress will be in identifying the relevant circuitry (which is the biological basis for those interventions); along with the more mature insights vis-á-vis the multifactorial, multilevel basis and its influence on treatment, this carries the promise to improve our knowledge, and to sharpen our conceptual layout.

The task ahead is to draw the 'big picture', choosing the right frame, the right brush and the right colours. The frame is defined by the borders of OCD, including the fundamental question regarding OCD and anxiety disorders (which most probably will be solved by separating OCD from anxiety). There are equally important questions in regard to OCD spectrum disorders, including body dysmorphic disorder (BDD), hypochondriasis, kleptomania, etc. The colours include, among others, genetics, brain imaging, neurocognitive measures and specific pharmacological challenge. The art would be to draw them on the board in harmony.

I hope that this volume provides an additional and worthy step to heighten the scientific and clinical level of this fascinating phenomenon called OCD.

REFERENCES

1. Zohar J, Insel TR. Obsessive-compulsive disorders; psychobiological approaches to diagnosis, treatment and pathophysiology. *Biol Psychiat* 1987;**22**:667–687 [winner of A.E. Bennett Award].
2. Albert U, Aguglia E, Maina G, Bogetto F. Venlafaxine versus clomipramine in the treatment of obsessive-compulsive disorder: a preliminary single-blind, 12-week, controlled study. *J Clin Psychiatry* 2002;**63**:1004–1009.
3. Weissman MM, Bland RC, Canino GJ *et al*. The cross national epidemiology of obsessive compulsive disorder. The Cross National Collaborative Group. *J Clin Psychiatry.* 1994;**55**(Suppl.):5–10.
4. Sasson Y, Zohar J, Chopra M, Lustig M, Iancu I, Hendler T. Epidemiology of obsessive-compulsive disorder: a world view. *J Clin Psychiatry* 1997;**58**(Suppl. 12):7–10.
5. Zohar J, Mueller EA, Insel TR, Zohar-Kadouch RC, Murphy DL. Serotonergic responsivity in obsessive-compulsive disorder. Comparison of patients and healthy controls. *Arch Gen Psychiat* 1987;**44**:946–951.
6. Zohar J, Insel TR, Zohar-Kadouch RC, Hill JL, Murphy DL. Serotonergic responsivity in obsessive compulsive disorder. Effects of chronic clomipramine treatment. *Arch Gen Psychiat* 1988;**45**:167–197.
7. Benkelfat C, Murphy DL, Zohar J, Hill JL, Grover G, Insel TR. Clomipramine in obsessive-compulsive disorder. Further evidence for a serotonergic mechanism of action. *Arch Gen Psychiatry* 1989;**46**:23–28.
8. Baxter LR Jr, Phelps ME, Mazziotta JC, Guze BH, Schwartz JM, Selin CE. Local cerebral glucose metabolic rates in obsessive-compulsive disorder. A comparison with rates in unipolar depression and in normal controls. *Arch Gen Psychiatry* 1987;**44**:211–218. Erratum in: *Arch Gen Psychiatry* 1987;**44**:800.
9. Murphy DL, Zohar J, Benkelfat C, Pato MT, Pigott TA, Insel TR. Obsessive-compulsive disorder as a 5-HT subsystem-related behavioural disorder. *Br J Psychiatry Suppl* 1989;**8**:15–24.

10. Zohar J, Insel TR, Zohar-Kadouch RC, Mueller EA, Murphy DL. Serotonergic role in obsessive compulsive disorder. In: Belmaker RH (ed.), *Progress in Catecholamine Research. Clinical Aspects.* Allen R. Liss Inc., 1989; pp. 385–391.

11. Zohar J, Zohar-Kadouch RC. Is there a specific role for serotonin in obsessive compulsive disorder? In: Brown SL, van Praag HM (eds), *The Role of Serotonin in Psychiatric Disorders.* New York: Brunner/Mazel, 1990; pp. 161–182.

12. Zohar J, Foa EB, Insel TR. Obsessive compulsive disorders: behavior therapy and pharmacotherapy. In: Karasu TB (ed.), *Treatment of Psychiatric Disorders. A Task Force Report of the American Psychiatric Association.* Washington, DC: American Psychiatric Press, 1989; pp. 2095–2104.

Index

Obsessive-Compulsive Disorder: Current Science and Clinical Practice, First Edition. Edited by Joseph Zohar.
© 2012 John Wiley & Sons, Ltd. Published 2012 by John Wiley & Sons, Ltd.